GOVERNING GLOBAL HEALTH

Global Environmental Governance Series

Series Editor: John J. Kirton

Global Environmental Governance addresses the new generation of twenty-first century environmental problems and the challenges they pose for management and governance at the local, national, and global levels. Centred on the relationships among environmental change, economic forces, and political governance, the series explores the role of international institutions and instruments, national and sub-federal governments, private sector firms, scientists, and civil society, and provides a comprehensive body of progressive analyses on one of the world's most contentious international issues.

Also in the series

A World Environment Organization
Edited by Frank Biermann and Steffen Bauer
ISBN 978-0-7546-3765-3

Sustainability, Civil Society and International Governance
Edited by John J. Kirton and Peter I. Hajnal
ISBN 978-0-7546-3884-1

Bilateral Ecopolitics
Edited by Philippe Le Prestre and Peter Stoett
ISBN 978-0-7546-4177-3

Governing Global Desertification
Edited by Pierre Marc Johnson, Karel Mayrand and Marc Paquin
ISBN 978-0-7546-4359-3

Participation for Sustainability in Trade
Edited by Sophie Thoyer and Benoît Martimort-Asso
ISBN 978-0-7546-4679-2

Governing Global Health
Challenge, Response, Innovation

Edited by
ANDREW F. COOPER
Centre for International Governance Innovation, Canada
JOHN J. KIRTON
University of Toronto, Canada
TED SCHRECKER
University of Ottawa, Canada

CIGI
The Centre for International Governance Innovation
Centre pour l'innovation dans la gouvernance internationale

ASHGATE

Published by
Ashgate Publishing Ltd.
Gower House
Croft House
Aldershot
Hampshire GU11 3HR
England

Ashgate Publishing Company
Suite 420
101 Cherry Street
Burlington, VT 05401-4405
USA

Ashgate website: http://www.ashgate.com

British Library Cataloguing in Publication Data
Governing global health : challenge, response, innovation.
- (Global environmental governance)
1. Group of Eight (Organization) 2. Public health -
International cooperation
I. Cooper, Andrew Fenton, 1950- II. Kirton, John J.
III. Schrecker, Ted
362.1

Library of Congress Control Number: 2006938318

ISBN: 978-0-7546-4873-4

Printed and bound in Great Britain by MPG Books Ltd, Bodmin, Cornwall.

Contents

PART IV THE CENTRAL INSTITUTIONS: THE G8 SYSTEM

PART V CONCLUSION

APPENDIX

List of Tables

List of Figures

List of Contributors

Obijiofor Aginam is Associate Professor in the Department of Law at Carleton University.

Chantal Blouin is Senior Researcher in Trade and Development at the North-South Institute.

Colin I. Bradford, Jr. is a non-resident Senior Fellow at the Brookings Institution, directing a global governance project co-sponsored by the Centre for International Governance Innovation.

Andrew F. Cooper is Associate Director of the Centre for International Governance Innovation and Professor of Political Science at the University of Waterloo.

Nick Drager is Senior Advisor in the Department of Ethics, Trade, Human Rights, and Health Law at the World Health Organization.

David P. Fidler is Professor of Law and the Harry T. Ice Faculty Fellow at Indiana University's School of Law and a Senior Scholar at the Center for Law and the Public's Health at Georgetown and Johns Hopkins universities.

Lee-Nah Hsu is a Health and Community Development Consultant and Visiting Professor at Mahidol University in Bangkok. She is also a member of the Technical Review Panel of the Global Fund to Fight AIDS, Tuberculosis, and Malaria.

John J. Kirton is Director of the G8 Research Group and Associate Professor of Political Science at the University of Toronto.

Ella Kokotsis is Director of Analytical Studies of the G8 Research Group.

Ronald Labonté is Canada Research Chair in Globalization and Health Equity at the Institute of Population Health at the University of Ottawa.

Jenevieve Mannell is a researcher with the G8 Research Group and a social communication specialist with a background in private enterprise, the Canadian mental health system, and international public health.

Colleen O'Manique is Associate Professor of Women's Studies at Trent University.

James Orbinski is a Research Scientist and Associate Professor of Family and Community Medicine at St. Michael's Hospital in Toronto and Associate Professor in the Department of Political Science at the Munk Centre for International Studies, both at the University of Toronto.

David Sanders is founding director of the School of Public Health at the University of the Western Cape in South Africa.

Ted Schrecker is a scientist with the rank of Associate Professor at the Institute of Population Health at the University of Ottawa.

Laura Sunderland is Senior Researcher with the G8 Research Group.

Jessica White is an intern in the Ecosystems Approaches to Human Health Programme Initiative at the International Development Research Centre.

Mark W. Zacher is Acting Director of the Centre of International Relations at the University of British Columbia.

Preface and Acknowledgements

This volume was inspired by the contemporary health crisis in the world and the manifest failure of the existing galaxy of global governance arrangements to cope. It thus takes as its central theme the need for innovation, in both the ideas and institutions of global health governance that have dominated for so long, still stand in first place today, but are being rapidly being reformed and potentially even replaced by new entrants in the field.

This twelfth book in Ashgate Publishing's Global Environmental Governance series continues the series' tradition of exploring the central issues and contemporary challenges of global governance in areas where the stable single issue areas of old are coming together in today's more intensely integrated, interconnected world. Nowhere is this fusion greater than in the field of health. Here the environmental causes and consequences of health are quickly becoming more understood. The broader socioeconomic determinants and results of health are becoming a dominant paradigm in the health field. And the link between trade and health is moving to centre stage. Such interwoven issues now stand at the core of the global health policy agenda and thus of this book. But they and their components are still largely governed by the single-issue international organisations of old. Only a few integrative bodies — the United Nations, the G8, and new multi-stakeholder bodies — are called upon to forge the needed connections and coherence in an effective way. That is why the need for innovation in global governance, and the contribution of the UN and G8 systems, along with civil society organisations provide the focus points for this work.

To address the critical challenges, global governance responses, and needed innovations in ideas and institutions in the world of health, this volume brings together the resources of three scholarly research programmes. The first is that of the Centre for International Governance Innovation (CIGI) and the University of Waterloo, under the direction of John English and Andrew F. Cooper. The second is that of the University of Ottawa's Canada Research Chair on Globalization and Health Equity, under the leadership of Ronald Labonté. The third is the University of Toronto's G8 Research Group's research programmes on 'Global Governance and the G8' and 'Strengthening Canada's Environmental Community Through International Regime Reform' (EnviReform), under the direction of John Kirton. The results of these research programmes were further developed in the autumn of 2005 in intensive workshops at the University of Ottawa and the University of Waterloo, and then taken through more revisions, both before and after anonymous peer review, to form the chapters in this work.

Acknowledgements

In producing this volume, we have enjoyed the exceptional support of those who have contributed so much in so many different ways. We are grateful in the first instance to CIGI. It provided the major funding for the second workshop, ensured that this effort moved from the initial stage of several research projects and papers into this polished, published book, and organised and hosted the culminating workshop at the University of Waterloo. CIGI also took the lead in bringing in the multi-stakeholder community, led by Rotary International, to enrich the effort.

We are grateful to the Institute of Population Health at the University of Ottawa, which organised and hosted our first workshop and recruited scholars and practitioners, including several from the developing world, during the annual Canadian Conference on International Health, which took place at the same time.

We also owe much to the G8 Research Group, particularly to Ella Kokotsis, Director of Analytical Studies, Laura Sunderland, Senior Researcher, and the many hard-working and dedicated researchers who have contributed so much to this volume. We appreciate, too, the contributions of Hana Dhanji, Sally Elliott, and Zaria Shaw. We are also grateful to the Social Sciences and Humanities Research Council of Canada, under its strategic grant programme on 'Social Cohesion in a Globalizing Age', for its award to the University of Toronto's EnviReform project and its standard research grant to John Kirton for its project on 'After Anarchy: G8 Governance in a Globalizing World'.

Institutionally, we also appreciate the loyal support of our colleagues, administrators, and staff at our home institutions. At CIGI these are Caroline Khoubesserian, former Senior Research Officer, Kelly Jackson, Research Project Manager, and Karen Daniel for her help with logistics. As with all projects at CIGI, we are indebted to the support of Jim Balsillie, chair and co-CEO of Research in Motion, and chair of CIGI's operational board of directors.

At the University of Waterloo our thanks go to Bob Kerton, former Dean of Arts, and Amit Chakma, Vice-President and Provost.

At the University of Ottawa we appreciate the support of the Institute of Population Health and research assistants Caitlin Burley (now at Ryerson University) and Joëlle Walker, who provided indispensable assistance in organising the Ottawa workshop.

At the University of Toronto we are thankful to the Centre for International Studies at the Munk Centre for International Studies, and its director, Professor Louis Pauly, who oversees the G8 Research Group's programme on 'Global Governance and the G8' and the EnviReform project, served as a member of the latter's scholarly project team, and imparted wisdom and collegiality that have been a constant and indispensable source of sound advice and support. At the Centre for International Studies Tina Lagopoulos and her colleagues worked tirelessly in support of our work.

We also thank Robert Scott, Wilfrid Wilkinson, and John Eberhard of Rotary International.

We owe a particular word of thanks to one individual, Madeline Koch, who as Managing Editor of the Global Environmental Governance Series, worked with her usual superb skill and dedication to produce this book.

We are also most grateful to Peter I. Hajnal, who supervised the anonymous referee process of this manuscript. We are most grateful to the dedication, thoroughness, and insight of those referees, whose important comments have been taken fully into account.

As always we reserve a special word of thanks for Kirstin Howgate and her colleagues at Ashgate for recognising the value of producing this volume and for working so effectively, and with generous understanding, to ensure the smooth adoption and speedy publication of this book.

We thank our students for their endless enthusiasm, constructive criticism, intellectual contributions and challenges, and continuing commitment to the causes and issues dealt with in this book. We acknowledge, as always, the patience and support of our families as we laboured to organise our conference, produce our own initial papers, and convert rough drafts into finished chapters. It is to them, Sarah Maddocks and Mary Kirton, that we dedicate this work.

Andrew F. Cooper, John J. Kirton, and Ted Schrecker
November 2006

List of Abbreviations and Acronyms

ACP	Africa, the Carribean, and the Pacific
AfDB	African Development Bank
AoA	World Trade Organization's Agreement on Agriculture
APEC	Asia-Pacific Economic Cooperation
ART	antiretroviral therapy or treatment
BINGO	business-initiated nongovernmental organisation
BMENA	Broader Middle East and North Africa
CIS	Commonwealth of Independent States
CPTech	Consumer Project on Technology
DfID	Department for International Development (United Kingdom)
FAO	Food and Agriculture Organization
FDI	foreign direct investment
G7	Group of Seven (Canada, France, Germany, Italy, Japan, the United Kingdom, and the United States)
G8	Group of Eight (G7 plus Russia)
G20	Group of 20 finance ministers and central bank governors (G8 plus Argentina, Australia, Brazil, China, India, Indonesia, Mexico, Saudi Arabia, South Korea, and Turkey)
GATS	General Agreement on Trade in Services
GATT	General Agreement on Tariffs and Trade
GAVI	Global Alliance for Vaccines and Immunization
GDP	gross domestic product
GHSI	Global Health Security Initiative
GNI	gross national income
GOARN	Global Observation Alert and Response Network
GPHIN	Global Public Health Intelligence Network
HIPC	heavily indebted poor country
HIV	human immunodeficiency virus
IAVI	International AIDS Vaccine Initiative
ICPD	International Conference on Population and Development
ICTSD	International Centre for Trade and Sustainable Development
IFF	International Financing Facility
IFIs	international financial institutions
IHR	International Health Regulations (formerly known as the International Sanitary Regulations of 1903)
IHR(2005)	Revision of the International Health Regulations (issued in 2005)
ILO	International Labour Organization
IMF	International Monetary Fund
IMR	infant mortality rate
INGO	international nongovernmental organisation

IOPH	International Organization for Public Hygiene
L20	Leaders 20 (proposed grouping of the G20 [finance ministers and central bank governors] at the leader's level)
LDC	least developed country
LINGO	little nongovernmental organisation
LONGO	labour-organised nongovernmental organisation
MDG	Millennium Development Goal
MDRI	Multilateral Debt Relief Initiative
MNC	multinational corporation
MSF	Médecins Sans Frontières
NCDO	National Committee for International Cooperation and Sustainable Development
NEPAD	New Partnership for Africa's Development
NGO	nongovernmental organisation
NIEO	New International Economic Order
ODA	official development assistance
OECD	Organisation for Economic Co-operation and Development
OHCHR	Office of the High Commissioner for Human Rights
OIE	World Organisation for Animal Health
PAHO	Pan American Health Organization
ProMED-mail	Program for Monitoring Infectious Diseases
PRSP	Poverty Reduction Strategy Paper
R&D	research and development
S&DT	special and differential treatment
SAP	structural adjustment programme
SARS	severe acute respiratory syndrome
SPS Agreement	Agreement on the Application of Sanitary and Phytosanitary Measures
TB	tuberculosis
TBT	technical barriers to trade
TRIPS	Trade-Related Aspects of Intellectual Property Rights
UNAIDS	Joint United Nations Programme on HIV/AIDS
UNCTAD	United Nations Conference on Trade and Development
UNDP	United Nations Development Programme
UNESCO	United Nations Educational, Scientific, and Cultural Organization
UNFPA	United Nations Fund for Population Activities
UNGA	United Nations General Assembly
UNICEF	United Nations International Children's Fund
UNSC	United Nations Security Council
WEO	World Environment Organization
WHO	World Health Organization
WMD	weapons of mass destruction
WSSD	World Summit on Sustainable Development
WTO	World Trade Organization

PART I
Introduction

Chapter 1

Governing Global Health in the Twenty-First Century

Andrew F. Cooper, John J. Kirton, and Ted Schrecker

Global health is in a crisis. The international community, at all levels, has now begun to respond. Once a technical field residing in the narrow domain of health ministers and their departments, global health issues are now an everyday concern of leaders and their publics around the world. These issues bombard citizens. They feature in front-page stories and newscasts. And sometimes they possess the power to push those with significant resources into action.

This crisis reflects the fact that in the post–Cold War, rapidly globalising, 21st-century world, the war for global health is being waged and lost on many fronts. The already massive body count is mounting fast. At least 25 million global citizens have died of HIV/AIDS. Many more have died from the much older chronic killers of malaria and tuberculosis (TB). They are joined by a long list of emerging and re-emerging deadly infectious diseases with exotic properties and names such as Marburg and Ebola. The shock of the terrorist assault on America on 11 September 2001 and the anthrax attacks that came in its wake have raised the spectre of bioterrorism. The swift spread in 2002–03 of severe acute respiratory syndrome (SARS) from its Asian incubator to the homes and hospitals of North America has shown how vulnerable a now tightly interconnected world is to new deadly diseases. The infection of Europe by the avian influenza from Asia in 2005 and the arrival of human deaths on Europe's doorstep in Turkey within a year confirm that even regions with ready access to the most advanced research and treatment technologies are vulnerable to certain internationally transmitted infectious diseases. And behind these clear and present dangers from diseases primarily afflicting the poor lie chronic killers such as cancer, obesity, cardiovascular disease, and asthma. Once regarded mainly as hazards for the rich, their toll is now rising very quickly in many countries outside the industrialised world in response to rapid changes in incomes, lifestyles, and living conditions.

This onslaught on health in a world of wealth highlights the limits of the global health governance system that has been created over the past 150 years. The world has constructed an ever more elaborate edifice of intergovernmental global health institutions, from a fragile start in the mid 19th century, to realise its current ideal of producing Health For All. At its centre stand the World Health Organization (WHO) and its fellow organisations of the United Nations system, including the World Bank.

Reinforcing them are powerful regional organisations such as the Pan American Health Organization (PAHO) and the European Union. Joining them in response to the assaults of the 21st century have been more informal, plurilateral bodies, notably the G8 major democracies and the Global Fund against AIDS, Tuberculosis, and Malaria. They have been accompanied by a growing array of multi-stakeholder networks, public-private partnerships, and committed action by civil society actors such as Rotary International and Médecins Sans Frontières (MSF).

So far, all have failed to control the crisis. The proud promise of the WHO and the Joint United Nations Programme on AIDS (UNAIDS) to put 3 million AIDS victims into treatment by 2005 through its '3 by 5' initiative has now been sidelined, with that target still far from being met. Three of the UN's Millennium Development Goals (MDGs) are directly concerned with health and the others relate to key social determinants of health; they are on track to fail as well, as the target date of 2015 for their realisation approaches fast. In September 2005 the UN World Summit in New York failed to include health in its outcome document as one of the values to which the organisation was devoted as a priority (United Nations General Assembly [UNGA] 2005). That same month the Global Fund mobilised barely half the money needed to fund existing and new initiatives for the next two years. Powerful regional organisations such as the EU have been unable to prevent avian influenza from infecting humans in countries on its borders. And civil society actors have often been hampered by inadequate resources, multiple constituencies, and multidimensional causes and solutions that lie well beyond their medically focussed mandates and professional capacities.

To be sure, amidst the many setbacks there have been some successes. These provide a foundation, a model, and an inspiration on which to build. But it is now clear that innovations in global health governance, rather than merely increasing investments or incremental improvements in the old systems, are needed to meet the deadly crisis of the new age. These innovations will need to come in the realm of ideas, as the prevailing principles and norms that guide global health governance are redefined and reinvented for a comprehensively and instantaneously interconnected, complex world. They will be needed in the realm of institutions, where new rules, decision-making procedures, resources, and participants are required if the expectations and behaviour of the world's countries and citizens are to converge on the reality, rather than just the ideal, of health for all. In both cases, the still dominant Westphalian model — now almost half a millennium old — of sovereign territorial states engaging in limited international cooperation for particular purposes is fast approaching the end of its useful life. Designing, developing, and delivering the successor system will require the talents of many from national and sub-national governments, international institutions, healthcare professionals, philanthropists, the private sector, local communities, nongovernmental organisations (NGOs), faith groups, committed individuals, and victims from around the world. Furthermore, expanded understanding of the social determinants of health underscores the fact that new ideas and institutions will need decisively to move beyond the focus on providing medical care and traditional public health interventions to address such risk factors as poverty, economic and physical insecurity, and undernutrition as well as the social arrangements that allow them to persist (Albrecht *et al.* 2000; Evans *et al.* 2001; Kim *et al.* 2000; Labonté and Schrecker 2005).

To contribute to this effort, this book addresses three central questions. First, what are the major health challenges the global community confronts in the 21st-century world? Second, how, how well, and why are the current ideas and institutions of global governance responding to the challenge? Third, what innovations are required to the current governance arrangements to meet the challenge in the years ahead?

To answer these questions, this volume has assembled the contributions of leading experts from major academic, research, intergovernmental organisations, civil society, and professional communities involved in governing global health. Together they offer a multidisciplinary analysis, embracing the fields of medicine, public health, law, political science, economics, women's studies, and development studies. This volume also brings together the perspectives, insights, and priorities of analysts, civil society activists, and global governors, all of whom are united by concern with understanding how global health governance operates and how it can be improved to stop the avoidable human slaughter the *status quo* is on course to make in the coming years.

The Analytical Framework

To address these tasks, this book follows a general analytical framework based on a model of stimulus-response-innovation. In keeping with the accumulating literature on global health governance (Cooper 1989; Lee, Buse, and Fustukian 2001; Kawachi and Wamala 2006), it conceives of intergovernmental institutions, national governments, civil society organisations, and citizens as essentially reactive, constrained learners and reluctant innovators, rather than as farsighted, creative, proactive strategic actors who routinely correctively anticipate and successfully act in advance to prevent. To be sure, there have been some supply-driven successes, such as the eradication of smallpox, resulting from new medical breakthroughs. But mostly the main actors innovate when new demands arise from severe shocks or crises. In response to such shocks, these actors respond in the first instance by trying to do more of the same, on the basis of their existing missions, mandates, organisational routines, and resources, and their dominant understanding of cause-and-effect relationships as a guide to how best to solve the expanded old or new problem at hand. The initial instinct is to replicate past successes from old approaches in new areas. The first defence when failure comes is to plead for more money and other resources to solve the challenge at hand. Yet in response to the failure of old approaches and actors to meet new demands, even when equipped with additional resources, there arises competition from new actors and new approaches. From these challenges and competition come ideas and innovation in the dominant institutions that govern global health.

Driving successive stages of this stimulus-response-innovation dynamic is the process of globalisation as it has intensified, despite major interruptions and reverses, from the mid 19th century to the present. Most broadly, globalisation in its successive stages has strengthened the scale, speed, scope, simultaneity, and domestic intrusiveness of disease and illness, driving the demand for global health governance to centre stage in many countries (Scholte 2000; Nye and Donahue 2000). Globalisation has also intensified the economic, social, and physical interconnectedness and complexity that give added force to contemporary global health challenges. Yet the scientific and information revolutions fuelled by globalisation have also brought new insights and resources through which many more actors can respond to the challenge in innovative and effective ways.

To capture these changes, the analysis herein draws on a wide range of major theories of global governance. In the field of political science, these include the perspectives of realism, liberal-institutionalism, epistemic community, political economy, constructivism, and multi-level governance. Here the purpose is not to test competing theories against the evidence to crown a winner, but to mobilise the insights of several traditions in an improved synthetic understanding of how global health governance does, could, and should work in the contemporary world. Thus many of the contributions are explicitly and centrally normative, while others flow from a more traditionally positivist approach. Yet all are aimed at identifying needed and effective innovations, including specific recommendations for actions that can be taken by many actors now.

The Authors' Arguments

Part II, 'Global Challenges and Responses', explores how the demand for and supply of global health governance has changed over the past two centuries, and how the transformations of the 21st century are generating innovative responses.

In Chapter 2, 'The Transformation in Global Health Collaboration since the 1990s', Mark Zacher focusses on the major strengthening of global health governance that started in the 1990s. Beginning with the emergence of regular institutionalised intergovernmental cooperation in health in the mid 19th century, he looks at the reasons for the weakness of earlier international cooperation and the subsequent strengthening of collaboration in four policy areas: disease surveillance, control of the transnational spread of diseases, emergency responses, and health assistance. Zacher argues that there was very little cooperation in surveillance until the 1990s because states, especially developing ones, did not want to report disease outbreaks on their territory for fear that other countries would impose embargoes on the entry of their goods and citizens. However, the multifaceted revolution in information technology led states to cooperate in promoting surveillance because they could do little to stop the outward flow of information. There was also little emergency assistance for a good part of the 20th century because information on the character of outbreaks was poor and there was a marked decrease in serious disease outbreaks — especially new or emerging diseases. But serious outbreaks of traditional diseases such as TB, cholera, and yellow fever in recent decades have forced the WHO to become quite active. From the mid 20th century to the 1980s, there were rather extensive international regulations directed at controlling the spread of diseases in ports and airports, but state compliance was poor. Today, however, states are now more willing to implement international regulations because of the development of new diseases and the speed of their spread. The most dramatic change in international health collaboration since the 1990s has come in increasing international health assistance to improve national health systems. This is due to a serious fear of the emergence and transnational spread of diseases that did not exist before, a strong perception of an impact of diseases on economic development and global commerce, and an explosion in the number and financial resources of nongovernmental actors.

In Chapter 3, 'Global Health, Social Movements, and Governance', James Orbinski is the first of several authors to address the 'securitisation' of public health, its meaning for global health, and the importance of civil society movements, particularly social justice movements, in redefining public health and global health norms to make them more just, fair, and equitable. In economics and finance, the term 'securitisation' refers to the bundling together of a group of assets (such as mortgages, car loans, or credit card balances) in order to use them as backing for bonds or other kinds of tradable debt instruments. In global health discourse, however, the term has come to denote recasting various health and illness prevention challenges in terms of their implications for national (or global) security. Orbinski argues that civil society organisations and social movements essentially react to changes in formal governance and government structures. They can do so in a manner that realigns those structures with a broader, more inclusive, community-oriented conception of governance and the broad polity in general. They can also do so in an ongoing relationship with the structure of governance and government that centres on a dialectic dynamic. This process can gradually alter the architecture that exists to govern global health in a polity or to engage government where an architecture does not exist. To shape this architecture in the intended desirable ways, civil society organisations must act by not deferring to any sacred cows, understanding the global context, forming advocacy coalitions, assembling reliable evidence, and seizing opportunities when they arise.

In Chapter 4, 'A Pathology of Public Health Securitism: Approaching Pandemics as Security Threats', David Fidler expands on the securitisation paradigm by noting that the past decade has seen public health problems increasingly framed as security threats. This new paradigm is evident, for instance, in the WHO's pursuit of global health security; the UN Security Council's [UNSC] consideration of HIV/AIDS as a threat to international peace and security, the integration of health issues into the concept of human security, and the elevation of public health in national security strategies. This activity has established the health-security link in conceptual and policy discourse. It is thus imperative to impose more analytical order and rigour on the health-security relationship. Fidler first outlines a pathology of 'public health securitism', defined as the policy belief that public health can be improved through security-related strategies and tactics. He then identifies four frameworks that can bring greater analytical rigour to the discourse on health and security; these involve bioweapons, communicable diseases, the use of decision trees, and 'epidemiological elasticity', which combines assessments of the mobility of a public health threat and its potential material impact. He then illustrates the application of each of these frameworks to the HIV/AIDS pandemic, the potential for pandemic influenza, and the pandemic of tobacco-related diseases.

Part III, 'The Central Institutions: The Multilateral System', explores how well the multilateral organisations of the UN, a galaxy created in the 'big bang' of international institutionalisation in the 1940s, are meeting the health needs of the global community now.

In Chapter 5, 'Public Health in a Globalising World: The Perspective from the World Health Organization', Nick Drager and Laura Sunderland examine the new characteristics of contemporary global health. They suggest that domestic action is no longer sufficient to deal with outbreaks of both infectious and non-communicable diseases. Collective action is crucial. The WHO has thus taken up a central role in the emerging global health architecture, by focussing on new issues and challenges, strengthening leadership and governance, and engaging the language of human rights to harness knowledge. Based on the WHO's work, they first suggest that the social determinants of health and economic issues as well as issues of accountability must be addressed. There must be a consensus on ethical principles — universalism, justice, dignity, human rights — that are concerned not only with states and sovereignty, but also with generating sufficient resources and defensible resource distributions. The existing two-track health budgeting and monitoring system is problematic, given that local and federal systems coexist and often conflict. Drager and Sunderland illustrate the institutional challenges presented by these new characteristics with reference to the WHO's work in achieving health and trade policy coherence.

In Chapter 6, 'Reaching the Millennium Development Goals', Colin Bradford argues that the central challenge is how to galvanise global action on health in such a way that it addresses the current health crisis through measures that strengthen public health systems in poor countries and catalyse policies and institutional changes that put countries on a trajectory of long-term sustainability. He argues that responses to global health crises need first to maintain the centrality of investment in public health systems and to reflect the multisectoral approach embodied in the MDGs. A global action plan for health set in motion simultaneously with global action plans for education, the environment, and water and sanitation would be critical to the success of global health and long-run sustainability. Such initiatives require, he argues, the support of a broader coalition than the G8 — notably, a group of 20 at the leaders level (L20) — if the necessary resources are to be moblised and the requisite continuous visibility for global health issues is to be maintained.

In Chapter 7, 'Can the World Trade Organization Help Achieve the Health Millennium Development Goals?', Chantal Blouin focusses on two modes of supply of health services — health tourism and foreign investment in the health sector. She uses research undertaken in 2003–04 under the aegis of the WHO to document the extent and impact of trade in health services in Argentina, Chile, China, Indonesia, Senegal, South Africa, and Thailand. Blouin's analysis raises many doubts about the contribution of trade in health services to the achievement of the health MDGs in general and the reduction of maternal mortality in particular. Health tourism is especially problematic: as it increases the patient load in developing countries, it drains physicians and nurses away from the local population, especially among rural patients. She recommends that national governments in developing countries fully assess the impact of health tourism before promoting and supporting it as a key export sector, and adjust their strategies in response.

In Chapter 8, 'Partnerships for Health, the Environment, and Governance', Lee-Nah Hsu and Jessica White focus on the link between environment and health. They argue that because of the interdependent nature of the MDGs — 'for example, health improvements cannot be achieved without certain levels of education or of food security' — the MDGs cannot sensibly be approached in isolation from one another. MDG No. 8, to develop a global partnership for development (see Appendix A), has been neglected thus far but is crucial. Hsu and White identify an urgent need for cross-sectoral policies exemplified by those that build on the links among the environment, development, and health. They further suggest the value of good governance principles including strategic vision, participation, consensus, responsiveness, accountability, equity, efficiency, effectiveness, transparency, and the rule of law.

Part IV, 'The Central Institutions: The G8 System', focusses specifically on the G8-centred system of global health governance that has emerged since the mid 1970s.

In Chapter 9, 'The G8 and Global Health Governance', John Kirton and Jenevieve Mannell present a comprehensive, systematic analysis of the G8's performance in global health governance. They argue that since the onset of rapid globalisation in 1996, the G8 has emerged as an effective, well-performing centre of global health governance across the board. In 1996 and 1997, the leaders at the G8 summits started discussing and deciding on global health issues in a substantial way. Since 2000, the G8 has more than doubled its health deliberations and decisions, delivered its decisions to a high degree, and mobilised new money to this end. In 2006 infectious disease was one of the three priority areas at the St. Petersburg Summit. This effective action by the G8 has been driven by those forces highlighted by the concert equality model of G8 governance. The old UN organisations, led by the WHO, have proven increasingly ineffective in mobilising resources or in meeting their targets and timetables. Kirton and Mannell argue that the G8's core common principles of open democracy and social advance bring its members close to their newly democratic African partners and make them comfortable with the multi-stakeholder approaches most appropriate to combat the new generation of disease.

In contrast, in Chapter 10, 'Diplomatic Rhetoric or Rhetorical Diplomacy: The G8 and Global Health Governance', Obijiofor Aginam critically assesses the actual and potential contributions of the G8. He finds 'an appalling disconnect with other normative and multilateral mechanisms on global health'. Although the G8 summits in Okinawa in 2000 and Genoa in 2001 catalysed the establishment of the Global Fund as a public-private partnership, the G8s' commitments to global health governance fail to align with existing global health mechanisms in mutually reinforcing ways. As a case study Aginam uses the impediments to access to essential medicines created by the Agreement on Trade-Related Aspects of Intellectual Property Rights (TRIPS). To date, he argues, the G8 summit has not functioned as a forum for incubating humane global health governance norms, but rather as a diplomatic forum for rhetoric with not enough real results.

In Chapter 11, 'Keeping Faith with Africa's Health: Catalysing G8 Compliance', John Kirton and Ella Kokotsis ask what the G8 leaders can do at their annual summit to ensure that their countries comply with their health-related African summit commitments after the G8 summit concludes. In an effort to establish a theoretically informed, empirically supported, and policy-relevant explanation of members' compliance, Kirton and Kokotsis examine whether compliance improves when summit commitments contain compliance-inducing catalysts. They examine compliance with G7/8 commitments over all issue areas from 1996 to 2006 to determine in aggregate fashion if the presence of each of the specified compliance-inducing catalysts in an individual commitment increases its compliance score. They then explore more closely compliance with African-related health commitments from 1996 to see which compliance catalysts work in this field. Kirton and Kokotsis conclude that G8 leaders can make a difference in fostering compliance with their overall commitments by giving them priority placement, specifying the agents to implement them, and setting targets. In the field of health, specifying timetables for implementation also helps. Conversely, mobilising large amounts of new money and, especially, relying on other established international institutions to take care of implementation constitute a recipe for failure to deliver real results.

In Chapter 12, 'Breaking Faith with Africa: The G8 and Population Health after Gleneagles', Ted Schrecker, Ronald Labonté, and David Sanders emphasise the social determinants of health as well as access to health care. They argue that this perspective requires a critique of the effects on the social determinants of health of the dominant development policy model that has been applied to Africa. Because of the G7's dominant role in the world economy and in governance institutions such as the World Bank, the International Monetary Fund (IMF), and the World Trade Organization (WTO), it is assigned a major share of the responsibility for trends in population health outside the developed world. Like Bradford and Aginam, Schrecker and his colleagues address not only the extent to which the G7/8 has lived up to its commitments, but also the adequacy and appropriateness of those commitments as they relate to health. Drawing on previous research on G7/8 commitments from 1999 to 2004, they argue that many commitments have been inadequate or incommensurate with the scale of the need for new resources (Labonté *et al.* 2004; Labonté and Schrecker 2005). Some (such as those promoting rapid import liberalisation) were actually destructive of health. While noting the real potential benefits of the many commitments related to African development and health that were made at the 2005 Gleneagles Summit, Schrecker, Labonté, and Sanders conclude with concern about the ability of health issues and health-related development policy to retain their newly won prominence on the G8 agenda. They wonder whether it is reasonable to expect leadership on global health from the G8.

In Chapter 13, 'Global Health and Universal Human Rights: The Case for G8 Accountability', Colleen O'Manique notes that the human right to health has been recognised in a range of conventions and declarations, including the Universal Declaration of Human Rights, the 1978 Declaration of Alma-Ata, the International Covenant on Economic, Social, and Cultural Rights, and the Convention on the Rights of the Child. O'Manique asks: What is a human right to health, and how is it understood in practice? What are the specific features of the current global order that can be linked to the violation of people's exercise of their basic human right to health, and what is the value system underpinning this order? Where does responsibility lie in ensuring that all humans have access to the basic constituents of human health? Returning to the theme of securitisation, she argues that there has been an elevation of the power of private actors that are not subject to restraints on their violations of people's exercise of basic human rights. National security doctrines and the 'war on terrorism' justify the extension of multiple practices of political domination to the global economic South. Like Aginam and Schrecker and his colleagues, O'Manique adopts an explicitly normative perspective on the accountability of the G8, in this case viewing their actions through the prism of international human rights norms.

As noted earlier, the authors in this book adopt a multiplicity of perspectives — a prerequisite for healthy debate on the urgent challenges that have been identified. Part V, with Chapter 14 on 'Toward Innovation in Global Health Governance', attempts to identify some common findings and directions for innovation according to the challenge-response-innovation model that formed the analytical foundation for this book. Amidst the many disagreements and uncertainties, there is general agreement that the challenges are proliferating, that the dominant ideas and institutions that guide current global health governance are not keeping pace, and that a wide range of innovations, from the incremental to the revolutionary, is required as a result. The book concludes with a set of recommendations for immediate action to catalyse the process of transformational innovation in global health governance that the global community badly needs to cope with the crisis now confronting it.

References

Albrecht, Gary L., Alfred Fitzpatrick, and Susan Scrimshaw, eds. (2000). *Handbook of Social Studies in Health and Medicine* (London: Sage Publications).

Cooper, Richard N. (1989). 'International Cooperation in Public Health as a Prologue to Macroeconomic Cooperation'. In R.N. Cooper, ed., *Can Nations Agree? Issues in International Economic Cooperation,* pp. 183–190 (Washington DC: Brookings Institution).

Evans, Timothy, Margaret Whitehead, Finn Diderichsen, *et al.*, eds. (2001). *Challenging Inequities in Health: From Ethics to Action* (New York: Oxford University Press).

Kawachi, Ichiro and Sarah Wamala, eds. (2006). *Globalization and Health* (Oxford: Oxford University Press).

Kim, Jim Yong, Joyce V. Millen, John Gershman, *et al.*, eds. (2000). *Dying for Growth: Global Inequality and the Health of the Poor* (Monroe ME: Common Courage Press).

Labonté, Ronald, Ted Schrecker, David Sanders, *et al.* (2004). *Fatal Indifference: The G8, Africa, and Global Health* (Cape Town: University of Cape Town Press).

Labonté, Ronald and Ted Schrecker (2005). *The G8, Africa, and Global Health: A Platform for Global Health Equity for the 2005 Summit* (London: Nuffield Trust).

Lee, Kelley, Kent Buse, and Suzanne Fustukian, eds. (2001). *Health Policy in a Globalising World* (New York: Cambridge University Press).

Nye, Joseph S. and John Donahue, eds. (2000). *Governance in a Globalizing World* (Washington DC: Brookings Institution Press).

Scholte, Jan Aart (2000). *Globalization: A Critical Introduction* (Houndsmills: Palgrave).

United Nations General Assembly (2005). '2005 World Summit Outcome'. 15 September. <www.un.org/summit2005/documents.html> (September 2006).

PART II
Global Challenges and Responses

Chapter 2

The Transformation in Global Health Collaboration since the 1990s

Mark W. Zacher

Global health collaboration has evolved through three historical regime periods: the mid 19th century to the early 20th century, the early 20th century through the 1980s, and the 1990s to the present. The first period witnessed arduous negotiations to conclude a treaty to control the international spread of epidemic diseases. It led to the acceptance of the International Sanitary Regulations of 1903. During the second period, for the most part, states tended to ignore the International Health Regulations (IHR), as the 1903 regulations came to be called. They thus had a very limited impact. The decade and a half since 1990 has seen quite a dramatic expansion in multilateral health cooperation. The trend is likely to continue.

There is an irony in this historical pattern. One would think that international collaboration would have been stronger in the second era, when medical science was developing in significant ways and at least some traditional diseases were quite widespread. But this was not the case for a number of reasons. From the early years of the 20th century there was a growing optimism that infectious diseases could be handled with increasing ease. It took the emergence of new diseases starting in the 1980s and a growing literature on the multiple negative impacts of infectious diseases to trigger a new outlook. In addition, the industrialised countries developed an increasing fear of the consequences of infectious diseases in the developing world (Commission on Macroeconomics and Health 2001; Smolinski, Hamburg, and Lederberg 2003; Heymann 2003; Heymann and Rodier 2001; National Intelligence Estimate 2000).

The Nineteenth-Century Regime

Throughout the millennia of human history there has been very little politics of international health. For a long time, humans did not have sufficient medical knowledge to understand disease pathogens and propose remedial and preventive measures. Nevertheless, states felt compelled to explore the possibility of international action when cholera pandemics spread from South Asia to most areas of the world during the 19th century. The first international conference to address the cholera problem occurred in 1851. But it and subsequent conferences until the end of the 19th century failed to reach agreement. There were serious differences between the countries of the Mediterranean and northern Europe, because the former group of states suffered much more than did those of northern Europe. This, quite naturally, made the former countries more concerned to achieve international disease controls than were the latter states.

While the differences in damages from the spread of pandemic diseases undermined the frequent attempts to achieve accords in the late 19th century, what had an equally, and perhaps more, important impact on the diplomatic failures was inadequate medical knowledge of cholera as well as other diseases such as plague, yellow fever, malaria, and tuberculosis (TB). It was not until the revolution in medical knowledge that started in the 1880s that it became possible for states to agree on some international controls. This revolution is often associated with the French scientist Louis Pasteur and the German scientist Robert Koch (Goodman 1971; Howard-Jones 1975; Cooper 1989).

The Twentieth-Century Multilateral Health Regime

The first major disease control convention, the IHR, was adopted in 1903. It required that states report disease outbreaks, and that ships and port authorities adopt a number of practices that would reduce the likelihood of the spread of diseases. It also specified that states could not implement regulations in excess of those specified in the IHR. The reason for this provision was that the developed states did not want developing countries to apply measures that would hinder the flow of commerce. The convention at first covered only cholera and the plague, but in 1912 and 1926 yellow fever, typhus, relapsing fever, and smallpox were added. In 1907 the International Organization for Public Hygiene (IOPH) was created to review the adequacy of the IHR and to revise them. Then, in 1922, the League of Nations Health Organization was created to provide technical assistance and medical advice to some developing countries. The United States refused to join the organisation, as it was not a member of the League. Thus most states did not support the transfer of the IOPH's functions to the League body.

Despite all the diplomatic efforts that had gone into developing the IHR and the continued existence of serious disease-related problems in many areas of the world, most states gave little attention to the regulations. Developing countries were reluctant to report disease outbreaks for fear of embargoes on their goods and citizens. They were also opposed to the stricture not to impose regulations in excess of those included in the IHR. This latter policy is quite understandable as many developing countries did not have strong healthcare systems that could deal with outbreaks without exceeding the limits set in the IHR (Howard-Jones 1978; Fidler 1999).

Developed countries lost interest in the IHR because they found that they could prevent and control outbreaks on their own in their territories. They did not need to rely on international rules. New public health measures and vaccines prevented diseases. New medicines helped doctors cure many people with diseases. Also, states were able to legislate their own rules for their ports if they wanted, and these rules were often better suited to local problems. The IHR did have some impact in shaping states' health practices in ports, but they did not have a prominent influence.

In 1946 a major institutional change occurred in the realm of global health governance when the United Nations created the World Health Organization (WHO) as a specialised UN agency. Its decisions are made by majority vote and are not legally binding. The one exception is the WHO's power to approve international conventions such as the IHR, although even in this case WHO member states have been able to opt out of a convention or specific provisions of it.

There was little dispute over the functions and the decision-making procedures of WHO. One modest innovation was the creation of six regional commissions that were particularly responsible for administering the WHO's economic assistance programmes (including the Pan American Health Organization [PAHO], which had been created in 1902). The WHO approved a revised version of the IHR in 1951, but it differed only slightly from the previous version. State compliance also differed little from practices during the pre–World War II era. Diplomatic discussions of the IHR from the 1950s through the 1970s focussed more on developed countries' concerns about excessive measures than they did with measures to prevent the spread of diseases. They regarded the IHR more as a vehicle for facilitating commerce than as a vehicle of disease control.

A further innovation in global health collaboration after World War II was the launch of a multilateral programme of financial assistance for controlling diseases. The magnitude of the funding for WHO programmes was modest; funds came from the WHO's general budget and were distributed among six WHO regional commissions that were staffed largely by personnel from regional states. The developed countries soon became very disenchanted with the spending practices of WHO regional commissions and rejected proposals to provide additional funds for financial assistance from the regular budget. The developed states provided some modest extra-budgetary accounts within WHO that they could control. Most health assistance funds were directed through bilateral transfers and organisations other than WHO and its regional commissions.

One notable aid initiative in the late 1960s and early 1970s was the WHO's campaign to abolish smallpox. The funding and technical assistance came largely in the form of a coordinated effort by the developed countries, including the Soviet Union. The political decision making and funding were largely a coordinated effort among developed countries rather than an effort of financial pooling and collective decision making. The effort was led by a prominent U.S. health official, Dr. Donald Henderson, who benefited from strong backing by the United States. The coordination approach to smallpox eradication came close to the kind of health collaboration that has dominated health assistance since the 1990s. In part because smallpox is the only disease to have been completely eliminated, states and international health organisations have drawn many lessons from the campaign to eliminate it (Fenner 1988).[1]

Nevertheless, the record of global health collaboration during the greater part of the 20th century shows that all of the three strategies attempted were largely unsuccessful. Surveillance failed largely because developing countries feared retribution if they announced outbreaks on their territories. Transnational controls on the spread of disease in ports and airports had little impact because developed countries were able to take care of most of their citizens who contracted diseases from foreigners and because developing countries wanted to avoid any reactions against 'excessive measures'. There was also steady progress in the post-war era in the reduction of deaths from diseases. On the whole, states did not fear widespread economic, social, and political damages from infectious diseases until the end of the 20th century. Furthermore, multilateral financial assistance did not develop significantly because developed countries did not trust the ability of developing countries to use such funds; in the colonial and Cold War eras, developed countries were oriented toward bilateral funding, and humanitarian nongovernmental organisations (NGOs) were very weak.

The Global Health Governance Regime from the 1990s to the Present

Since 1990 there has been a dramatic expansion in global health collaboration. There is no simple explanation for this development. Key factors have been the emergence of new pandemic diseases, a broader understanding of the negative effects of disease in the developing world, a greater transparency with regard to disease outbreaks (influenced in particular by improved information technology), an expansion of NGOs committed to improving social and economic conditions in the developing world, and improvements in international institutions.

When WHO members turned their attention to the revision of the IHR in the early 21st century, the developed countries dropped their insistence on a ban on measures in excess of the IHRs' standards. Given the emergence of new and lethal diseases, the industrialised states (particularly the United States) wanted a high degree of latitude in dealing with the diseases. Because the developing countries were unlikely, in any case, to comply with a stricture against excessive measures, insistence on such a provision was unlikely to have any positive effects for developed countries (WHO 2006b).

In 2005, a revision of the IHR was adopted, to come into force in June 2007. IHR(2005) contained as many regulations relating to sanitary practices on international carriers and at points of entry as did the previous versions of the convention. Most states, and particularly most developed countries, continued to consider it worthwhile to have health rules in an international treaty that allowed WHO bodies to hold states and commercial carriers accountable for pursuing particular health practices. An increasing fear of infectious diseases starting in the 1990s led to increasing concern about compliance. However, it is unclear whether rules concerning carriers and activities at points of entry (such as ports) would be more effective than they were in the past.

The WHO had also always been involved in prescribing proper medical practices in specific disease outbreaks and different types of outbreaks. In the past the World

Health Assembly and the occasional WHO expert group approved recommendations concerning the management of specific outbreaks or types of outbreaks. But the WHO has become much more active in prescribing medical practices. In 2000, it created the Global Observation Alert and Response Network (GOARN), which links about one hundred networks of health experts to advise ministries of health and health NGOs (WHO 2006a). It has grown and become more active since 2000. In addition, the IHR(2005) specified the right of new WHO committees (namely the Emergency Committee and the Review Committee) and the World Health Assembly to approve temporary recommendations for specific outbreaks and standing recommendations for types of infectious disease problems (WHO 2005). The WHO secretariat, particularly the director general, has become more important in providing recommendations and is now quite willing to threaten public criticisms if states do not comply. During the 2003 outbreak of severe acute respiratory syndrome (SARS), the WHO resorted to travel advisories, recommending that individuals not travel to certain areas (including the city of Toronto). Here the WHO was targeting individuals rather than governments — something that was quite unusual for an intergovernmental institution. Overall, the WHO has moved closer to becoming a ministry of health for the world (Fidler 1999, 2004, 2005; WHO 2002; Lederberg, Shope, and Oaks 1992; Smolinski, Hamburg, and Lederberg 2003; Brower and Chalk 2003).

One of the most important areas of strategic change has involved surveillance. As noted previously, developing countries had been reluctant to report disease outbreaks from the earliest days of health multilateralism in the early 20th century. They justifiably feared embargoes on their goods and citizens. They insisted that any reporting of diseases on their territories come from their governments. It was the transformation of information technology in the 1990s that primarily changed their views and, consequently, WHO practices. The internet, in particular, gave health professionals and the media the ability to report disease outbreaks to the outside world, and deprived governments of the ability to block such reporting. Thus governments soon began to report outbreaks on their own, and the transformation in transparency with regard to disease outbreaks has clearly been based on technological change more than on any other factor.

One example of international health reporting dependent on the internet is a system of reporting called the Program for Monitoring Infectious Diseases (ProMED-mail), launched by a group of doctors and the Rockefeller Foundation in 1994 (International Society for Infectious Diseases 2006). Medical professionals could report outbreaks to a central website in the U.S.; ProMED-mail then distributed the information to international organisations and governments. Another case is the Global Public Health Intelligence Network (GPHIN), created by Canada with the cooperation of the WHO in 1997 (Public Health Agency of Canada 2004). An office at Health Canada sifts through a large number of websites that provide information on disease outbreaks. It then collates lists of disease outbreaks and sends these lists to the WHO and a number of governments, who then corroborate the claims of disease outbreaks. The WHO reports the findings on its website. GPHIN now reports more disease outbreaks than any other organisation.

A number of important normative and legal changes have followed from these changes in technology and reporting practices. In the first years of the 21st century the World Health Assembly passed recommendations that approved the WHO's reporting of outbreaks on the basis of information from nongovernmental sources. In the 2003 SARS crisis the WHO secretariat reported information from such sources in China and threatened that it would publicise the information if China did not admit the existence of the outbreaks. In other words, an intergovernmental organisation was circumventing governments to control certain behaviour of their citizens (Fidler 2004; National Advisory Committee on SARS and Public Health 2003; Knobler *et al.* 2004; United States General Accounting Office 2004). Finally, in 2005 the World Health Assembly revised the IHR to make it legal for the WHO to receive and publicise reports from nongovernmental sources. In fact, the IHR(2005) provides detailed guidelines for reporting on outbreaks (Heymann and Rodier 1998; Zacher 1999; Grein *et al.* 2000; Fidler 2004, 2005; National Advisory Committee on SARS and Public Health 2003; WHO 2002; WHO 2006b).

Perhaps the most dramatic change in global health collaboration since the 1990s has been the expansion of multilateral health assistance — and more particularly public-private partnerships. Before 1990 there was little multilateral health aid. It now dominates the health aid field. Since the mid 1990s the World Bank has become the largest donor among international organisations. A surfeit of NGOs active in the health aid field has developed. These organisations comprise humanitarian bodies such as Médecins Sans Frontières (MSF) and Oxfam and foundations such as the Bill and Melinda Gates Foundation and the United Nations Foundation. In addition, multinational pharmaceutical firms such as Merck and Roche have clearly felt that their reputations would suffer if they did not offer some significant contributions to the reduction of infectious diseases in the developing world. Most new health assistance institutions now include a mixture of states, intergovernmental bodies, and NGOs (including foundations). Aid donors exert considerable pressure on recipient governments to cooperate with all donors and their own domestic agencies to produce more efficient aid enterprises. 'Coordination' is the key word today, and it generally involves collaboration among states, state agencies, intergovernmental organisations, and NGOs. There are a host of public-private partnerships in the health aid field. The best known is the Global Fund to Fight AIDS, Tuberculosis, and Malaria (World Bank 1993; Keck and Sikkink 1998; Widdus 2001; Lucas 2002; Reich 2002; Lee, Walt, and Haines 2004; Initiative on Public-Private Partnerships for Health 2006; Global Fund to Fight AIDS 2006).

One form of health assistance that sometimes receives a great deal of publicity is emergency interventions to control pandemic outbreaks. The WHO and its regional commissions have been involved in providing assistance since they were established, but the frequency and magnitude of such interventions have changed. Most emergency interventions in the past involved simply the provision of medical advice to ministries of health and local medical staff. Today, the number of WHO-sponsored staff in some operations is close to a hundred as opposed to five. The WHO has also established formal ties with more than a hundred laboratories with specialised expertise — formally known as WHO collaborating centres. Since 2000 these centres, as well as other types of assistance offered by states and occasionally the WHO secretariat, have been coordinated by GOARN, which facilitates getting staff into the field more quickly. Also states are willing to contribute staff because governments, and especially their health officials, are much more concerned about pandemic outbreaks since the dramatic expansion of new or emerging diseases in the last two decades. Some of the more notable emergency responses have involved the Ebola outbreak in the Congo in 1995–96, SARS in China and other states in 2003, and the avian influenza outbreaks in a number of countries in Southeast Asia from 2000 to 2004. The emergency responses (particularly since the 1990s) are multi-state and multi-organisation enterprises. The WHO was basically a facilitator in that it had very few of its own staff in the field (Garrett 1994, 2000; Knobler *et al.* 2004).

In these recent emergency responses there have been some additional marked departures from the past. Even though they were relatively minor in scale, they are symbolically quite significant. For the first time the WHO relied on NGOs for a great deal of its intelligence. This was particularly notable in the SARS crisis. It occurred in the avian influenza crises as well. In both of these international health crises the WHO secretariat told states that they would be formally accused of lying if they did not accurately report the scope of the problems. It is hard to imagine the WHO secretariat telling this to the Chinese government — and then the Chinese government firing its minister of health and the mayor of Beijing as a way of showing that it would conform with WHO requests. Also of particular note was the WHO's issuance of travel advisories during the SARS crisis. These advisories recommended that individuals not travel to certain countries or areas of countries. A final strategic approach toward reducing deaths and illnesses from infectious diseases has been allowing developing states to manufacture and trade essential medicines, permitting them to acquire medicines at lower prices. The cost of drugs has been high because of international trade laws and international intellectual property rights laws, and because pharmaceutical manufacturers often do not manufacture drugs for tropical diseases for which there are very small markets in the developed world. This latter problem is often referred to as the '10/90 gap' in that only about 10 percent of the global drug research and development focusses on diseases that account for 90 percent of global problems. Profits are made from drugs developed for the wealthiest 10 percent of the world's population.

In the international trade realm, the central norm is the principle of nondiscrimination in the General Agreement on Tariffs and Trade (GATT) and the World Trade Organization (WTO) — that is to say, states must apply the same trade restrictions to all member states. There was, however, a proviso to this principle, allowing restrictions to be altered for certain states if people's health is at stake and the regulations do not unnecessarily hinder international trade (GATT 1947, art. XX[b]). A comparable provision exists in the 1995 Agreement on Trade-Related Aspects of Intellectual Property Rights (TRIPS). Under TRIPS, all WTO member states are to establish minimum standards for protecting and enforcing intellectual property rights (WTO 1994, art. 7). The basic rationale is that such standards and their enforcement for a particular time (20 years) encourages technological innovation. However, TRIPS does stipulate that members may 'adopt measures necessary to protect public health' (art. 8[1]). Also, article 30 provides that members can provide limited exceptions to patent rights 'provided that such exceptions do not unreasonably prejudice the legitimate interests of the patent owner' (art. 30). Article 31 stipulates conditions under which a product that is under a patent can be produced by an entity other than the right holder. In cases where a member state issues a license to a third party ordering the production of a patented product, this is referred to as compulsory licensing. A severe restriction was, however, placed on the issuing of such licenses. Article 31(f) states that compulsory licensing shall be authorised predominantly for the supply of the domestic market of the member authorising such use. This means that developing countries without an advanced domestic pharmaceutical industry could not take advantage of this clause.

It was not until 2003 that a solution to this problem was reached, prompted by two crises involving Brazil and South Africa (Abbott 2002; Grabowski 2002; Koivusalo 2003). In 1996 Brazil launched a programme of supplying antiretroviral therapy (ART) to HIV/AIDS patients free of charge. It also produced generic drugs that were patented in other countries and justified their production under article 31 and threatened to order Brazilian firms to produce the drugs under compulsory licensing. The threat was enough to pressure international pharmaceutical firms to reduce the prices of drugs for import into Brazil. In February 2001 the United States threatened to challenge Brazil in a WTO suit, but the U.S. backed off under pressure from NGOs. In 1997 the South African government passed legislation that revoked patents on drugs to treat AIDS, issued compulsory licences for the production of generic drugs, and imported generic versions of patented drugs from Brazil and India. In 1998 a coalition of 39 pharmaceutical firms challenged the South African legislation under South African law (not TRIPS). They were backed by the United States and European Union. However, a coalition of NGOs led by MSF induced the lawyers for the drug manufacturers to withdraw their opposition to the legislation in 2001.

Within the WTO a major innovation occurred in November 2001 at a WTO ministerial meeting in Doha, Qatar. The developing countries secured a provision in the Doha declaration on the TRIPS Agreement and Public Health that it should be interpreted in a way that supported their ability to protect public health and to provide access to essential medicines (WTO 2001, art. 4). Every member was given the right to grant compulsory licenses (art. 5[b]). A weakness of the Doha declaration was that it did not clarify the previously mentioned domestic market issue regarding compulsory licensing. An accord was finally reached by the TRIPS council in August 2003 that allowed a member state to produce a patented medicine under a compulsory licence and then export it to a least developed country that did not have domestic capacity to produce the drugs itself. A state must however receive approval from the TRIPS council (WTO 2001; Sykes 2002; Matthews 2002, 2004; WTO and WHO 2002; t'Hoen 2002)

The key factor that brought about these changes was the pressure exerted by NGOs — led by MSF. They strongly criticised the pharmaceutical firms and the developed countries that supported their positions on patent rights. There is no doubt that the position of the western industrialised interests and their allied states collapsed because they feared the impacts of the criticisms from their NGOs, which had considerable influence over national public opinions. There are few cases where concessions by firms and governments have been so clearly attributable to NGO pressure.

Conclusion

Contrary to the beliefs of many, global health collaboration was very weak from the beginning of the 20th century through to the 1980s. The inadequacies of early international collaboration were due to a number of factors. One was the weaknesses in the health systems of developing countries in that they often could not detect disease outbreaks, and they could not implement disease control policies on carriers and in ports and inland areas. They also feared embargoes against goods and individuals if they reported outbreaks.

Ironically, it was the increasing strength of the medical and public health systems in the developed world that promoted a lack of interest in international collaboration among the industrialised states. The incidence of diseases declined in these countries, and the success of curative intervention increased. Thus, over the decades of the 20th century, people of the industrialised world became confident that infectious diseases were a problem of the past. In fact, developed countries were interested in international health collaboration only because they opposed health interventions by developing countries that impeded the flow of commerce.

Since the 1990s, there has been a dramatic strengthening in multilateral approaches to the control of infectious diseases. Surveillance improved dramatically because of improvements in information technology. States could seldom block the reporting of diseases via the internet. Reponses to emergency outbreaks became quicker and more effective because of linkages among national health institutions — often through WHO coordination. Multilateral aid expanded dramatically because of increased fears of the health, economic, and social costs of infectious diseases, as well as because of the dramatic growth of health NGOs and the improvements in international institutions. The great majority of international health assistance programmes are now public-private partnerships. This can be significantly attributed to the increasing resources and normative influence of NGOs.

The involvement of the global community in promoting health through revising intellectual property rights law is a relatively recent development. It occurred because of the increasing development and legal status of intellectual property rights law with the acceptance of the TRIPS Agreement in 1995. It also came because NGOs made this issue a central one in their drive to improve health conditions in the developing world.

Overall there has been a marked strengthening in global health collaboration in the last 15 years. There is no indication that this trend will change. Fears of pandemics (for example, avian influenza) have increased; the strength of transnational medical and humanitarian NGO networks has grown; and there has been an increasing recognition of the multiple costs of infectious diseases — especially in the developing world. Of these factors special attention should be given to the growing normative commitments to health assistance in many areas of the world. It has only been because of these normative commitments that NGOs and public-private partnerships have altered decision making on global health.

Note

1 The last naturally occurring case of smallpox was in Somalia in 1977. Thanks to a world-wide vaccination programme, the disease is considered eradicated; however, there remains concern that smallpox could be used as an agent of bioterrorism (Centers for Disease Control and Prevention 2006).

References

Abbott, Frederick M. (2002). 'The Doha Declaration on the TRIPS Agreement and Public Health: Lighting a Dark Corner at the WTO'. *Journal of International Economic Law,* vol. 5, no. 2, pp. 469–505.

Brower, Jennifer and Peter Chalk (2003). *The Global Threat of New and Reemerging Infectious Diseases: Reconciling U.S. National Security and Public Health Policy* (Santa Monica CA: Rand).

Centers for Disease Control and Prevention (2006). 'Smallpox Disease Overview'. Atlanta. <www.bt.cdc.gov/agent/smallpox/overview/disease-facts.asp> (September 2006).

Commission on Macroeconomics and Health (2001). 'Macroeconomics and Health: Investing in Health for Economic Development'. World Health Organization, Geneva. <www.cid.harvard.edu/cidcmh/CMHReport.pdf> (September 2006).

Cooper, Richard N. (1989). 'International Cooperation in Public Health as a Prologue to Macroeconomic Cooperation'. In R.N. Cooper, ed., *Can Nations Agree? Issues in International Economic Cooperation,* pp. 183–190 (Washington DC: Brookings Institution).

Fenner, Frank, ed. (1988). *Smallpox and Its Eradication* (Geneva: World Health Organization).

Fidler, David P. (1999). *International Law and Infectious Diseases* (Oxford: Oxford University Press).

Fidler, David P. (2004). *SARS: Governance and the Globalization of Disease* (New York: Palgrave Macmillan).

Fidler, David P. (2005). 'From International Sanitary Conventions to Global Health Security: The New International Health Regulations'. *Chinese Journal of International Law,* vol. 4, no. 2, pp. 325–392.

Garrett, Laurie (1994). *The Coming Plague: Newly Emerging Diseases in a World Out of Balance* (New York: Farrar, Strauss and Giroux).

Garrett, Laurie (2000). *Betrayal of Trust The Collapse of Global Public Health* (New York: Hyperion).

General Agreement on Tariffs and Trade (1947). <www.wto.org/english/docs_e/legal_e/gatt47_01_e.htm> (September 2006).

Global Fund to Fight AIDS, Tuberculosis, and Malaria (2006). Geneva. <www.theglobalfund.org/en> (September 2006).

Goodman, Neville M. (1971). *International Health Organizations and Their Work,* 2nd ed. (London: Churchill Livingston).

Grabowski, Henry (2002). 'Patents, Innovation, and Access to New Pharmaceuticals'. *Journal of International Economic Law,* vol. 5, no. 4, pp. 849–860.

Grein, Thomas W., Kande-Bure O. Kamara, Guénaël Rodier, *et al.* (2000). 'Rumors of Disease in the Global Village: Outbreak Verification'. *Emerging Infectious Diseases,* vol. 6, no. 2, pp. 97–102. <www.cdc.gov/ncidod/eid/vol6no2/grein.htm> (September 2006).

Heymann, David L. (2003). 'Evolving Infectious Disease Threats to National and Global Security'. In L. Chen, J. Learning, and V. Narasimhan, eds., *Global Health Challenges for Human Security,* pp. 105–124 (Cambridge MA: Harvard University Press).

Heymann, David L. and Guénaël Rodier (1998). 'Global Surveillance of Communicable Diseases'. *Emerging Infectious Diseases,* vol. 4, no. 3, pp. 362–365. <www.cdc.gov/ncidod/eid/vol4no3/heymann.htm> (September 2006).

Heymann, David L. and Guénaël Rodier (2001). 'Hot Spots in a Wired World: WHO Surveillance of Emerging and Re-emerging Infectious Diseases'. *Lancet,* vol. 1, no. 5, pp. 345–353.

Howard-Jones, Norman (1975). *The International Scientific Background of the International Sanitary Conferences* (Geneva: World Health Organization).

Howard-Jones, Norman (1978). *International Public Health between the Two Wars: The Organizational Problems* (Geneva: World Health Organization).

Initiative on Public-Private Partnerships for Health (2006). Geneva. <www.ippph.org> (September 2006).

International Society for Infectious Diseases (2006). 'ProMED-mail'. Brookline MA. <www.promedmail.org> (September 2006).

Keck, Margaret E. and Kathryn Sikkink (1998). *Activists Beyond Borders: Advocacy Networks in International Politics* (Ithaca: Cornell University Press).

Knobler, Stacey, Adel Mahmoud, Stanley Lemon, *et al.*, eds. (2004). *Learning from SARS: Preparing for the Next Disease Outbreak* (Washington DC: National Academies Press).

Koivusalo, Meri (2003). 'Assessing the Health Policy Implications of WTO Trade and Investment Agreements'. In K. Lee, ed., *Health Impacts of Globalization,* pp. 161–176 (London: Palgrave Macmillan).

Lederberg, Joshua, Robert E. Shope, and Stanley C. Oaks, eds. (1992). *Emerging Infections: Microbial Threats to Health in the United States* (Washington DC: National Academies Press).

Lee, Kelley, Gill Walt, and Andy Haines (2004). 'The Challenge to Improve Global Health: Financing the Millennium Development Goals'. *Journal of the American Medical Association,* vol. 291, no. 2, pp. 2636–2638.

Lucas, Adetokunbo O. (2002). 'Public-Private Partnerships: Illustrative Examples'. In M.R. Reich, ed., *Public-Private Partnerships for Public Health,* pp. 19–39 (Cambridge MA: Harvard Center for Population and Development Studies).

Matthews, Duncan (2002). *Globalizing Intellectual Property Rights: The TRIPS Agreement* (London: Routledge).

Matthews, Duncan (2004). 'WTO Decision on Implementation of Paragraph 6 of the Doha Declaration on the TRIPS Agreement and Public Health: A Solution to the Access to Essential Medicines Problems?' *Journal of International Economic Law,* vol. 7, no. 1, pp. 73–107.

National Advisory Committee on SARS and Public Health (2003). 'Learning from SARS: Renewal of Public Health in Canada'. Health Canada, Ottawa. <www.phac-aspc.gc.ca/publicat/sars-sras/naylor> (September 2006).

National Intelligence Estimate (2000). 'The Global Infectious Disease Threat and Its Implications for the United States'. NIE 99-17D. National Intelligence Council, Washington DC. <www.ciaonet.org/wps/dod109/dod109.pdf> (September 2006).

Public Health Agency of Canada (2004). 'Global Public Health Intelligence Network'. Ottawa. <www.phac-aspc.gc.ca/media/nr-rp/2004/2004_gphin-rmispbk_e.html> (September 2006).

Reich, Michael R. (2002). 'Introduction'. In M.R. Reich, ed., *Public-Private Partnerships for Public Health,* pp. 1–16 (Cambridge MA: Harvard Center for Population and Development Studies).

Smolinski, Mark S., Margaret A. Hamburg, and Joshua Lederberg, eds. (2003). *Microbial Threats to Health: Emergence, Detection, and Response* (Washington DC: National Academies Press).

Sykes, Alan (2002). 'TRIPS, Pharmaceuticals, Developing Countries and the "Doha Solution"'. *Chicago Journal of International Law,* vol. 3, no. 1, pp. 47–68.

t'Hoen, Ellen (2002). 'TRIPS, Pharmaceutical Patents, and Access to Essential Medicines: A Long Way from Seattle to Doha'. *Chicago Journal of International Law,* vol. 3, no. 1, pp. 27–46.

United States General Accounting Office (2004). 'Emerging Infectious Diseases: Asian SARS Outbreak Challenged International and National Responses'. GAO-04-564. Report to the Chairman, Subcommittee on Asia and the Pacific, Committee on International Relations, House of Representatives. United States General Accounting Office, Washington DC. <www.gao.gov/cgi-bin/getrpt?GAO-04-564> (September 2006).

Widdus, Roy (2001). 'Public-Private Partnerships for Health: Their Main Targets, Their Diversity, and Their Future Directions'. *Bulletin of the World Health Organization,* vol. 79, no. 8, pp. 713–720.

World Bank (1993). *World Development Report 1993: Investing in Health* (Washington DC: World Bank).

World Health Organization (2002). *Global Crisis, Global Solutions: Managing Public Health Emergencies of International Concern through the Revised International Health Regulations* (Geneva: World Health Organization).

World Health Organization (2005). 'Revision of the International Health Regulations'. WHA58.3. Geneva. <www.who.int/entity/csr/ihr/IHRWHA58_3-en.pdf> (September 2006).

World Health Organization (2006a). 'Global Outbreak Alert and Response Network'. Geneva. <www.who.int/csr/outbreaknetwork/en/> (September 2006).

World Health Organization (2006b). 'International Health Regulations'. Geneva. <www.who.int/csr/ihr/en> (September 2006).

World Health Organization and World Trade Organization (2002). 'WTO Agreements and Public Health: A Joint Study by WHO and the WTO Secretariat'. Geneva. <www.wto.org/English/res_e/booksp_e/who_wto_e.pdf> (September 2006).

World Trade Organization (1994). 'Trade-Related Aspects of Intellectual Property Rights'. Annex IC of the Marrakesh Agreement Establishing the World Trade Organization. 15 April, Marrakesh. <www.wto.org/english/docs_e/legal_e/27-trips_01_e.htm> (September 2006).

World Trade Organization (2001). 'Declaration on the TRIPS Agreement and Public Health'. WT/MIN(01)/DEC/2. 14 November. <www.wto.org/English/thewto_e/minist_e/min01_e/mindecl_trips_e.htm> (September 2006).

Zacher, Mark W. (1999). 'Global Epidemiological Surveillance: International Cooperation to Monitor Infectious Diseases'. In I. Kaul, I. Grunberg, and M.A. Stern, eds., *Global Public Goods: International Cooperation in the 21st Century,* pp. 266–283 (New York: Oxford University Press for the United Nations Development Programme).

Chapter 3

Global Health, Social Movements, and Governance

James Orbinski

'The health of people is the foundation upon which all their happiness and all their powers as a state depend.' So said the conservative 19th-century British prime minister Benjamin Disraeli. In the same century, and a mere half-continent away, Rudolph Virchow (1848) — a German politician, physician, and a father of public health — said that 'medicine is a social science, and politics nothing but medicine on a grand scale'. Both Disraeli and Virchow implicitly recognised that health is both an indicator and an outcome of politics writ large. What were discerning insights then would be equally prescient today had they been made in relation to an emergent and equity-oriented understanding of global health. Theirs was a time when government and intergovernmental agreements alone could influence the practice of public health both within and between nations. Today, beginning with the end of the Cold War and then accelerated by the events of 11 September 2001, public health is in the midst of a revolution, one that is being forced from above by states and from below by non-state actors as it tries to adapt to new global forces and factors, not the least of which is a widening array of actors each in some way concerned with health. Among these are social movements that are driving key changes in the discourse and practice of global health. While such forces cannot be easily named, they can be described with powerful effect in achieving a new understanding of the actors and dynamics at play (Sen 2005). Social movements can be loosely defined as collective challenges to existing arrangements of power and distribution by people with common purposes and solidarity, in sustained interaction with elites, opponents, and authorities (Meyer and Tarrow 1998). To be effective, these largely informally legitimate forces require a formally legitimate political process in which and with which to engage. In a post-modernist 21st century, this requires governance. This chapter does not attempt an exhaustive theoretical examination of global health, social movements, and governance, but does attempt to describe their importance to contemporary conceptions of global health through an examination of the process by which nongovernment organisations (NGOs), such as the small Dignitas International and the transnational NGO Médecins Sans Frontières (MSF), are engaging the issue of access to health care and medicines for people living with HIV/AIDS in the developing world. In doing so, it challenges a securitised conception as a singularly useful lens for global health — or public health writ large — and reveals a more complex and dialectical process in emerging conceptions of global health and governance.

In Chapter 4, David Fidler outlines a securitised conceptualisation of global heath. His arguments and analysis are prescient and cogent, and will not be repeated here. However, one question lingers: Is global health simply a security concern — one that is driven largely by legitimate concerns regarding biochemical, nuclear, or 'low tech' bomber terrorism, economic security in the trade in food and the goods associated with intellectual property, and emergent and re-emergent infectious diseases such as severe acute respiratory syndrome (SARS) and avian influenza, HIV/AIDS, tuberculosis (TB), and malaria? Or is global health best conceptualised as pursuing equity, justice, and fairness, and as fundamentally considering public health measures and access to health care and healthcare technologies, such as drugs, as a basic human entitlement? If it is the latter, then social movements matter, and matter a lot. There is no question that in response to September 11 and the very real threat of terrorism, the shear volume and power of political, scientific, military, intellectual, financial, and material capital that are now focussed on what have traditionally been public health capacities will reshape the global public health enterprise. There is also no question that the interplay between health and security concerns related to state practice itself is not new. Indeed, the first embassies were established in medieval Italy to provide city-states with information about disease outbreaks arising in neighbouring areas (Merianos and Peiris 2005). Security issues today — however more complex today than in medieval Italy — are a key force, but they are not the only forces in the dynamic shaping public health as both a state policy practice and a professional discipline, academic or otherwise. Global health today is a complex phenomenon, requiring a broader more organic viewpoint than that allowed by a highly linear securitised analysis.

In the fall of 2005 I was in a small hamlet of houses some 40 kilometres from the main hospital in the Zomba district of Malawi, where Dignitas International, a new Canadian NGO, is working with the government's ministry of health in a programme that puts people on treatment for HIV, targets prevention, and seeks to empower community to contain and control the HIV/AIDS epidemic (Dignitas International 2006). I was talking to a woman who has AIDS, and because of this also has TB and who, unsurprisingly, wants to live. As we sat on a small carpet outside her house, she was breathless and embarrassed about a cancerous tumour that had started to appear on her face — both the breathlessness and the tumour are indirect and direct effects of AIDS. There is some irony in that her name is Charity, and she has two children — a little girl aged six and a boy aged twelve. Her son's name is Mpwele — it means 'gift'. And he is a gift to her. Without the US$1 he earns for a twelve-hour day of back-breaking work tending the corn fields of neighbours, Charity's small family would starve, and she would have no money to get to the local clinic where she gets treatment for HIV and TB. She hopes to get newly available generic drugs — vastly cheaper than patented versions of the same life-saving drugs — for the treatment of HIV/AIDS. Dignitas International supports the ministry of health's clinic because the government's entire social services budget is a meagre US$15 per capita per annum (including all health, education, and spending in other social services as well as all foreign aid) (Dimbleby 2005). In Malawi, as elsewhere in the developing world, health systems are unable to hire new workers and have had their policy choices constrained by World Bank and International Monetary Fund (IMF) structural adjustment conditionalities (Cheru 2002).

As we talked, three other women gathered, and within minutes a clutch of some 21 curious, giggling children also collected around us. I asked her where all the men were. 'They are all dead', she said. They have all died of AIDS. Many women have died too, she told me. In fact in sub-Saharan Africa, more than half — or 55 percent — of all people living with HIV/AIDS are women (UNAIDS 2006). I asked the children to raise their hands if both their parents were dead. Seven of the 21 children raised their hands — that is, 33 percent of the children in that village alone are now without parents. It is an imperfect sample of the effects of an epidemic that is so rapacious, so wide in the swath that it is cutting through all of Africa, that today, for example, there are 500 000 children orphaned by AIDS in Malawi — a fraction of the 13 million similarly orphaned children on the continent of Africa alone ('Malawi: AIDS Deaths Fuelling Orphan Numbers' 2005). In five years, there will be more than 1 million children orphaned because of HIV/AIDS in Malawi, and today the average life expectancy in Malawi is 36 years — which as, it happens, is Charity's age (UNICEF 2005).

The orphans in this hamlet live on the tenuous kindness of the four women who are still alive in the village — tenuous because these women have their own children to feed, and there is never enough for them. Of a population of 12 million, 5 million people needed food assistance in Malawi in 2005 and the early part of 2006. Why? Because drought has struck for the fifth year in a row. It is, according to the Food and Agriculture Organization (FAO), part of an emerging pattern of severe droughts that could become permanent due to climate change (Vidal and Radford 2005). The same is true for Central America and Southeast Asia. As well as drought due to climate change, AIDS has left at least 15 percent of the workforce in Malawi dead. AIDS has also killed an inordinate number of healthcare professionals, and their number has dwindled further thanks to the phenomenon of 'brain drain' — for example, between 23 percent and 28 percent of all doctors working in the United Kingdom, Canada, the United States, and Australia are foreign-trained medical graduates, 75 percent of whom are trained in developing nations such as Malawi (Mullan 2005). Today in Malawi, with a population of 12 million people, the country struggles with only one third of its required nursing workforce (Kober and Van Damme 2004), and there are fewer than 100 doctors working in the public health system (One World 2005). It is a standing joke and a matter of fact, that there are more Malawian doctors working in Manchester, England, than in all of Malawi (Broadhead and Muula 2002). AIDS has also left women with the burden of caring for the sick and unable to work the fields in adequate force to yield a minimal crop. If Charity does not get treatment, then seven orphans will become nine orphans (42 percent of children in that village), and how they will survive is anyone's guess. So many people have died of AIDS in Malawi that now 10 percent of all families are headed by a child, and half of all families are headed by a person over 65 — and most often by a grandmother ('AIDS Creating a Generation of African Orphans: Experts' 2003).

Six years ago, I was in South Africa, at an MSF clinic. MSF was about to publicly begin treatment with illegally imported antiretroviral therapy (ART). I was examining a 20-year-old man. If he were virtually anywhere in the western world, he would be just starting his life. But there his life was nearly over. He was so weak that two friends had to help him onto the examining table. As he sat gasping for air, he asked me among the most simple yet profound set of questions — questions of justice that get to the heart of the inequity of the HIV/AIDS epidemic. He asked me: 'Why do you come here with only kindness when what I need is medicine to stop this AIDS? Your kindness is good but it will not help this AIDS. They have such medicine in your countries, why not here in South Africa for people like me?' Even now, six years later, the HIV/AIDS pandemic is devastating countries, communities and families; it is robbing Africa, disproportionately, ruinously, of its women; it is creating generations of orphans and is shredding sector after sector of socioeconomic infrastructure. Health, education, agriculture, the police, the army, the private sector — nothing is immune. It is unleashing a brutal pattern of sexual violence, often against children. It is causing political leaders — balanced, sombre political leaders such as the president of Swaziland — to use words such as 'extinction' and 'annihilation' when describing to their people what is in store if AIDS is not defeated (Lewis 2006).

Since the beginning of the pandemic, at least 25 million are dead, between 2.4 million and 3.3 million people now die every year of AIDS, between 3.4 million and 6.2 million people are newly infected every year, and some 40 million now people live with HIV world-wide (UNAIDS 2006). Despite some minor advances, the Caribbean, India, China, and much of Asia continue to struggle with an HIV explosion. It is not just another epidemic. Richard Feacham, the director of the Global Fund to Fight AIDS, Tuberculosis, and Malaria, has said that 'HIV/AIDS is the greatest disaster in recorded human history. It is already worse than the black death in Europe in the middle of the 14th century, and the word "already" is important because the epidemic will get far worse before it gets better, even if we did all the right things tomorrow. There is no chance that we will do all the right things tomorrow' (Feacham 2004). And yet unlike the black plague, HIV/AIDS is a treatable infectious disease.

The factors defining the health of people like those in this little hamlet in Malawi and much of the developing world are a microcosm of a similar complexity when considering global health in the macrocosm. Some of the factors that combine to create egregious inequities in health outcomes are inadequate health systems, the poor availability of overpriced drugs, diagnostics, and vaccines, co-infection with other emerging and re-emerging infectious diseases, climate change, and the disempowerment of vulnerable groups such as women and orphaned children. Final examples of a vastly incomplete list are the lack of an equitable medical research and development agenda and the absence of a needs-driven priority-setting policy exercise that considers the most vulnerable first. Such inequities accrue potentially uncontainable risks not just for 'them' but for all of us.

There have been tremendous public health advances in many parts of the world and many current initiatives to improve health are important and effective. And yet poverty continues to be a main driver (if not the main driver) of poor health in much of the world (Commission on Macroeconomics and Health 2001). It was 25 years ago that the aspiration of Health For All was declared at Alma-Ata by the governments of the world (International Conference on Primary Health Care 1978). Today, health systems in much of the developing world are policy rich and capacity poor, and world-wide, more people live in poverty than ever before (Pogge 2006). Life expectancy in Africa is 39 years, or 27 years less than the average of 66 years in the developed world. In our world of about 6.5 billion people, 2.8 billion people live on less than US$2 per day. This is a rise of 10 percent over the past 18 years. Every day 840 million go to bed hungry (15 percent), and 1.3 billion (21 percent) do not have access to safe drinking water. One in three people around the world and half of all people in Africa and Asia have no access to essential medicines; chronic diseases (for example, diabetes, asthma, cardiovascular disease, cancer) are flourishing everywhere; half of all mortality in sub-Saharan African and Asia is due to preventable or treatable infectious disease; the '10/90 gap' in health-related research and development (R&D) — that is, only 10 percent of all drug R&D focusses on diseases that account for 90 percent of global problems — means that many diseases that occur largely in the developing world among poor people are neglected and thus the diseases themselves thrive. Because of a virtual absence of drug R&D, millions continue to suffer and die from diseases such as malaria, TB, sleeping sickness (trypanosomiasis), Chagas disease, or leishmaniasis. As well, much-needed adaptations of treatments for diseases such as HIV/AIDS to developing world conditions remain largely unaddressed. And in much of the developing world, health systems are collapsing, meaning that the capacity to deal with diseases such as SARS and avian influenza is increasingly a phantom capacity, so that diseases like these will invariably spread — and the absence of a viable public health capacity in much of the developing world is a security threat globally. And yet, despite this dire state of global health, forces from below are reshaping the global health enterprise.

Health systems are vital in the fight against disease and poverty. As well as offering access to health care, they can, if properly designed and managed, reduce the financial burden of illness, build social cohesion, and mitigate the feelings of powerlessness that are at the heart of vulnerability. They are also the primary means by which epidemics can be contained and controlled, and they work best in achieving this pragmatic end when they are most inclusive and respectful of human dignity and rights (Gostin and Lazzarini 1997).

In Malawi, public health practice is in the midst of a quiet revolution, and is a microcosm of a broader quiet revolution talking place globally. It is not security concerns that are driving this revolution, but social justice concerns. Today in Malawi, in less than two years, the ministry of health in conjunction with a small legion of NGOs has managed to put some 33 000 people on treatment for HIV/AIDS. The national number is now 37 840 on treatment (Harries et al. 2006). The ministry of health plans to have more than 245 000 on treatment for HIV/AIDS by 2010 — within a mere four years. While this is only half of the projected need, the ministry is working to redefine its health system capacity to deliver treatment to even more people. It is working with NGOs such as Dignitas International in training low-literacy home-based care workers and community-based care workers to monitor and deliver treatment effectively and efficiently. Prevention and care strategies are being researched and modified with an equal, if not more intense, vigour. What is happening in Malawi is also happening all over the developing world, under the World Health Organization's (WHO) '3 by 5' initiative, which now has more 1.3 million people on treatment for HIV (UNAIDS 2005).

None of this would have been possible without an earlier not-so-quiet revolution driven largely by MSF, which launched its Campaign for Access to Essential Medicines in 1999 (MSF 2006). Rooted in a social justice ethic, the campaign grew out of the direct experience of MSF nurses and doctors watching their patients die of poorly or partially treated infectious diseases in the developing world. MSF asked a very simple question: Why? To answer, MSF established its own internal research capacity and began a careful policy analysis of the problem of lack of access to medicines in the developing world. The analysis proceeded on the assumption that there could be no 'sacred cows' in that pragmatism — not dogmatism — would drive the analysis, that equity-oriented principles rather than ideology would guide it, and that all players and policies would be open to scrutiny. The analysis included MSF itself, other NGOs, national governments, the WHO and other UN agencies, other international government organisations such as the World Trade Organization (WTO) and the World Bank, the pharmaceutical industry (for both patent-protected and generic drugs), and foundations concerned with pharmaceutical issues. It soon became obvious that existing treatments were less and less available as production was being cut because markets for some tropical diseases were not viable from a profit perspective, that many treatments were decreasingly effective because of drug resistance, that there was a lack of R&D of new or adapted drugs for many tropical diseases as well as global diseases, and that many new drugs were patented and thus priced well beyond the reach of too many people in the developing world. Even when the newly available triple therapy of antiretrovirals for people living with HIV/AIDS was declared at the opening of the 1996 Vancouver International AIDS Conference as being able to 'convert deadly AIDS into a chronic, manageable disorder like diabetes' (MacInnis 2006), it was not until MSF began its Campaign for Access to Essential Medicines in earnest that access to ART and other drugs in the developing world began to change.

The internal MSF policy examination process began in 1998. At the launch of the campaign in 1999 MSF invited more than a hundred NGOs, pharmaceutical industry representatives, WHO representatives, government representatives, academics, and health policy specialists from around the world first to Geneva to examine compulsory licensing options for pharmaceuticals, and then to Amsterdam to establish a broader but highly specific agenda on access to medicines. A coalition was formed, and key partners including MSF, Health Action International, and the Consumer Project on Technology (CPTech) set out a clear set of values and policy objectives, and agreed to work informally with other members of the coalition to achieve these (MSF 1999). The coalition then worked to bring the issues relating to lack of access to medicines in the developing world to a global public and political stage. Elements of the coalition worked to argue for an '*exception sanitaire*' for essential medicines at the 1999 Seattle WTO ministerial meeting ('Sleep Less in Seattle' 1999). The coalition also worked to pool the procurement of generic drugs and reveal the pricing policies and discrepancies for patent-protected medicines around the world, bringing the price of ART down from US$13 400 for patent-protected versions of antiretroviral drugs to less than US$300 for generic versions of the same drugs. It also worked to negotiate price reductions and ensure production of a variety of other drugs used in the treatment of tropical diseases and drug-resistant tuberculosis (MSF 2006). MSF also launched pilot treatment programmes all over the world to demonstrate that HIV/AIDS treatment is possible in developing world settings. MSF now has more than 60 000 people on treatment for HIV/AIDS in 32 countries around the world (MSF 2006). In 2001, the coalition successfully challenged 39 multinational pharmaceutical companies in South Africa that sought to block the government's right to import generic medicines (CPTech 2006). Also in 2001 the Global Fund to Fight AIDS, Tuberculosis, and Malaria was created, partially in response to pressure from this coalition. This global coalition also was successful in getting the WTO to acknowledge that health interests trump trade interests in its declaration issued at the 2001 ministerial in Doha, Qatar (WTO 2001). It fought for the Perez Motta text of 2003 that now allows in principle for generic export of patented medicines to countries without pharmaceutical manufacturing capacity. It has led to Bill C-9 in Canada to allow generic production of certain medicines for export to developing countries and to similar bills now under consideration in other countries. It has pushed the WHO to launch a commission on innovation, public health, and intellectual property rights. It has cajoled the WHO to assume its responsibility in actively pursuing people's health through for example, the 3 by 5 initiative. None of these outcomes has been perfect — some, like the Doha and Motta declarations and Bill C-9, are far from perfect. But they do demonstrate, however imperfectly, that change is possible. And, most importantly, people who were going to die a terrible death now can at least hope that they can live with HIV and other neglected diseases in the developing world.

MSF has also launched a global not-for-profit drug R&D initiative — the Drugs for Neglected Diseases Initiative (2006) — that is now creating new affordable treatments for diseases that primarily affect poor people in the developing world. The initiative began in 2003. It now has 20 drugs in its development pipeline. The goal is not to singularly assume the responsibility for neglected disease R&D, but to demonstrate that alternatives to the current system are possible, and to insist on political responsibility in achieving a needs-driven, equity-oriented global R&D agenda as a public responsibility.

This principled and pragmatic approach has worked well, coupled with a loosely organised coalition that capitalises on situation-specific opportunities and is flexible enough to allow organisations to join and leave it. It has used communications technology including the internet and mobile phones as well as formal and informal meetings effectively to maintain its agenda and to coordinate simultaneous policy initiatives and demonstrations around the globe. This approach has allowed the campaign both to attack unjust policies, practices, and outcomes and simultaneously to negotiate specific agreements with industry, government, and others such as foundations to achieve major equity-oriented outcomes that are concrete, sometimes imperfect, and in many cases emergent. It has also spawned or emboldened other movements or global health coalitions, such as the effort to achieve a new open-source global R&D framework for neglected diseases (Dentico and Ford 2005). It has also pushed for numerous concrete government initiatives such as the French government's Tobin tax on international travel, which is now directed at creating children's formulations of medicines for the developing world ('France's Parliament Approves Airline Tax to Fund HIV/AIDS Programs' 2006). Finally, as in Malawi and elsewhere in the developing world, it has had and may yet continue to have a significant positive effect on access to medicines and on access to health care.

These outcomes — actual and emergent — have developed from a respect for basic human dignity and an equity-oriented conception of global health. These point to what have been conceived as social justice issues posed by forces from below that must be resolved in an ongoing dialectic with forces from above.

Health-oriented social movements like the Campaign for Access to Essential Medicines have emerged in reaction to the material impact of the policy choices of global political and economic actors. Such social movements have reacted in a manner that seeks to realign those policy choices with a broader, more inclusive equity-oriented conception of global health. They do so in an ongoing relationship that centres on a dialectic point-counterpoint dynamic that is both public and rooted in sound analysis and evidence. To be successful in moving a social justice agenda forward, these interactions are most fruitful when focussed on issue-specific points of dissonance and approached in a manner that highlights the practical and material implications of normative ideas that challenge current policy practices. This process can gradually alter the architecture that governs global health or to engage government where that architecture does not exist. To shape this architecture in intended or desirable ways, such health-oriented social movements must act by not deferring to any sacred cows, by understanding the global context, by forming advocacy coalitions, and by seizing opportunities when they arise.

Social movements can respond to and can shape their social and political environments in many ways, and must be clear about their roles, their responsibilities, their capabilities, and their limits. Here the history of social movements can be instructive. In the most general of terms, in looking at the history of social movements — the 300-year-long movement against slavery, the labour rights movement, the movement against child labour, the women's suffrage movement, the civil rights movement, the human rights movement, and the environmental movement — it is evident that each of these began in an articulation of principled ideas from within communities and then moved to confront those who hold power, for example political or economic actors that have particular visions on the exercise of power. This confrontation then moved on to include interaction with sources of power, to partnership, and then usually to legitimate and appropriate co-optation of the material ends that codify (in law) and materialise (in practice) the principles and values that gave birth to the movement in the first place. But social change is rarely if ever a straight, linear process, nor can its process be easily located on the overly simplistic continuum of articulation, confrontation, interaction, partnership, and co-optation. Material convergence does not necessarily mean a convergence of values, so that rights achieved must be defended and constant vigilance is required to maintain hard-won gains. Here the status of African Americans in the United States today and the rights of women that are not yet won the world over are examples where gains must be constantly reasserted or demanded.

Vital to this dialectical process today is governance, rather than simply government. It will be central to the form that global health takes both as a state practice and as an academic or professional discipline. And governance is a messy, uncertain business. Ramesh Thakur and Thomas Weiss (forthcoming) have defined governance to mean 'efforts to bring a more orderly and reliable response to social and political issues that go beyond the capacities of states to address individually'. Like the apparently inchoate universe of actors now engaged with global health issues, governance implies the absence of a central authority and the need for collaboration or cooperation among governments and others to seek common practices and goals in addressing global issues. Today the myriad of actors requiring governance in global health include not simply states and their individual ministries of health, but also intergovernmental UN organisations such as the WHO and the United Nations Development Programme (UNDP); international institutions that lie outside the UN system such as the World Bank, the International Monetary Fund (IMF), and the WTO; NGOs — so diverse now in their nature and number they are sometimes categorised as INGOs (international NGOS), BINGOs (business-initiated NGOS), LINGOS (little NGOs), or LONGOs (labour-organised NGOs); health foundations such as the Rockefeller and Bill and Melinda Gates foundations; transnational public-private partnerships focussed on health issues, such as the International AIDS Vaccine Initiative (IAVI) and the Medicines for Malaria Venture; multinational corporations (MNCs) that seek to sell heath services in a global marketplace; philanthropists such as George Soros, whose Open Society Institute supports innovative approaches to health systems and democracy in the former Soviet Republics and in much of the developing world; and, of course, one-person states such as Bono, whose public appeal can influence, if not shape, international political agendas.

Today public health is in the midst of a revolution. It is being subsumed under the new reality of global health, an emergent concept of health where governance is central to what government can do to develop meaningful policy frameworks that can deal effectively with a myriad of issues. Even still, public health is struggling to emerge from a Westphalian conceptual trap, a 350-year-old view that sees the world as discrete sovereign nation-states that, properly secured, can remain impermeable and impervious to the threats and considerations that others may suffer or seek to impose. And yet, like governments, the public health establishment has moved at glacial speed in response to an ever-accelerating interdependence defined not simply in terms of trade in goods and services, nor simply in the vastly increased international movement of people over the last quarter century, but also in terms of a shared environment, infectious diseases, terrorism, and a growing and codifying set of international normative equity-oriented ideas about what is and is not just. Global health is a complex phenomenon that requires a more nuanced conception that incorporates but moves beyond security concerns.

Public health internationally has been reshaped since the end of the Cold War by a securitisation from above and, simultaneously, by an ever-growing normative power from below. Surely the more materially powerful of these forces is from above, but the reactive nature of forces from below are reshaping the meaning of public health to an intentional and actual social justice conception of global health. Social movements for health — be these local or global — can challenge state, institutional, and cultural authorities in order to enhance public participation in social policy and regulation, and to democratise the production and dissemination of scientific knowledge in medical science and public health (Brown and Zavestoski 2004). Globally, the self-imposed participation of civil society groups and transnational civil society movements from below is also reshaping public health itself as a practice and as an academic discipline. It is being pushed to adapt to new global factors and forces that are changing its basic concepts or, perhaps more accurately, are calling public health back to where it began.

That social justice is the foundation on which public health is built is not a new idea, nor is it uncontested (Krieger and Birne 1988). It emerged about 150 years ago, in the same century that Virchow proclaimed that public health is simply politics by other means, as public health itself was emerging as both a social movement and as a profession. The political context was not unimportant — it was a time of great social unrest, of social movements, counter-movements, and political choices that have shaped conceptions of both the polity and of public heath ever since. It was a period not unlike now. In today's contemporary context, health-oriented social movements are not minor considerations in an emerging conception of global health, but major forces that have redefined global health and may yet redefine it further.

References

'AIDS Creating a Generation of African Orphans: Experts'. (2003). *Agence France Press,* 26 February. <www.aegis.com/news/afp/2003/AF030281.html> (September 2006).

Broadhead, Robert L. and Adamson S. Muula (2002). 'Creating a Medical School for Malawi: Problems and Achievements'. *British Medical Journal,* vol. 325, no. 7360, pp. 384–387.

Brown, Phil and Stephen Zavestoski (2004). 'Social Movements in Health: An Introduction'. *Sociology of Health and Illness,* vol. 26, no. 6, pp. 679–694.

Cheru, Fantu (2002). 'Debt, Adjustment, and the Politics of Effective Response to HIV/AIDS in Africa'. *Third World Quarterly,* vol. 23, no. 2, pp. 299–312.

Commission on Macroeconomics and Health (2001). 'Macroeconomics and Health: Investing in Health for Economic Development'. World Health Organization, Geneva. <www.cid.harvard.edu/cidcmh/CMHReport.pdf> (September 2006).

CPTech (2006). 'Court Case between 39 Pharmaceutical Firms and the South African Government'. Washington DC. <www.cptech.org/ip/health/sa/pharma-v-sa.html> (September 2006).

Dentico, Nicoletta and Nathan Ford (2005). 'The Courage to Change the Rules: A Proposal for an Essential Health R&D Treaty'. *PLoS Medicine,* vol. 2, no. 2. <medicine.plosjournals.org/perlserv/?request=get-document&doi=10.1371/journal.pmed.0020014> (September 2006).

Dignitas International (2006). 'Harnessing the Power of Community to Fight AIDS'. <www.dignitasinternational.org> (September 2006).

Dimbleby, Jonathan (2005). 'Our Last Chance'. *Observer,* 11 September.

Drugs for Neglected Diseases Initiative (2006). <www.dndi.org> (September 2006).

Feacham, Richard (2004). 'Financing Global Public Health: Innovation and Investment'. Speech given to the World Federation of Public Health Associations Congress and the UK Health Association's Annual Public Health Forum on Sustaining Health in a Changing World: Vision to Action, 20 April, Brighton UK. <www.theglobalfund.org/en/media_center/speeches/speech_feachem_040411.asp> (September 2006).

'France's Parliament Approves Airline Tax to Fund HIV/AIDS Programs'. (2006). *Medical News,* 4 January. <www.medicalnewstoday.com/medicalnews.php?newsid=35687> (September 2006).

Gostin, Laurence O. and Zita Lazzarini (1997). *Human Rights in Public Health in the AIDS Pandemic* (London: Oxford University Press).

Harries, Anthony D., Erik Schouten, and Edwin Libamba (2006). 'Scaling Up Antiretroviral Treatment in Resource-Poor Settings'. *Lancet,* vol. 376, pp. 1870–1872.

International Conference on Primary Health Care (1978). 'Declaration of Alma-Ata'. 12 September, Alma-Ata, Kazakhstan. <www.euro.who.int/AboutWHO/Policy/20010827_1> (September 2006).

Kober, Katerina and Wim Van Damme (2004). 'Scaling Up Access to Antiretroviral Treatment in Southern Africa: Who Will Do the Job?' *Lancet,* vol. 364, pp. 103–107.

Krieger, Nancy and Anne-Emanuelle Birne (1988). 'A Vision of Social Justice as the Foundation of Public Health: Commemorating 150 Years of the Spirit of 1848'. *American Journal of Public Health,* vol. 88, no. 11, pp. 1603–1606.

Lewis, Stephen (2006). 'Press Conference by Stephen Lewis on HIV/AIDS in Africa'. 17 March, United Nations, New York. <www.un.org/News/briefings/docs/2006/060317_Lewis.doc.htm> (September 2006).

MacInnis, Ron (2006). 'The International AIDS Conference: A Retrospective'. Global AIDS Link. <www.internews.org/articles/2006/20060800_aidslink_macinnis.htm> (September 2006).

'Malawi: AIDS Deaths Fuelling Orphan Numbers'. (2005). *IRIN News,* 5 October. <www.irinnews.org/AIDSreport.asp?ReportID=5286&SelectRegion=Southern_Africa&SelectCountry=MALAWI> (September 2006).

Médecins Sans Frontières (1999). 'Amsterdam Statement to WTO Member States on Access to Medicine'. 26 November, Amsterdam. <www.accessmed-msf.org/prod/publications.asp?scntid=17122001173935&contenttype=PARA&> (September 2006).

Médecins Sans Frontières (2006). 'Campaign for Access to Essential Medicines'. <www.accessmed-msf.org> (September 2006).

Merianos, Angela and Malik Peiris (2005). 'International Health Regulations'. *Lancet,* vol. 366, pp. 1249–1251.

Meyer, David S. and Sidney Tarrow (1998). 'A Movement Society: Contentious Politics for a New Century'. In D.S. Meyer and S. Tarrow, eds., *The Social Movement Society: Contentious Politics for a New Century* (New York: Rowman and Littlefield).

Mullan, Fitzhugh (2005). 'The Metrics of the Physician Brain Drain'. *New England Journal of Medicine,* vol. 353, no. 17, pp. 1810–1818.

One World (2005). 'Malawi Guide'. <uk.oneworld.net/guides/malawi/development> (September 2006).

Pogge, Thomas (2006). 'Human Rights and Global Health: A Research Program'. In C. Barry and T.W. Pogge, eds., *Global Institutions and Responsibilities: Achieving Global Justice,* pp. 190–217 (Oxford: Blackwell Publishing).

Sen, Amartya (2005). 'Foreword'. In P. Farmer, ed., *Pathologies of Power: Health, Human Rights, and the New War on the Poor* (Berkeley: University of California Press).

'Sleep Less in Seattle' (1999). *Lancet,* vol. 354, no. 9194, p. 1917.

Thakur, Ramesh and Thomas George Weiss (forthcoming). *The United Nations and Global Governance: An Idea and Its Prospects* (Bloomington IN: University of Indiana Press).

UNAIDS (2005). 'AIDS Epidemic Update: December 2005'. <www.unaids.org/epi/2005/doc/EPIupdate2005_html_en/epi05_00_en.htm> (September 2006).

UNAIDS (2006). '2006 Report on the Global AIDS Epidemic'. Geneva. <www.unaids.org/en/HIV_data/2006GlobalReport/default.asp> (September 2006).

UNICEF (2005). 'Children under Threat: The State of the World's Children 2005'. <www.unicef.org/sowc05> (September 2006).

Vidal, John and Tim Radford (2005). 'One in Six Countries Facing Food Shortage'. *Guardian,* 30 June.

Virchow, Rudolph (1848). 'Die offentliche gesundheitspflege' [The Public Health Service]. *Medizinische Reform,* vol. 5, pp. 21–22.

World Trade Organization (2001). 'Declaration on the TRIPS Agreement and Public Health'. WT/MIN(01)/DEC/2. 14 November. <www.wto.org/English/thewto_e/minist_e/min01_e/mindecl_trips_e.htm> (September 2006).

Chapter 4

A Pathology of Public Health Securitism: Approaching Pandemics as Security Threats

David P. Fidler

One of the most interesting and controversial features of the discourse on public health governance in the past decade concerns the proliferation of attempts to approach public health problems as security threats. These diverse efforts have formed part of the process that experts call the securitisation of public health. The securitisation process has raised many challenging issues and questions, including disagreements over the prudence of the governance strategy of securitising public health. Is the securitisation paradigm the best way forward with respect to pandemic preparedness and response?

Public health governance has now entered a post-securitisation phase. Viewing public health through the lens of security has become an integral aspect of public health governance in the 21st century. In short, securitisation has happened, and analysis should direct its attention to sorting out the implications of this sea change in public health governance. Entering into the post-securitisation phase means that the policy belief that public health can be improved by framing and approaching problems through security-related tactics and strategies has become a leading driver of public health governance.

The emergence and intensifying strength of this belief in 'public health securitism' represents a significant change for public health governance nationally and internationally. The coming of age of this belief in the power of linking public health and security adds a new element to thinking about the structure and dynamics of public health governance. Given its significance, it is important to deepen our understanding of this phenomenon and its implications for the future.

This chapter presents a pathology of public health securitism in order to outline the causes, processes, and consequences of this seminal development for the world of public health policy. This pathology reveals that the securitisation of public health has some unfinished business. Although the belief in the need to connect public health to concepts of security is strong, it has not been characterised by analytical rigour. A leading challenge in the post-securitisation phase is to strengthen the analytical content of public health securitism. This chapter reviews possible ways to bring clarity and stability to thinking about the relationship between public health and security. These approaches share the objective of providing a way to determine what public health threats are security issues and thus deserve the policy priority such a designation creates.

The chapter also examines three pandemics through the focus provided by analysing the different ways of defining how public health and security relate to each other. These pandemics are the continuing HIV/AIDS pandemic, mounting fears about pandemic influenza, and the growing global spread of tobacco-related diseases. These case studies shed light on how approaching pandemics as security threats illustrates the current and future importance of public health securitism for public health governance.

Public Health Governance's Post-Securitisation Phase

As a policy matter, thinking about public health in terms of security is a recent phenomenon, emerging only since the mid 1990s. Public health and security concepts were linked earlier. The preamble of the constitution of the World Health Organization (WHO) proclaimed in 1946 that 'the health of all peoples is fundamental to the attainment of peace and security' (WHO 1994). Such earlier linkages did not, however, feature in the manner in which either national or international governance on public health developed in the post–World War II period.

The securitisation phase for public health governance began in the mid 1990s in response to three major developments: heightened fears about the proliferation of bioweapons, especially among terrorist groups; the continued global spread of HIV/AIDS and the pandemic's increasingly devastating political, economic, and social implications in the developing world; and growing awareness about deepening vulnerabilities of populations in rich and poor countries caused by the globalised spread of disease risks, be they pathogens, products, or pollutants. These developments stimulated analysts to begin to frame public health problems as security threats.

These attempts to securitise public health concerns attracted attention, as new paradigms tend to do. A significant literature developed as more people participated in the debate. Indeed, the securitisation debate remains lively. However, the securitisation process is now over. Efforts to approach public health challenges through security concepts have prevailed in a way that constitutes a transformative development for public health governance.

The most compelling evidence that the securitisation of public health has occurred, and now constitutes part of the public health governance landscape, can be found in the diverse ways security concepts have been used to draw attention to public health problems. The use of security as a trope has become ubiquitous in how experts frame public health governance. The prominence of security concepts in debates about public health threats and governance is historically unprecedented.

Academic literature and policy advocacy on security and public health include arguments that elevate the importance of public health with respect to the security of individuals, the nation-state, the international system of states, and the global community. The concept of human security holds that individuals are the proper subject matter for thinking about security (United Nations Development Programme [UNDP] 1994), and those interested in human security have attempted to integrate the threat that diseases pose to individuals and their communities into the human security approach (Commission on Human Security 2003).

More traditional notions of security focus on the nation-state and concern themselves with threats to national security (Princeton Project on National Security 2005). In this realm, too, public health has frequently appeared, in connection both with the threat posed by weapons of mass destruction (WMD), particularly bioweapons, and with the damage to a state's material power that naturally occurring communicable diseases could inflict (United States 2002; Fidler 2003). Public health problems have also been framed as indirect threats to national security, as illustrated by analysis that points to the ability of HIV/AIDS to contribute to the destabilisation of 'countries of strategic concern' to the United States (Eberstadt 2002; Garrett 2005).

A broader, but still traditional, perspective on security concerns international security, or the security relationships that exist among sovereign states. Although questions of war and armed conflict have dominated the study of international security, public health has appeared increasingly frequently on the international security agenda. The United Nations Security Council (UNSC) has, for example, twice addressed the HIV/AIDS pandemic as a threat to international peace and security (UNSC 2000, 2005). Proposals for UN reform have included recommendations that the UNSC use its mandate to maintain international peace and security in cases involving overwhelming outbreaks of communicable diseases (UN 2004, 2005).

Still more expansive concepts of security, such as those that focus on the security of the community of states and non-state actors, or global society, also incorporate public health considerations. The WHO (2001) described its efforts to improve global communicable disease surveillance and response capabilities as the pursuit of 'global health security'. The UN secretary general and the high-level panel he appointed to advise him on UN reform placed improving national and global public health at the centre of a new vision for collective security, a vision that went beyond the state-centric perspective that dominated the UN's post–World War II activities (UN 2004; UNSC 2005). The extent to which public health is central to this vision of 'comprehensive collective security' is remarkable in both the annals of public health and UN thinking on collective security.

To be sure, these diverse perspectives on what security means do not reveal consensus on the meaning of security or what the appropriate level of analysis is for security policy. What is common among these different, often antagonistic frameworks is that they all have made efforts to address public health problems. These activities across such a broad range of security outlooks demonstrate an increasing awareness about the political and governance importance of public health not seen in previous decades of security discourse. More importantly, these activities reveal a strong belief in a two-sided policy relationship: public health can be improved through a security focus, and security can be enhanced by incorporating public health concerns.

The strength of the policy belief in public health securitism across the range of security concepts has made such securitisation a permanent feature of public health governance in the 21st century. Arguments may still rage about whether it is good or bad for public health governance. But securitisation has happened at every conceivable level of security and public health analysis, even some not mentioned above (for example, the concept of ecological security) (Pirages 1997).

Some may doubt the sincerity of some efforts to connect public health and security, such as the cynical playing of the 'security card' by public health officials and advocates desperate for more political attention and economic resources. The deeper the cynicism the stronger the argument about the triumph of public health securitism becomes. Such cynicism reflects a coldly calculated decision that public health can be improved by appealing to security concepts and considerations. Similarly, some may find novel concepts, such as human security, hopelessly naive. However, the deep commitment to human security by many communities, and their integration of public health into this commitment, provides evidence of the power of the belief that security-related thinking can improve public health (Commission on Human Security 2003). When the United States Central Intelligence Agency and human rights advocates both agree that security needs mandate improvements in public health nationally and internationally, something interesting and perhaps profound has taken place (Fidler 2004).

Paradigm Aggregation: Public Health Securitism and Public Health Governance

The emergence of public health securitism has produced paradigm aggregation rather than a paradigm shift. Post-securitisation public health governance involves three frameworks that converge to produce the political, economic, and moral context in which public health policy operates. The sea change that public health securitism represents is best viewed in light of security considerations entering into a governance context previously oriented by concerns involving economic considerations and aspirations grounded in concepts of human dignity.

As historians of international health diplomacy have made clear, international cooperation on public health originated in the concerns of the European great powers with the economic burdens their trade and commerce suffered through the application of disparate, uncoordinated, and often irrational national quarantine systems (Goodman 1971; Howard-Jones 1950, 1975). The threat of the international spread of communicable diseases was thus constructed predominantly as a threat to the economic opportunities that trade and commerce provided states. This template dominated how states approached international health cooperation in the first century of such cooperation.

The focus of international health efforts slowly drifted away from national economic self-interest as humanitarian concerns about health in other countries gradually emerged prior to World War II. The establishment of the WHO in 1948 accelerated this trend because the organisation directed most of its energies toward trying to improve public health in developing countries (Pannenborg 1979). Animating this concern with health conditions in poor countries was the vision for health proclaimed in the preamble of the WHO constitution (WHO 1994). The idea that the enjoyment of the highest attainable standard of health was a fundamental human right was central to this vision.

The humanitarian and rights-based framework taking shape through WHO activities was connected to efforts in development being pushed by developing countries in the aftermath of decolonisation. The Declaration of Alma-Ata in 1978, which launched the Health for All by the Year 2000 initiative, captured the convergence of humanitarianism, the right to health, and the new thinking on development (International Conference on Primary Health Care 1978). The declaration reaffirmed the right to health, asserted that health inequalities between developed and developing countries were unacceptable, and linked health for all to the economic and social development strategies found in the so-called New International Economic Order (NIEO).

The emergence of linkages between security and public health since 1995 adds yet another governance template to the economic-based and human dignity–based frameworks that prevailed in earlier periods. Some concerns expressed about the securitisation of public health involved fears that security-based attitudes are eclipsing or subordinating the human dignity template that prevailed in international health governance from the WHO's establishment. As explored below, the securitisation process does create tensions with the human dignity agenda; but this process has not been a zero-sum game among the economic, human dignity, and security templates of public health governance.

Without question, security-based arguments have contributed to a new emphasis on the material self-interests of states with respect to public health governance. These arguments resonate with the original governance template for international health cooperation that reflected the economic concerns of the great powers. The security-related perspectives also help highlight the increasing economic costs that countries face from the globalisation of disease, especially with respect to their export interests. With disease rising as a threat to the state's material power and well-being, states have started to engage public health governance with more intensity.

Human dignity has not, however, dropped off the agenda. The securitisation process has included security concepts, especially human security, that conceive of security more broadly than the traditional narrow emphasis on the material power and interests of states. In addition, one of the dominant themes of the securitisation process has been that international cooperation and the national and global involvement of non-state actors are essential in public health governance to achieve security, whether the concept of security in question is narrow or broad. The commonalities of the strategies required to engage in successful public health governance in the early 21st century allow the economic, human dignity, and security templates to coexist, held together by the epidemiological requirements of addressing diseases effectively in an intensely globalising environment.

Pathology of Public Health Securitism

Understanding that public health securitism has taken public health governance into a post-securitisation phase is important, but it is not sufficient for comprehending the seminal nature of this change in attitudes, strategies, and tactics concerning public health governance. This section provides a pathology of public health securitism, or an exploration of the causes, processes, and consequences of this important development in public health governance.[1] This brief examination supports the belief that security-based arguments have utility for public health policy.

Causes

The rise of public health securitism has many causes. But cutting across these causes is the realisation that the danger presented by diseases to states, peoples, and individuals has increased in the last decades of the 20th century and early stages of the 21st century. The *Oxford English Dictionary* defines security as 'the condition of being protected from or not exposed to danger'. The trend toward using security-based thinking and concepts in a time of increasing disease danger makes sense, at a basic level. The key to understanding the causes of public health securitism involves the scrutiny of the reasons why diseases are more dangerous in the early part of the 21st century than they were in the post–World War II period.

Analyses of communicable disease emergence provide insight into the increasing dangers these diseases present. In its well-known report, the U.S. Institute of Medicine's Committee on Microbial Threats to Health in the 21st Century identified 13 factors that produce microbial dangers for the U.S. and other countries (see Table 4-1) (Smolinski, Hamburg, and Lederberg 2003). Similarly, public health experts argue that dramatic changes in patterns of product consumption, stimulated

Table 4-1 Factors in the Emergence of Communicable Diseases

1 Microbial adaptation and change
2 Human susceptibility to infection
3 Climate and weather
4 Changing ecosystems
5 Human demographics and behaviour
6 Economic development and land use
7 International travel and commerce
8 Technology and industry
9 Breakdown of public health measures
10 Poverty and social inequality
11 War and famine
12 Lack of political will
13 Intent to harm (e.g., bioterrorism)

Source: Smolinski, Hamburg, and Lederberg (2003).

by the globalisation of trade and lifestyle choices, significantly increase risks to health, as evidenced by growing pandemics of chronic diseases related to tobacco use and obesity (Beaglehole and Yach 2003).

Increasing risks and dangers from diseases arise in an environment in which public health governance has proved ill equipped to respond. The turn to security-based arguments involves the perception that the human dignity and economic templates that prevailed in earlier historical periods are insufficient bases, on their own, for the kind of robust governance required in the early 21st century. With disease dangers rising, the rallying cries of the right to health and Health For All no longer carry the weight they previously did. Framing disease dangers in terms of security has proven to be attractive across political and ideological spectrums as an approach that can motivate states and communities to strengthen national and global public health.

Processes

In order to understand how the belief that security-related arguments could provide policy traction for public health governance developed as rapidly and strongly it is necessary to look at various processes through which this transformation occurred. These processes can be divided into practical, tactical, and strategic categories. At the practical level, many people concerned about growing disease dangers in a context of weak to non-existent public health capabilities used every argument available to raise policy attention about this governance challenge. Thus, security-based arguments were intermingled with economic rationales and appeals to humanitarian impulses in a melange that reflected a call for urgent action rather than a desire for theoretical coherency.

At the tactical level, there have been modifications made to accommodate public health concerns in traditional security concepts and practices. Thinking on U.S. national security attempted to graft public health into its priorities. This grafting process involved two aspects. First, the traditional Cold War definition of national security as security against the military power and potential military violence from other states began to look anachronistic when the U.S. felt threatened by potential violence from non-state actors, notably terrorists. Although national security was still defined in terms of threats of exogenous violence, the range of potential actors that could pose a security threat expanded in light of the terrorist threat. Part of that terrorist threat involved the possible use of bioweapons against the U.S., a threat that came to pass with the anthrax attacks of October 2001. This threat against the U.S. meant that the quality of public health systems in the U.S. and in other countries grew in national security importance.

Second, the post–Cold War period also encouraged policy makers and policy thinkers to question the narrow perspective on U.S. national security that prevailed during the long conflict with the Soviet Union. This questioning involved experts analysing whether U.S. national security policy should consider transnational phenomena, such as environmental degradation and communicable diseases, as threats to the material power, interests, and well-being of the United States. Part of this approach posited whether naturally occurring communicable diseases could directly cause such material damage to the U.S. as to be a threat akin to a violent attack. Another facet of this outlook focussed on how transnational phenomena might present indirect national security problems for the United States. Could, for example, environmental degradation or communicable diseases contribute to the violent destabilisation of important countries or regions and thus damage U.S. interests and power overseas?

At the strategic level, the process involved fundamentally rethinking the concept of security. Here, the rapid development of human security as a rival to the traditional, state-centric perspectives on security is the most important innovation. Human security's focus on the individual as the core subject of security policy opened more space in security thinking for public health issues. The tactical process described above allowed public health to have some national security significance, but the centre of policy attention remained the security of the nation-state in terms of its material power. Human security challenged the assumptions of the traditional national security template and thus created greater possibilities for states and the international community to consider public health more seriously as a security issue.

These practical, tactical, and strategic processes do not mesh into each other to produce a harmonised process that generated public health securitism. Each individually contributed to the politics that has gradually led to public health securitism's emergence. The messiness of the processes is one reason why public health governance faces some unfinished business in its post-securitisation phase.

Consequences

The last element of the pathology of public health securitism concerns its consequences. One consequence has already been highlighted — the aggregation of templates informing public health governance. This aggregation is not without competition and friction. The increased dangers that diseases present have reconnected the security and economic self-interests of states with public health governance. This reality has created tension with the governance template focussed on human dignity, with its concerns about the right to health and equitable social and economic development.

At one level, these tensions merely indicate that public health governance is returning to normality in international relations. Most issues involving international politics and foreign policy experience friction between interest-based approaches and value-based approaches. Public health governance after World War II witnessed the withering of great power interest in international disease control and prevention largely because these states enjoyed steadily improving national public health outcomes. International health activities devolved to the 'low politics' of 'mere humanitarianism' in international relations, allowing the human dignity template to appear dominant in the ethos of international health cooperation. The securitisation of public health has made what appeared to be a fundamental transformation look more like a transitory mirage.

The consequences of the securitisation of public health are not, however, exclusively about the potential fragmentation of public health governance into a rivalry between interests and values. The epidemiological requirements of addressing mounting disease dangers do not change according to whether an interest-based approach or a value-based perspective dominates. Surveillance remains critical under the framework of either public health securitism or human dignity. Vaccines and antibiotics do not change their physiological effects depending on whether the impetus behind their use is based on security or rights. Thus the nature of public health governance allows a degree of convergence between interest-centric and value-centric perspectives on solutions to disease dangers.

This convergence of interests and values forces both sides of the debate to think about public health security in depth. Thinking of disease threats as security dangers requires understanding not only disease-specific epidemiology but also the broader determinants of disease dangers. Public health securitism does not, by definition, imply that concern with the social determinants of health is jettisoned because security becomes an organising policy framework. Seeing diseases as security dangers actually forces interest-based approaches to appreciate the depth of the policy needs required to address disease dangers.

Where public health securitism has its greatest consequences for public health governance is in the area of priority setting. The attractiveness of security-related arguments flows from the priority policy attention that security threats are perceived to receive. The process of securitisation was a process of prioritisation in public health governance. This dynamic helps explain why virtually everybody has jumped on the security bandwagon since 1995. Like the various processes that produced public health securitism, the bandwagoning did not represent a coherent sorting out of priorities but rather a pluralistic endeavour that privileged security arguments without producing policy coherency on prioritisation.

A theme in the untidy bandwagoning process concerns priority setting between communicable and non-communicable diseases. Security-based arguments tend to cluster around communicable diseases. National security concerns identified bioweapons as the threat, especially those that might use contagious pathogens. The international security discourse has also centred on communicable diseases, as illustrated by the UNSC's work on HIV/AIDS. Initiatives informed by the concept of human security have gravitated toward communicable disease dangers, as evidenced by the focus on communicable disease problems in the Millennium Development Goals (MDGs) (WHO 2006a).

Public health securitism need not be restricted to communicable disease problems. Rather, the securitisation of public health governance makes it more difficult to elevate many non-communicable disease problems. The nature of some of the leading problems, such as tobacco-related diseases and obesity, makes the effort to use security-based arguments more difficult both in a conceptual sense and in terms of common sense. A similar difficulty arises with respect to tobacco-related and obesity-related diseases and the human rights framework because the spread of such non-communicable diseases requires, in most cases, voluntary participation in behaviour that is bad for one's own immediate health and the health of others. The difficulties experienced within the security and human rights frameworks perhaps explain the efforts made to cast non-communicable diseases as material burdens on the economic interests of countries and corporations.

Unfinished Business: Toward Greater Analytical Rigour in the Relationship between Security and Public Health

Thus the dawn of the post-securitisation phase for public health governance does not mean that public health securitism has produced a clear and coherent consensus on the relationship between security and public health. Public health securitism has proved to be a powerful but promiscuous idea that will not disappear any time soon from the landscape of public health governance. The pathology of public health securitism points to some unfinished business, especially with respect to bringing more analytical clarity to the identification of security problems within public health governance.

There are four different ways to bring order to the process of identifying what public health problems pose security threats. Each of these frameworks shares the common goal of providing parameters for deciding what public health concerns should be labelled security threats and given the policy priority such threats require. These four contribute to more rigorous analysis of the security-public health relationship.

Bioweapons Framework

Traditional notions of security have been based on the violence paradigm — the threat of exogenous violence against the state, its military power, or its people (Princeton Project on National Security 2005). The violence paradigm continues to have significant power because 1) threats of violence clearly fall within any definition of security and 2) states have to remain vigilant against potential violent threats. The bioweapons framework maintains that securitisation of public health should only involve public health's relationship to the identification of, and responses to, bioweapons threats. This approach produces a very narrow perspective because it rejects treating, for example, naturally occurring communicable diseases as security concerns.

The legitimacy of the bioweapons framework depends on the appropriateness of relying on the violence paradigm as the exclusive basis for thinking about security nationally or internationally. This framework is parsimonious and provides clear direction in terms of how public health governance should be securitised. Although some actions taken to improve security against bioweapons violence have general public health benefits (such as surveillance), these positive externalities for public health governance are not the intended security objective.

The bioweapons framework is unlikely to carry the day in the post-securitisation phase of public health governance. It recommends a drastic retrenchment in public health securitism that essentially throws every other perspective on security off the securitisation bandwagon. More fundamentally, this perspective rejects the broader thrust of the securitisation of public health governance — that disease dangers of multiple varieties have emerged that threaten individuals, populations, the state, and the international community. The 'back to the future' approach counselled by the bioweapons framework does not respond to the globalisation of disease threats that public health governance must address.

Communicable Disease Framework

A second approach involves limiting securitisation to communicable diseases. As noted earlier, the securitisation of public health governance has gravitated toward communicable diseases as the most prominent dangers to public health in the early 21st century. Limiting public health securitism to communicable diseases would also provide a bright-line rule for distinguishing what public health problems should be accorded security status. With such a limitation in place, securitising public health could focus on what communicable diseases are sufficiently dangerous to warrant heightened governance attention. Unlike the bioweapons framework, the communicable disease approach does not exclude looking at communicable disease problems through security perspectives that are broader than the violence paradigm.

The communicable disease framework may, however, be under-inclusive in terms of disease threats and over-inclusive in terms of concepts of security. The choice to exclude all non-communicable disease threats from public health securitisation neglects the acute dangers that can be posed by some such diseases. International legal regimes in trade and environmental protection have long recognised that pollutants and contaminants can pose extraordinary dangers to public health and should be prevented, protected against, and, if necessary, controlled. For example, states have used international law to address transboundary pollution generally and transboundary pollution caused by industrial or nuclear accidents specifically (Birnie and Boyle 2002). To leave these types of situations outside an understanding of public health's relationship with security appears arbitrary in light of all the diplomatic activity and international law devoted to dangerous non-communicable disease threats.

In terms of concepts of security, the communicable disease framework might be over-inclusive because the framework does not contain any parameters for determining which communicable disease problems deserve security status and which do not. Not all communicable diseases should be considered security threats. Some methodology is required for determining when a communicable disease becomes a security threat. The communicable disease framework does not provide this methodology. Without such a methodology, the concept of security could become little more than a rhetorical device used to bring more policy attention to a wide variety of communicable diseases.

Decision Tree Frameworks

A more sophisticated approach to bringing some conceptual order to the relationship between security and public health has appeared in decision tree frameworks. These break the question of a public health issue as a security threat into a series of factors that lead analysis to specific conclusions. Decision tree frameworks have appeared in the scholarship of Henry Feldbaum and Kelley Lee (2004) and of Colin McInnes (2004), as well as in the approach used by the WHO (2005) in the new International Health Regulations (IHR[2005]) adopted in May 2005.

The work of Feldbaum and Lee and of McInnes focusses on the need to improve analytical approaches to deciding what health problems are global health security issues. Figure 4-1 provides the Feldbaum-Lee decision tree, and Figure 4-2 provides the McInnes decision tree. Both construct a way to determine whether a health issue is a risk to the individual national security threat or is a global health security issue. The decision trees allow their analytical frameworks to be applied to bioweapons, communicable diseases, or non-communicable diseases. Unlike the communicable disease framework, the decision trees include a methodology for deciding whether a given problem is a security threat and what type of security threat it represents.

In the IHR(2005), a decision instrument guides states parties in determining what disease events may constitute a 'public health emergency of international concern' for the purposes of notifying the WHO (see Figure 4-3). Public health emergencies of international concern are not defined in the IHR(2005) as security threats, but the concept of a public health emergency of international concern is not far removed from identifying dangerous disease events as security problems. According to the WHO, for example, the IHR(2005) is a core component of its strategy to improve global health security (Fidler 2005). Like the academic decision trees, the IHR(2005) decision instrument applies to communicable and non-communicable disease events (whether intentionally caused, accidental, or naturally occurring) and thus avoids the under-inclusiveness of the bioweapons and communicable disease frameworks.

These decision tree approaches share the common elements of identifying acute health risks that cause, or have the potential to cause, high levels of morbidity and mortality as either security threats or public health emergencies of international concern. The Feldbaum-Lee decision tree expressly lays out these factors as securitisation criteria. The IHR(2005) is concerned with emergency situations, which clearly includes acute, high-impact disease events. The McInnes decision tree centres on extreme events, which appear to be defined as acute disease risks that post a threat of significant death and illness.

If adopted as the key variables for securitising public health problems, the acute and high morbidity and mortality factors eliminate most non-communicable diseases that cause high levels of morbidity and mortality through chronic but not acute disease. For example, radioactive pollution from a nuclear reactor accident, such as Chernobyl, could not be defined as a security issue because the potential high morbidity and mortality would, beyond the immediate accident site, develop chronically over years rather than acutely over days. Feldbaum and Lee (2004) argue, however, that tobacco-related diseases are acute threats that cause significant morbidity and mortality. They also argue that childhood obesity does not become securitised because it is not an acute health risk. Both tobacco-related and obesity-related diseases are chronic not acute health risks, as those concepts are understood by epidemiologists. Why tobacco but not obesity gets included in the Feldbaum-Lee securitisation process is not clear.

The common approach discernable from the decision trees raises questions about what constitutes an acute threat. From an epidemiological perspective, some communicable diseases, such as HIV/AIDS and tuberculosis (TB), damage health

Figure 4-1 Feldbaum-Lee Decision Tree for Defining a Global Health Security Issue

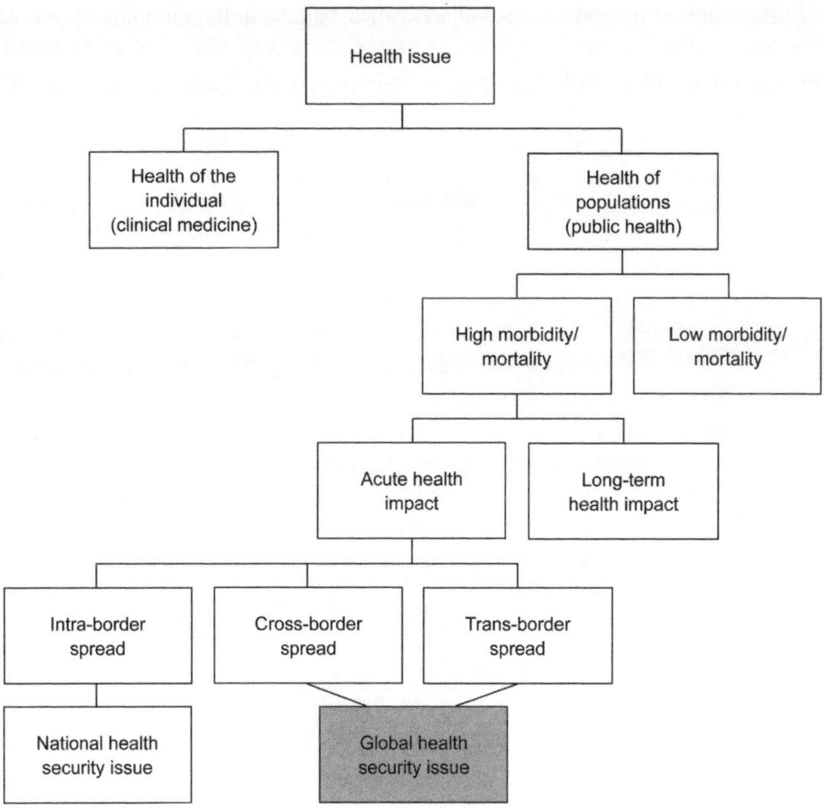

Source: Feldbaum and Lee (2004, 25).

over lengthy periods of time, more akin to a chronic disease than an acute infection, such as influenza, severe acute respiratory syndrome (SARS), or haemorrhagic fever viruses (such as Ebola and Marburg). HIV/AIDS produces high levels of morbidity and mortality but not through physiological means that fit the traditional notion of an acute infection. In fact, the non-acute nature of HIV infection is part of what has made AIDS such a global public health problem.

Loosening the acute factor to open up securitisation to more non-communicable disease problems and to address infections that are chronic may, however, produce a one-branch decision tree that securitises public health problems that generate high levels of morbidity and mortality. Such a move risks equating security with public health rather than creating a framework for prioritising some public health problems as security threats.

Epidemiological Elasticity Approach

Another approach to identifying which public health problems constitute security issues involves assessing the level of danger posed by health risks by determining the propensity of the risks to spread and cause damage in human populations, or the

Figure 4-2 McInnes Decision Tree for Defining a Global Health Security Issue

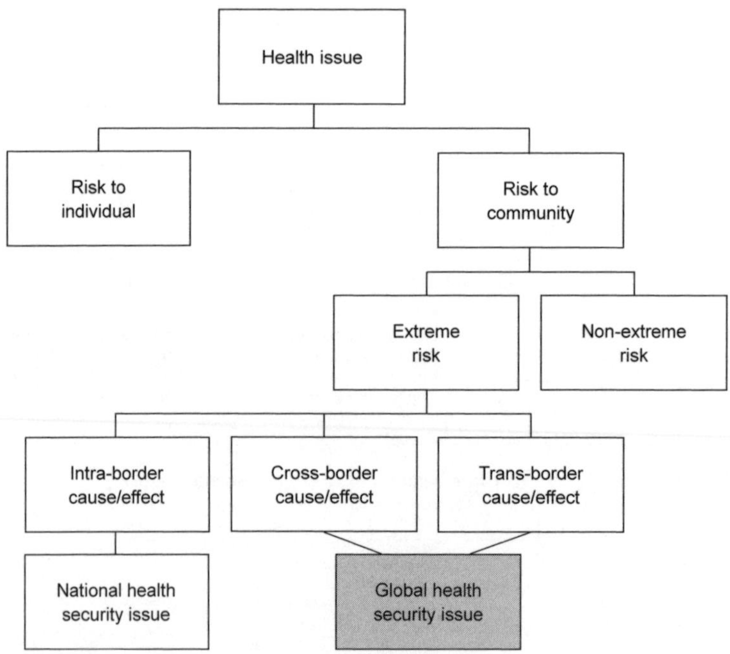

Source: McInnes (2004, 55).

Figure 4-3 Decision Instrument of the Revised International Health Regulations

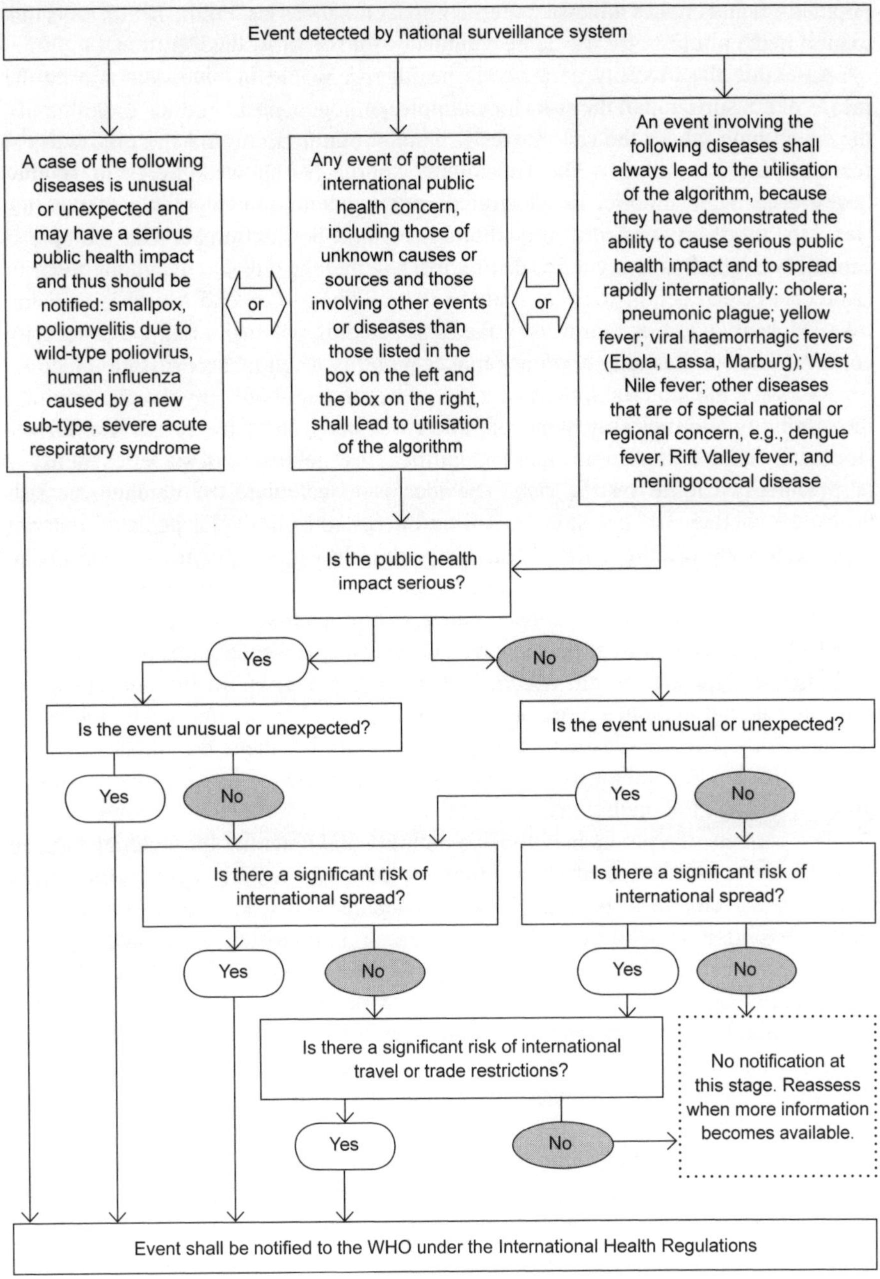

Source: WHO (2005, 45).

epidemiological elasticity (epi-elasticity) of a public health threat. A public health risk would have a high epi-elasticity if the risk demonstrates mobility within human populations and creates adverse material impact for societies. Public health risks that exhibit high epi-elasticity would be candidates for security consideration.

Assessing the mobility of a public health risk would involve determining the means of transmission of the risk (for example, pathogen, pest, product, or pollutant), the speed with which the risk moves in human populations, and the geographical reach of the risk's mobility. The decision tree approaches showed interest in whether health risks were mobile, as illustrated by the attention paid to whether a risk was capable of cross-border, trans-border, or intra-border spread. But the spread capability of a risk only served to distinguish whether the risk was a national security issue or a global health security issue in the Feldbaum-Lee and McInnes decision trees. Mobility was not, therefore, a factor in deciding whether a risk was a security concern. The epi-elasticity approach makes mobility a central securitisation factor.

Assessing the material impact of a public health risk would involve determining the morbidity and mortality, the economic costs, and other adverse material effects (for instance, reduction in military capabilities, fear generated in societies) actually or potentially caused by the risk. The idea is to calculate the damage the risk poses to societies. The decision trees were interested in limited aspects of material damage, namely whether a risk threatened high or low morbidity and mortality. The Feldbaum-Lee decision tree does not accommodate a low morbidity or mortality risk that otherwise causes, or threatens to cause, enormous material damage to affected countries, such as a limited bioweapons attack with a non-contagious pathogen. The McInnes decision tree might accommodate such a risk within the concept of an extreme risk, but without a more precise definition of extreme, such accommodation is guesswork. The epi-elasticity approach expressly broadens the impact analysis in securitisation beyond morbidity and mortality statistics to include other forms of material damage to populations.

Assessments of a public health risk's mobility and potential for material damage will involve consideration of other important factors. One such factor is the means of response available to be brought to bear against the risk, such as surveillance and intervention capabilities. The existence or non-existence of public health infrastructure can affect the mobility of a public health risk and the material damage it can inflict on a population. For example, a population universally vaccinated against a highly mobile, contagious pathogen will not, in all likelihood, suffer high morbidity and mortality from that pathogen's spread. The vaccine — the means of response — has a material impact on the epi-elasticity of the pathogen's overall risk to public health.

Another factor that flows into both mobility and material impact is the mutability of the public health risk, or its ability or potential to change, or be changed, as it enters human populations or in response to intervention efforts. The most obvious example of the importance of mutability is the development of antimicrobial resistance in communicable pathogens, such as malaria and TB, which make resistant microbes more dangerous public health risks because the propensity to spread and to cause damage is enhanced. The mutability factor is not, however, limited to communicable diseases. The routes by which non-communicable disease vectors affect human populations can change, or be changed, in response to public health interventions. Raising taxes and increasing regulatory burdens on tobacco and alcohol, for example, may produce an increase in smuggling and other forms of illicit trade.

The epi-elasticity approach is not a decision tree because the assessment of the mobility and material impact factors produces an objective picture of the level of danger the public health risk poses. Concluding that a risk has a high epi-elasticity does not mean that it is automatically a security problem. The epi-elasticity approach leaves open a margin of discretion in the securitisation process because, as McInnes (2004) argued, how security is defined in most situations involves both objective and subjective considerations. This outcome is really no different from the definitional choices that have to be made in the decision tree approaches, such as whether a public health risk is acute or extreme. However, the epi-elasticity approach's focus on mobility and material damage provides a more robust methodology for using empirical data to aid the determination through the securitisation process of what public health problems should be prioritised as security threats.

Three Pandemics: HIV/AIDS, Pandemic Influenza, and Tobacco-Related Diseases

The rise of public health concern about pandemics provides an interesting lens through which to look at public health securitism, its pathology, and its unfinished business. The three pandemics involving HIV/AIDS, influenza, and tobacco-related diseases provide rich case studies for analysing the belief that public health can be improved through the use of security-based policies. Collectively, the developments related to these pandemics support the argument that public health governance has entered a post-securitisation phase. Public health securitism appears with respect to the policy discourse on each pandemic, illustrating the power of this policy belief today in public health and other circles. The pandemics also help illustrate the various parts of the pathology of public health securitism and underscore the importance of greater analytical rigour in the relationship between security and public health.

Pandemics and Public Health Securitism

The ubiquity of thinking about public health problems in terms of security that has developed since 1995 owes much to the re-emergence of pandemic and potentially pandemic diseases. The threat of global disease as a public health concern diminished during the post–World War II period, particularly with respect to developed countries that dramatically reduced their vulnerability to communicable diseases. In addition, for much of this period, increased morbidity and mortality caused by non-communicable diseases remained largely a rich country concern and thus did not have global implications.

The re-emergence of pandemic potential for communicable diseases and the emergence of pandemic possibilities for non-communicable diseases since 1995 are directly connected to the fundamental cause behind the rise of public health securitism — the awareness that the dangers presented by diseases have significantly increased from the local to the global level. Pandemics are not, by definition, dangerous because whether a disease is dangerous involves other considerations. But pandemics can be dangerous, and mounting concerns about the dangers to public health posed by pandemics involving HIV/AIDS, influenza, and tobacco-related diseases have stimulated policy to gravitate toward security-based arguments as a strategy to motivate public health governance on these global disease threats.

The pandemic threat has acted as a counterweight to the bioweapons threat's tendency to produce narrow conceptions of the relationship between security and public health. But for the threat of pandemic communicable diseases, it is unlikely that the U.S. would have been willing to move the security–public health relationship beyond bioweapons. The grim progress of the HIV/AIDS pandemic and the emergence of conditions conducive to communicable disease pandemics have contributed to shattering the complacency many developed countries exhibited toward public health in the post–World War II period.

The rise of pandemic threats also supported the use of different kinds of security arguments in discourse about how to deal with these dangers. Pandemics provided a background against which concepts of national, international, and human security could be advanced and debated. The HIV/AIDS pandemic proved particularly powerful in attracting diverse security-related arguments in policy and academic debates about how to respond to this crisis. The continued use of these types of arguments in the frenzy of interest around avian influenza and its potential to trigger a global pandemic has reinforced the prominence of security-based thinking with respect to pandemic disease.

These observations suggest that the emergence and threat of pandemics have materially contributed to the securitisation of public health governance. This development is cold comfort because it means that diseases have emerged as global dangers for which past governance frameworks have proved inadequate. The security approach prioritises pandemic preparedness and response over other public health needs and aspirations.

Securitisation Claims and the Three Pandemics

The growth in the threat posed by pandemics generally also raises issues explored above concerning the identification of public health threats as security problems. Are the HIV/AIDS pandemic, the feared influenza pandemic, and the pandemic of tobacco-related diseases all security threats? The hardest to analyse in response to this question is the pandemic of tobacco-related diseases. Experts have frequently securitised the HIV/AIDS pandemic and the anticipated influenza pandemic. Security-based arguments are not as frequently made with respect to the global spread of tobacco-related diseases. As already argued, part of the unfinished business of public health securitism involves the development of greater analytical rigour in the relationship between security and public health. Application of the various frameworks described earlier to the three pandemics at issue here underscores the need for such rigour.

Clearly, none of these three pandemics ranks as a security threat under the bioweapons framework because none involves the intentional use of disease as a weapon. This conclusion merely reinforces the under-inclusiveness and narrowness of the bioweapons approach to the securitisation of public health problems. The communicable disease framework would cover HIV/AIDS and pandemic influenza but not the pandemic of tobacco-related diseases. Given the actual and anticipated scale of the death and illness caused globally by tobacco consumption, the exclusion of this pandemic entirely on the basis that it involves non-communicable diseases does not seem analytically justifiable.

The various decision tree approaches produce important questions that cast some doubt on their utility. Although the IHR(2005) clearly applies to events involving sources of non-communicable diseases, no one has argued that the concept of a public health emergency of international concern would apply in any context to the continued spread of HIV/AIDS or tobacco-related diseases.[2] Such continued spread of these established pandemics would not be considered unusual or unexpected within the meaning of the IHR(2005). This situation might change with respect to HIV/AIDS if, for example, multi-drug resistant strains of HIV/AIDS began circulating globally, thus significantly imperilling the efficacy of antiretroviral treatment (ART) efforts.

Under the Feldbaum-Lee and McInnes decision trees, pandemic influenza would be the only pandemic of the three under consideration here to merit clear security status. For HIV/AIDS to be securitised under these decision trees, it would have to be considered either an acute disease (Feldbaum and Lee 2004) or an extreme disease event (McInnes 2004). As mentioned earlier, whether HIV/AIDS is an acute infection is questionable. The problem faced by the 'acute health impact' factor in the Feldbaum-Lee decision tree is stretching 'acute' to cover both pandemic influenza and HIV/AIDS, which stand at opposite ends of acuteness in epidemiological terms. Feldbaum and Lee stretch the concept further, in fact, in arguing that tobacco-related diseases should be securitised, which must mean Feldbaum and Lee think they have acute health impact; this again strains epidemiological credulity.

In terms of the McInnes decision tree, HIV/AIDS and tobacco-related diseases would have to be perceived to be extreme health risks to be securitised pandemics. Aggregate morbidity and mortality statistics are not sufficient to achieve extreme status because, under that approach, tobacco-related diseases would be more extreme as a health risk than HIV/AIDS. The heavy securitisation of the HIV/AIDS pandemic and the lack of security-related claims for tobacco-related diseases reinforce this conclusion.

The McInnes decision tree, furthermore, seems to exclude tobacco-related diseases as security threats altogether because it is hard to argue that their spread over the course of decades constitutes an extreme health risk in the same way pandemic influenza. As with the concept of acute in the Feldbaum-Lee decision tree, the McInnes decision tree raises the question of whether the term 'extreme' needs to be defined more objectively. Both decision trees easily accommodate pandemic influenza, but they have both difficulty with HIV/AIDS, even though it is an intensively securitised pandemic.

In contrast to the awkward application of the decision trees to the HIV/AIDS and tobacco-related disease pandemics, the epi-elasticity approach assesses the level of danger presented by public health risks according to their respective propensities to spread and cause damage to human populations and societies. The mobility and material impact factors apply equally to all three pandemics, so the epi-elasticity approach does not exclude any pandemic for not satisfying a decision tree factor. This approach assesses the level of danger each of the pandemics presents, and policy makers can more objectively assess whether each pandemic poses a sufficient danger to warrant securitisation at the national or global level.

An epi-elasticity analysis of the three pandemics would lead to the conclusion that pandemic influenza would have the highest epi-elasticity and thus be the most dangerous public health risk of the three. This outcome means that pandemic influenza's combined mobility and material impact factors exceed those of HIV/AIDS and tobacco-related diseases. The next highest epi-elasticity would belong to HIV/AIDS, with tobacco-related diseases being third in terms of the level of danger posed to public health.

In terms of the mobility factor, pandemic influenza would exhibit mobility greater than the mobility of HIV or tobacco products. As an airborne virus, pandemic influenza's means of transmission is more efficient than that of HIV or tobacco products. Pandemic influenza would also have very high mobility because of the speed of virus transmission between humans and the potential of the virus to reach every corner of the earth very rapidly. HIV and tobacco products have also demonstrated impressive mobility locally, regionally, and globally in their respective spread and penetration of human populations.

In terms of material impact, pandemic influenza again would threaten to damage populations and societies on a scale and speed that HIV/AIDS and tobacco-related diseases could not currently generate. Projections about the impact of pandemic influenza often discuss the scale of morbidity and mortality, the economic harm, and the political and social disruption pandemic influenza could cause in both rich and poor countries (Russell 2005). The global handwringing about the lack of preparedness for pandemic influenza demonstrates that an adequate means of response is currently lacking. Prospects for mitigating the material impact of pandemic influenza are, at present, not good.

As between HIV/AIDS and tobacco-related diseases, HIV/AIDS is more dangerous in terms of its material impact in populations and societies. The morbidity and mortality and economic costs created by tobacco-related diseases are enormous in terms of aggregate numbers (WHO 2006b). But no one has argued that tobacco's material impact on societies has the potential to destabilise entire countries, decimate political elites and productive-age labour forces, harm peacekeeping efforts, and create legions of orphans, as HIV/AIDS is now doing in sub-Saharan Africa (Garrett

2005). Nor does contracting a tobacco-related disease involve the economic, social, and psychological costs associated historically with the stigma of HIV/AIDS.

There is also the ability of HIV to mutate in ways that may render existing ART ineffective and defeat attempts to create a vaccine. The means of response available for preventing tobacco-related diseases is, on the whole, easier and cheaper than HIV/AIDS prevention and control strategies. Thus the overall propensity of HIV/AIDS to cause material damage to a population is greater than that of tobacco.

This rough attempt to establish the level of danger these three pandemics respectively pose correlates with the way securitisation processes have unfolded. The epi-elasticity analysis supports the securitisation of pandemic influenza and HIV/AIDS because their combined mobility and material impact factors make them more dangerous risks than tobacco-related diseases. Thus pandemic influenza and HIV/AIDS deserve the public health governance priority that securitisation processes have accorded them as dangerous threats.

Although the epi-elasticity analysis does not rank tobacco-related diseases as a security threat, this approach acknowledges the possibility that a non-communicable disease could represent such a threat because of its mobility and material impact on the health of populations. In fact, the epi-elasticity of tobacco-related diseases may be higher than some communicable diseases, which helps underscore the emphasis that public health authorities nationally and globally have been placing on the importance of more vigorous action against tobacco consumption.

Conclusion

With respect to the war on terrorism, some have expressed the hope that one day terrorism will again be treated as a law enforcement problem rather than a threat to national security. Some in public health may long for the day when disease risks are again treated as public health problems rather than security threats. Desecuritisation would signal that the disease dangers that stimulated linkages between security and public health had been reduced. Ironically, the only way to desecuritise public health might be to increase political interest and policy attention on public health through securitisation. This reasoning supports this chapter's emphasis on the strength of securitism in public health governance today and the continuing importance of this policy belief in the future.

The pathology of public health securitism outlined in this chapter also highlights another reason why securitisation will not fade away any time soon as a feature of public health governance. Securitisation of public health has provided for convergences of narrow and broad conceptions of security and of interest-based and value-based approaches to health and security. In other words, the securitisation of public health creates a two-way street conceptually because it not only brings security into public health but also causes public health to inform security. The basis for a much deeper and broader governance transformation is now under construction in the post-securitisation phase of public health governance.

Notes

1 'Pathology' means the science of the causes and effects of diseases, especially the laboratory examination of blood and tissue samples for diagnostic or forensic purposes. The term is used very deliberately here. In the laboratory, a pathologist might determine that a health condition is benign or malevolent; pathology does not mean that something is sick. Many believe that the frequency of the use of security concepts marks a new 'condition' in the global health body politic that requires examination of its causes, effects, and consequences.

2 The IHR(2005) expressly applies to any new human influenza strain (WHO 2005).

References

Beaglehole, Robert and Derek Yach (2003). 'Globalisation and the Prevention and Control of Non-Communicable Disease: The Neglected Chronic Diseases of Adults'. *Lancet*, vol. 362, pp. 903–908.

Birnie, Patricia W. and Alan E. Boyle (2002). *International Law and the Environment*, 2nd ed. (Oxford: Oxford University Press).

Commission on Human Security (2003). 'Human Security Now: The Final Report of the Commission on Human Security'. New York. <www.humansecurity-chs.org/finalreport/English/FinalReport.pdf> (September 2006).

Eberstadt, Nicholas (2002). 'The Future of AIDS'. *Foreign Affairs*, vol. 81, no. 6, pp. 22–45. <www.foreignaffairs.org/20021101faessay9990/nicholas-eberstadt/the-future-of-aids.html> (September 2006).

Feldbaum, Henry and Kelley Lee (2004). 'Public Health and Security'. In A. Ingram, ed., *Health, Foreign Policy, and Security: Towards a Conceptual Framework for Research and Policy*, pp. 19–28 (London: Nuffield Trust).

Fidler, David P. (2003). 'Public Health and National Security in the Global Age: Infectious Diseases, Bioterrorism, and Realpolitik'. *George Washington International Law Review*, vol. 35, pp. 788–856.

Fidler, David P. (2004). 'Caught between Paradise and Power: Public Health, Pathogenic Threats, and the Axis of Illness'. *McGeorge Law Review*, vol. 35, pp. 45–104.

Fidler, David P. (2005). 'From International Sanitary Conventions to Global Health Security: The New International Health Regulations'. *Chinese Journal of International Law*, vol. 4, no. 2, pp. 325–392.

Garrett, Laurie (2005). 'HIV and National Security: Where Are the Links?' Council on Foreign Relations, New York. <www.cfr.org/content/publications/attachments/HIV_National_Security.pdf> (September 2006).

Goodman, Neville M. (1971). *International Health Organizations and Their Work*, 2nd ed. (Edinburgh: Churchill Livingstone).

Howard-Jones, Norman (1950). 'Origins of International Health Work'. *British Medical Journal*, vol. 1, no. 4661, pp. 1032–1037.

Howard-Jones, Norman (1975). *The Scientific Background of the International Sanitary Conferences, 1851–1938* (Geneva: World Health Organization).

International Conference on Primary Health Care (1978). 'Declaration of Alma-Ata'. 12 September, Alma-Ata, Kazakhstan. <www.euro.who.int/AboutWHO/Policy/20010827_1> (September 2006).

McInnes, Colin (2004). 'Health and Foreign Policy'. In A. Ingram, ed., *Health, Foreign Policy, and Security: Towards a Conceptual Framework for Research and Policy*, pp. 29–42 (London: Nuffield Trust).

Pannenborg, Charles O. (1979). *A New International Health Order: An Inquiry into the International Relations of World Health and Medical Care* (Alphen aan den Rijn, Netherlands: Sijthoff and Noordhoff).

Pirages, Dennis (1997). 'Ecological Theory and International Relations'. *Indiana Journal of Global Legal Studies*, vol. 5, no. 1, pp. 53–63.

Princeton Project on National Security (2005). 'Report of the Working Group on State Security and Transnational Threats'. Woodrow Wilson School of Public and International Affairs, Princeton. <www.wws.princeton.edu/ppns/conferences/reports/fall/SSTT.pdf> (September 2006).

Russell, Sabin (2005). 'Bird Flu Capable of Causing "Incalculable" Misery: 100-Nation Meeting Focuses on Plans to Contain Outbreak'. *San Francisco Chronicle*, 8 November. <sfgate.com/cgi-bin/article.cgi?f=/c/a/2005/11/08/MNGGAFKKU51.DTL &type=science> (September 2006).

Smolinski, Mark S., Margaret A. Hamburg, and Joshua Lederberg, eds. (2003). *Microbial Threats to Health: Emergence, Detection, and Response* (Washington DC: National Academies Press).

United Nations (2004). 'A More Secure World: Our Shared Responsibility'. Report of the Secretary General's High-Level Panel on Threats, Challenges, and Change. New York. <www.un.org/secureworld> (September 2006).

United Nations (2005). 'In Larger Freedom: Towards Security, Development, and Human Rights for All'. Report of the Secretary General of the United Nations for Decision by Heads of State and Government in September 2005. New York. <www.un.org/largerfreedom> (September 2006).

United Nations Development Programme (1994). *Human Development Report* (New York: United Nations Development Programme).

United Nations Security Council (2000). 'Resolution 1308 (2000) on the Responsibility of the Security Council in the Maintenance of International Peace and Security: HIV/AIDS and International Peacekeeping Operations'. <daccess-ods.un.org/access.nsf/Get?Open&DS=S/RES/1308%20(2000)&Lang=E&Area=UNDOC> (September 2006).

United Nations Security Council (2005). 'Security Council Presidential Statement Recognizes "Significant Progress" Addressing HIV/AIDS among Peacekeepers, But Says Many Challenges Remain'. Press release SC/8450, 18 July, New York. <www.un.org/News/Press/docs/2005/sc8450.doc.htm> (September 2006).

United States (2002). 'The National Security Strategy of the United States of America'. Washington DC. <www.whitehouse.gov/nsc/nss.html> (September 2006).

World Health Organization (1994). 'Constitution of the World Health Organization'. Geneva. <www.who.int/about/en » WHO Constitution> (September 2006).

World Health Organization (2001). 'Global Health Security: Epidemic Alert and Response'. World Health Assembly Resolution WHA54.14, 21 May, Geneva. <ftp.who.int/gb/pdf_files/WHA54/ea54r14.pdf> (September 2006).

World Health Organization (2005). 'Revision of the International Health Regulations'. WHA58.3. Geneva. <www.who.int/entity/csr/ihr/IHRWHA58_3-en.pdf> (September 2006).

World Health Organization (2006a). 'WHO and the Millennium Development Goals'. Geneva. <www.who.int/mdg/en> (September 2006).

World Health Organization (2006b). 'Why Is Tobacco a Public Health Priority?' Geneva. <www.who.int/tobacco/health_priority/en> (September 2006).

PART III
The Central Institutions: The Multilateral System

Chapter 5

Public Health in a Globalising World: The Perspective from the World Health Organization

Nick Drager and Laura Sunderland

In today's globalising world, the international global health context is changing rapidly. Governments must deal with health risks that spill in across their borders and that they themselves spill over into the rest of the world. Domestic action is no longer sufficient for countries to ensure public health security. Collective action is crucial. The new global health context requires new rules, new actors, and innovative responses.

This chapter starts with an overview of public health in today's globalising world. It sets out the context that the global health architecture must operate within and the issues it must address. It then focusses on the challenges faced in shaping the future global health architecture in the context of today's world. To illustrate some of the difficulties, the challenge of moving toward health and trade policy coherence at both the national and global levels is presented.

The Current Context: Public Health in a Globalising World

Globalisation is changing the public health landscape (Drager and Beaglehole 2001). Health is now front and centre on the global stage. The following cases illustrate the current public health context.

At the World Trade Organization's (WTO) ministerial meeting in Doha, Qatar, in 2001, members took the unprecedented step of adopting a special declaration on issues related to Trade-Related Aspects of Intellectual Property Rights (TRIPS) and public health. Mike Moore, then the director general of the WTO, emphasised the importance of this issue on the opening day of the conference, indicating that the agreement on public health and TRIPS was the 'deal-breaker' of the new round ('WTO Chief Says Drugs Row May Scuttle Trade Round' 2001). This is a clear example of a public health issue playing a crucial role in starting a new trade round.

United Nations secretary general Kofi Annan similarly raised the profile of health issues. He did this in 2001 by calling for and establishing the Global Fund to Fight AIDS, Tuberculosis, and Malaria. Annan explicitly linked improved health outcomes as critical to the achievement of the Millennium Development Goals (MDGs), which are driving today's development paradigm.

Health is used as a foreign policy currency by industrialised countries in their efforts to promote global health security after the tragedy of 11 September 2001. Current British foreign policy has recently been summed up in four words: Prevent conflicts, promote well-being. In the United Kingdom's white paper on 'Eliminating World Poverty: Making Globalisation Work for the Poor', improving health is a central component of its strategy (UK 2000).

By promoting health in the economic and foreign policy agenda, public health practitioners recognise that domestic action alone is not sufficient to ensure health locally. Increasingly, practitioners must look across other sectors and across borders to protect the health of citizens.

The new rules, markets, actors, and tools of today's globalisation are influencing the development of a new kind of public health practitioner, one with the knowledge and skills to make increased integration and interdependence work for health. This new context also requires new responses at the global level in terms of a review and reconceptualisation of the current global health architecture. The global health architecture must now be able to facilitate, support, and craft the necessary collective action to ensure that globalisation is harnessed to deliver better health for those currently left behind in the development process.

Globalisation and Health

Public health scientists are still in the early stages of gathering evidence on the effects of globalisation on population health. This evidence is required to inform policies and actions to protect and promote the health of poor and vulnerable populations.

To move this research forward the World Health Organization (WHO) has proposed a framework for considering the various channels through which economic globalisation affects population health status (Woodward *et al.* 2001). A summary of the framework is illustrated in Figure 5-1.

The WHO see the process of globalisation as being circular, with important feedback effects among three elements. The first element is increasing cross-border flows of people, goods, money, services, and ideas. The second element is stimulating the development of global rules and institutions. The third element, which is promoted by the other two elements, is the opening of economies.

Globalisation itself is influenced by a number of driving and constraining forces such as technological developments, political influences, economic pressures, changing ideas, and increasing social and environmental concerns. Population health status and its distribution are determined by population-level influences, including effects from health-related sectors, health risks at the individual level, and the healthcare system. These last two elements are strongly influenced by the household economy.

There are multiple linkages between globalisation and the proximal determinants of health. Effects on health systems include the impact of WTO agreements such as the General Agreement on Trade in Services (GATS) on the migration of health personnel and the TRIPS Agreement, which affects pharmaceutical prices in international markets and thus affects on health budgets.

More indirect effects operate through national income and include the price and income effects of macroeconomic shocks or trade and financial liberalisation. These types of shocks or changes to national income influence the availability of public resources for health and the price of inputs. This impact through household income has effects on nutrition and living conditions.

The WHO is using this conceptual framework, in conjunction with trade negotiators and health policy analysts, in order to trace potential effects of a particular policy proposal. Practical issues include analysing GATS commitments to open up the health sector to increased foreign direct investment (FDI) and its possible implications for access to healthcare services.

Figure 5-1 Globalisation

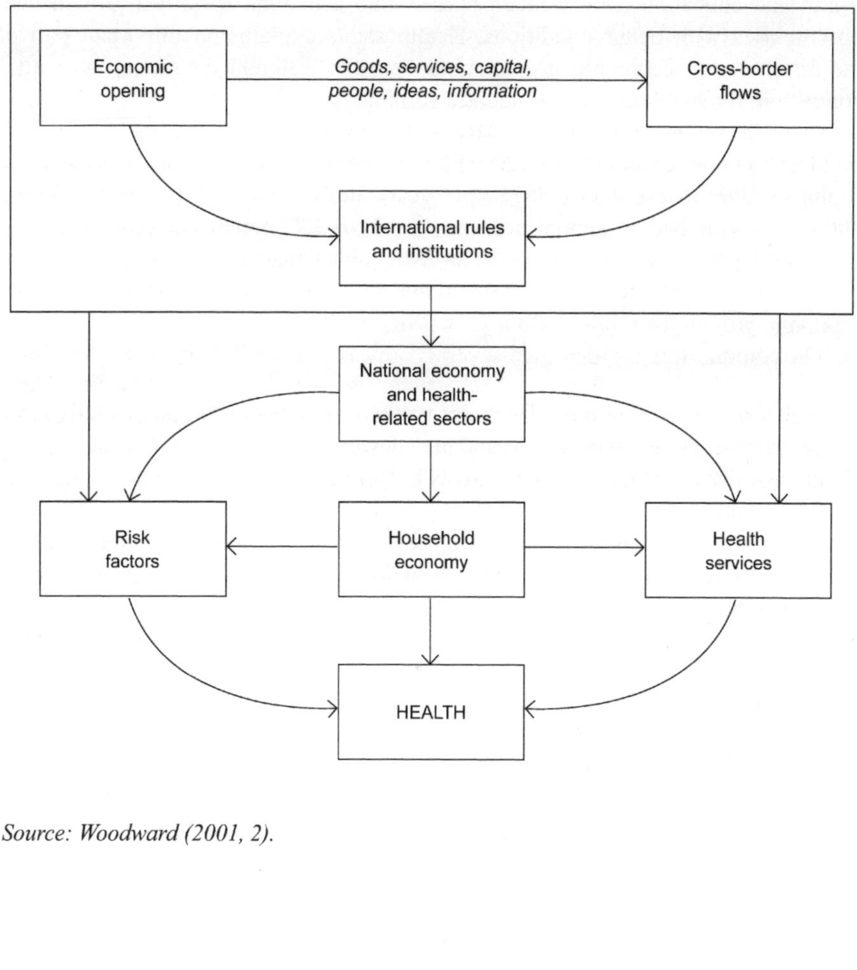

Source: Woodward (2001, 2).

Health and Growth

The pathways illustrated in Figure 5-1 show the effects of globalisation on health. Health also affects economic growth. Work by the WHO's Commission on Macroeconomics and Health provides compelling evidence that better health for the world's poor not only is an important goal in its own right, but also can act as a major force for economic development and poverty reduction. The analysis of the commission shows that disease is a drain on economies. Conversely, investment in health spurs economic growth.

The main message to emerge from the commission is that it is feasible and affordable to improve health outcomes dramatically among the poor. Targeted and effective interventions would save an estimated 8 million lives per year. The commission presents evidence that the wealth created will be many times greater than the costs of the interventions, potentially generating US$360 billion annually within 15 years.

Macroeconomic evidence shows that countries with the weakest conditions of health and education have a much harder time achieving sustained growth than do countries with better conditions. Health status explains an important part of the difference in economic growth rates between different countries, even after controlling for standard macroeconomic variables.

Using the infant mortality rate (IMR) as a proxy for health status, the Commission on Macroeconomics and Health (2001) found that of the poorest countries (with per capita income of less than US$750 per year), those with an IMR of 50–100 per 1000 live births had an annual average growth of 3.7 percent per year, compared to only 0.1 percent in countries with an IMR higher than 150. In other words, for poor countries with the same income, those with lower IMRs experienced higher economic growth than those with higher IMRs.

The commission has identified several pathways of health to growth, including:

- higher labour productivity: Healthier workers are physically and mentally more productive, earn higher wages, and miss fewer days of work than those who are chronically ill. This creates incentives for foreign companies to make long-term investments.
- higher rates of investment and savings: People who live longer are more likely to put away funds for retirement; increased domestic savings in turn provide funds for capital investment.
- higher educational attainment: Healthy children are better able to learn, and they miss fewer days of school. As health improves, parents and children invest more in education.
- demographic changes: Improvements in health lead to lower rates of mortality and fertility and to a reduced dependency ratio. This again allows for greater investment in the health and education of each child.

The Increasing Cross-Border Threats of Infectious and Non-Communicable Diseases

The UN Secretary General's High-Level Panel identified infectious diseases as a key threat to global security (UN 2004). Figure 5-2 shows the number of verified outbreaks of selected diseases from 2001 to 2005.

These outbreaks can have major macroeconomic implications. The lessons learned from severe acute respiratory syndrome (SARS) were significant. The gross domestic product (GDP) losses in 2003 that have been attributed to SARS are estimated at US$20 billion for Asia, with additional estimated business costs as high as US$60 billion of lost revenue. These financial shocks, however, are small when compared to estimates that propose that avian influenza may well pose a cumulative cost to Asia of between US$80 billion and US$100 billion, even if it remains confined to poultry and clears up by 2007–08. An added impact from the loss of tourism in Asia could raise the final bill to as high as US$150 billion by 2008. The impact of a serious human influenza pandemic would be even more damaging to tourism, the economy, and human life.

Figure 5-2 Verified Communicable Disease Outbreaks, 1 January 2001–30 September 2005

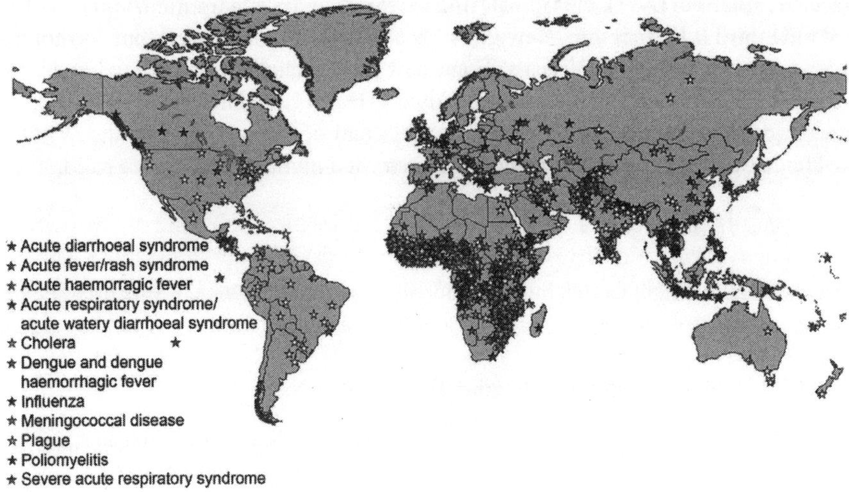

Note: The WHO has verified more than 1242 events between 1 January and 6 September 2006.

Sources: CSR Office for Alert and Response Operations, WHO Map Production, Public Health Mapping and GIS Communicable Diseases, World Health Organization.

Infectious diseases, while devastating to economies and societies, are not the only type of health problem to have macroeconomic implications. Threats to global health come from infectious diseases, but in many countries threats come even more prevalently from non-communicable diseases. For example, the number of deaths worldwide due to HIV/AIDS in 2005 is projected at 2 830 000, whereas the projection for the number of deaths from cardiovascular disease in 2005 is a staggering 17 528 000.

The Opportunities of Globalisation for Public Health

There are two sides to the globalisation coin. Despite the many risks addressed in this chapter, there are also significant opportunities that globalisation can bring in terms of public health. Knowledge, technology, and best practices for affordable and effective prevention and treatments are being shared more widely, and new research is under way to fill gaps in medical knowledge.

New market incentives are being created to spur more investment in research and development (R&D) of new drugs and vaccines for malaria, HIV/AIDS, and tuberculosis (TB) and better diagnostic tests for these diseases. New resources are being raised to increase access to existing drugs and vaccines and to provide more effective treatments to combat polio, measles, diarrhoea, and respiratory diseases. International partnerships between the public and private sector have launched campaigns, including the Roll Back Malaria Partnership, the International AIDS Vaccine Initiative (IAVI), the Global Alliance for Vaccines and Immunization (GAVI), and the Stop TB Partnership. New global health rules are being developed to control cross-border or global health risks. These new rules include improved global disease surveillance through the revised International Health Regulations (IHR[2005]), the Framework Convention on Tobacco Control, and collaboration with the WTO to ensure that public health is protected and promoted in multilateral trade rules.

The Global Health Agenda

The global health agenda that must be addressed by today's global health architecture can be summarised in ten key priority areas, as shown in Table 5-1. In shaping the

Table 5-1 A Global Health Agenda: Ten Priority Areas

1. Ensure universal coverage and promote equity and health.
2. Build individual and global health security.
3. Promote health-related human rights.
4. Reduce poverty and its effects on health.
5. Tackle the social and economic determinants of health.
6. Promote a healthier environment.
7. Build fully functional and equitable health systems.
8. Ensure an adequate health workforce.
9. Harness knowledge, science, and technology.
10. Strengthen governance and leadership.

future global health architecture, it is important to recognise the core functions of the WHO as the leader in global health.

Those functions are:

- to provide leadership on matters critical to health and to engage in partnerships where joint action is needed;
- to articulate ethical and evidence-based policy positions;
- to set norms and standards and to promote and monitor their implementation;
- to shape the research agenda and to stimulate the generation, translation, and dissemination of valuable knowledge;
- to provide technical support, to catalyse change, and to develop sustainable institutional capacity; and
- to monitor the health situation and to assess the health trends.

Shaping the Global Health Architecture for Global Health Governance

Given the current context, in terms of globalisation, threats to human security, and the global health agenda, it is important to examine more specifically the challenges of shaping the architecture for global health governance. The rapidly changing global situation, the shifts in patterns of disease, the improved understanding of the social and economic determinants of health, and the diversity of institutional actors are all integral to shaping the new architecture. Figure 5-3 highlights many of the actors involved in contemporary in health governance.

Health governance has three broad, central needs that must be addressed and resolved by the new global architecture. The first is to address factors that cross, and even ignore, the geographical boundaries of the state. The second is to define and address the determinants of health from a multisectoral perspective. The third is to involve, both formally and informally, a broader range of actors and interests. The global health architecture must bring together state and non-state actors and ensure accountability to the global health community.

In addition, there are four specific issues that the global health architecture must resolve. The first is to agree on the normative framework upon which global health governance can be built. A consensus must be reached on underlying moral and ethical principles that define global health cooperation, such as universalism, health as a human right, justice, and dignity. The second is to define the leadership and authority of global health governance and to determine the extent of the willingness of states to pool sovereignty and act collectively. The third is to generate sufficient resources (for example, using dual-track budgets) for global health cooperation and to distribute those resources appropriately according to agreed priorities, as seen through the lens of global public health governance. The fourth issue is to develop mechanisms to ensure effective monitoring, accountability, and incentives for complying with global health governance priorities.

Institutional Challenges: Developing Policy Coherence in Trade and Health

Moving to address the broad determinants of health, as well as including the diverse range of actors that are involved in these determinants, is a complex process. It presents numerous institutional challenges at both national and global levels. The example of developing policy coherence in trade and health is presented here to illustrate some of these challenges and begin to identify good practices in moving toward collective responses. The linkage of trade and health is a relatively new area that needs to be addresses by today's national and global heath architecture.

The liberalisation of trade promoted by the WTO can affect health in multiple ways. Sometimes the impact is direct and the effect is obvious, as when a disease crosses a border together with a traded good. Other times the effects are more indirect. For example, reducing trade tariffs may have an impact on prices for medical equipment and health-related products; changing international rules for patent protection influences access to essential medicines, diagnostic devices, and technology transfer; and liberalising trade in health services can affect national health systems. Conversely, national and international health standards and rules can

Figure 5-3 Global Health Governance Mapped

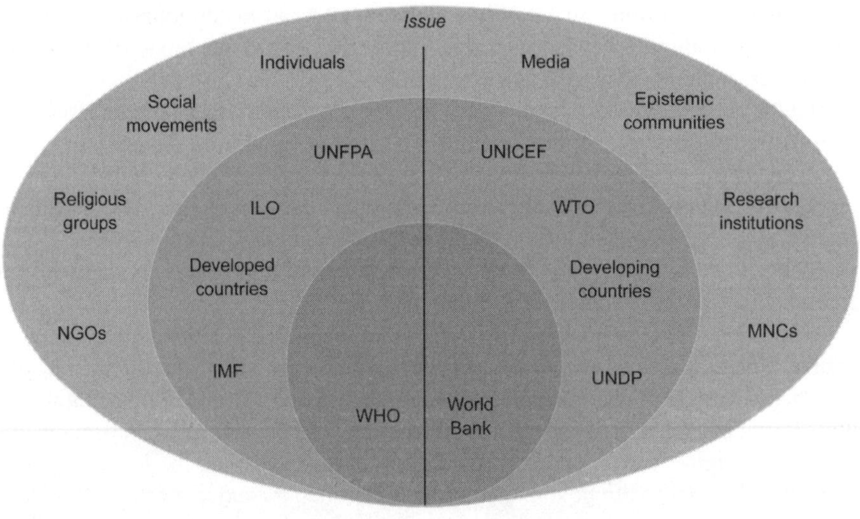

ILO = International Labour Organization; IMF = International Monetary Fund; MNCs = multinational corporations; NGOs = nongovernmental organisations; UNDP = United Nations Development Programme; UNFPA = United Nations Fund for Population Activities; UNICEF = United Nations International Children's Fund; WHO = World Health Organization; WTO = World Trade Organization

Source: Dodgson (2002).

have important implications for trade. For example, the standards, guidelines, and recommendations of the Codex Alimentarius can affect trade in foodstuffs, and the WHO's IHR(2005) can directly influence international travel and traffic in goods.

Four WTO multilateral trade agreements are particularly important to the WHO's member states. First, the GATS has a direct impact on the cross-border movement of patients and health professionals and the foreign ownership of health facilities. Indeed, health ministries around the world face a new challenge to assess the risks and respond to the opportunities of increasing openness in health services under the GATS, as shown in Table 5-2. Second, the Agreement on the Application of Sanitary and Phytosanitary Measures (SPS) affects food safety and the cross-border spread of infections. Third, the Agreement on Technical Barriers to Trade (TBT) is relevant to health norms and standards. Fourth, the TRIPS Agreement can affect the price and availability of essential medicines. Table 5-3 gives an overview of these four agreements and the relevant health issues.

The WHO works closely with the WTO and other international organisations involved in trade to support the efforts of its member states to develop policies on international trade and health that are mutually coherent and reinforcing, and that maximise the health benefits and minimise the risks, especially for poor and vulnerable populations. Work in this area is a major part of the WHO's response to the May 2006 World Health Assembly resolution on international trade and health (WHO 2006a). The resolution calls on the WHO to provide support to member states to frame coherent policies that address the relationship between trade and health, to respond to member states' requests for support of their efforts to build the capacity to understand the implications of international trade and trade agreements for health, and to address relevant issues through policies and legislation. It also

Table 5-2 Health Opportunities and Risk

	Opportunity	Risk
Mode 1: Cross-border supply of services	Increased care to remote and under-served areas	Diversion of resources from other health services
Mode 2: Consumption abroad	Foreign exchange earnings for generated health services of importing country	Crowding out of local population and diversion of resources to service foreign nationals
Mode 3: Commercial presence	New opportunities for employment and access to new technologies	Development of two-tiered health system with an internal brain drain
Mode 4: Presence of persons	Economic gains from remittances of healthcare personnel working overseas	Permanent outflows of health personnel, with loss of investment in educating and training such personnel

Source: Blouin, Drager, and Smith (2005).

requests the WHO work with competent international organisations to generate and share evidence on the relationship between trade and health.

The WHO's work in this field focusses on analysis and research to inform policy and practice on the development of tools and training to build capacity in member states to fully understand the public health implications of multilateral trade agreements. More specifically it aims to strengthen capacities in the ministries of health to enable them to work effectively with their colleagues in the ministries of trade, commerce, and finance in their efforts to shape and manage the trade policy environment for health. Countries are establishing and strengthening institutional mechanisms to foster trade and health policy coherence. Indeed, the WHO and WTO are moving toward policy coherence by engaging in seven specific forms of collaboration: high-level policy consultations, governance meetings, research and analysis, country missions, regional and national meetings, training courses, and informal consultations.

Current work points to seven key institutional challenges that must be addressed at the national level in order to achieve improved trade and health policy coherence. These seven key institutional challenges are as follows:

- achieving a common understanding of the key trade and health policy issues, through ongoing dialogue;
- articulating a clear commitment and ministry of health leadership in order to work toward trade and health policies that mutually support human development objectives;

Table 5-3 Specific Health Issues and Most Relevant World Trade Organization Agreements

Health Issue	Agreement on the Application of Sanitary and Phytosanitary Measures	Agreement on Technical Barriers to Trade	Agreement on Trade-Related Aspects of Intellectual Property Rights	General Agreement on Trade in Services
Infectious disease control	•	•		
Food safety	•			
Tobacco control		•	•	•
Environment	•	•		
Access to drugs			•	
Health services				•
Food security	•			
Emerging issues				
Biotechnology	•	•	•	
Information technology			•	
Traditional knowledge			•	

Source: WHO and WTO (2002).

- creating sustainable institutional mechanisms that enhance coherence and promote the use of innovative instruments and appropriate incentives;
- involving stakeholders early and effectively to build trust and transparency;
- getting the evidence right, working out costing and financing options, and proposing alternatives;
- measuring, tracking, and evaluating progress and course corrections; and
- developing negotiation skills.

By focussing on trade and health, this chapter has illustrated that 'getting it right' — in terms of rules, actors, institutions, mechanisms, and incentives that address the social, economic, and environmental determinants of health — is a complex and difficult task.

Conclusion

Globalisation is changing the public health landscape. In today's interdependent, interconnected world it is essential that countries take into account the risks to — and opportunities for — population health that are spilling over their borders. It is clear that domestic action alone cannot ensure population health. Increased collective action by countries is needed. This chapter has outlined the current context for global public health in terms of globalisation, threats to human security, and the global health agenda. It then provided an overview of the challenges faced in shaping a robust global health architecture and effective global health governance that will lead to collective action. The overall goal of global health governance and an effective global health architecture is to harness globalisation to meet the health and development needs of those currently left behind in the development process.

References

Blouin, Chantal, Nick Drager, and Richard Smith, eds. (2005). *International Trade in Health Services and the GATS: Current Issues and Debates* (Washington DC: World Bank and World Health Organization).

Commission on Macroeconomics and Health (2001). 'Macroeconomics and Health: Investing in Health for Economic Development'. World Health Organization, Geneva. <www.cid.harvard.edu/cidcmh/CMHReport.pdf> (September 2006).

Dodgson, Richard, Kelley Lee, and Nick Drager (2002). 'Global Health Governance: A Conceptual Review'. World Health Organization and London School of Hygiene and Tropical Medicine, Geneva.

Drager, Nick and Robert Beaglehole (2001). 'Globalization: Changing the Public Health Landscape'. *Bulletin of the World Health Organization,* vol. 79, no. 9, p. 803. <www.who.int/bulletin/pdf/2001/issue9/bu1488.pdf> (September 2006).

United Kingdom (2000). 'Eliminating World Poverty: Making Globalisation Work for the World's Poor'. White Paper on International Development. <www.dfid.gov.uk/pubs/files/whitepaper2000.pdf> (September 2006).

United Nations (2004). 'A More Secure World: Our Shared Responsibility'. Report of the Secretary General's High-Level Panel on Threats, Challenges, and Change. New York. <www.un.org/secureworld> (September 2006).

Woodward, David, Nick Drager, Robert Beaglehole, *et al.* (2001). 'Globalization and Health: A Framework for Analysis and Action'. *Bulletin of the World Health Organization,* vol. 79, no. 9, pp. 847–881. <www.who.int/bulletin/pdf/2001/issue9/bu1329.pdf> (September 2006).

World Health Organization and World Trade Organization (2002). 'WTO Agreements and Public Health: A Joint Study by WHO and the WTO Secretariat'. Geneva. <www.wto.org/English/res_e/booksp_e/who_wto_e.pdf> (September 2006).

World Health Organization (2006a). 'International Trade and Health'. WHA59.26, 27 May, Geneva. <www.who.int/gb/ebwha/pdf_files/WHA59/A59_R26-en.pdf> (September 2006).

World Health Organization (2006b). 'Globalization, Trade, and Health'. Geneva. <www.who.int/trade> (September 2006).

'WTO Chief Says Drugs Row May Scuttle Trade Round'. (2001). *Agence France-Presse,* 8 November.

Chapter 6

Reaching the Millennium Development Goals

Colin I. Bradford, Jr.[1]

Global health conditions are in a state of crisis. Not only are inadequate health conditions in poor countries ravaging lives and restraining development, but the HIV/AIDS pandemic is also threatening to undermine progress on all other fronts in developing countries and menacing the sense of health security in industrial countries.

A state of crisis can help galvanise action. But urgency can crowd out the systemic approaches needed for sustainability. The question is how to stimulate global action on health in such a way that it addresses the HIV/AIDS crisis through measures that strengthen public health systems in poor countries and catalyse policies and institutional changes that put countries on a trajectory of long-term sustainability.

This chapter makes three central arguments. First, the prioritisation of global health needs to maintain the centrality of investment in public health systems and follow the multisectoral approach embodied in the achievement of the Millennium Development Goals (MDGs) by 2015, which can generate higher yield results and long-run sustainability. Second, for this to succeed, a global action plan for health must be set in motion simultaneously with global action plans in education, environment, and water and sanitation, each of which is critical to the success of global health and sustainability for the long term. Third, the prioritisation of global health emanating from a political process, for example a mechanism such as a Leaders 20 (L20) summit, can mobilise resources, maintain continuous visibility, and monitor results while strengthening global governance in the process.

Global Health as a Multisectoral Issue

The MDGs represent a new consensus on development that is fundamentally different from the Washington consensus in the 1990s. The Washington consensus implied that sound economic policies are the *sine qua non* for development to occur. In contrast, the Monterrey consensus on the MDGs — from the United Nations International Conference on Financing for Development in Monterrey, Mexico, in March 2002 — embodies a new notion that poverty reduction is multidimensional and that progress depends not on a single-sector approach prioritising economics but on simultaneous actions across sectors.

This is certainly true in health. Three of the eight MDGs are health goals: reducing mortality among children under five, reducing maternal mortality, and reversing the spread of communicable diseases, specifically HIV/AIDS, malaria, tuberculosis (TB), and others (see Appendix). The other five MDGs are, in fact, critical to achieving these global and national health goals, namely universal education, gender equality, environmental balance, poverty reduction, and global partnerships. For the first time, the dominant development paradigm recognises a comprehensive set of interconnected imperatives as critical to progress. It goes beyond the notion that a selective set of financial keys is exclusively crucial to sustainable development.

Meeting the targets for child health, maternal health, and communicable diseases requires improvements in public health systems, not quick fixes or isolated technological interventions. For success in health, broad systemic and institutional changes are required in the health sector and comprehensive advances in education, gender, environment, and international cooperation are also required. That is the meaning of the MDGs. It is now inconceivable to think that a sustainable improvement in health for all in developing countries can occur if people cannot read, if women and girls do not have equal access to health clinics, schools, and water, if the environment is polluted, if poverty reduction is not a priority, and if scaled-up international cooperation is not forthcoming.

Furthermore, the MDGs have their roots in the series of UN summit conferences in the early to mid 1990s in which all members participated, and in which public officials, private sector leaders, and civil society advocates were involved. The MDGs are not UN goals; they are societal goals approved by nation-states in a long series of summit conferences from the World Summit for Children in New York in 1990 to the UN General Assembly (UNGA) — the Millennium Summit — in 2000 to Monterrey in 2002 and the World Summit on Sustainable Development (WSSD) in Johannesburg in 2003. In addition to this engagement and endorsement at the national level, the MDGs are now the primary framework for international cooperation used by the World Bank, the International Monetary Fund (IMF), the Organisation for Economic Co-operation and Development (OECD), the World Trade Organization (WTO), the World Health Organization (WHO), most UN development agencies, and all bilateral development agencies of industrial countries. The MDGs are now the universal framework for the broad global agenda that they embrace for all public and private actors across the globe.

Nonetheless, this unprecedented global consensus can be eroded by actions that fail to capture the new dynamic of multisectoral imperatives revealed by the MDGs. The so-called Copenhagen consensus illustrates the danger. A distinguished group of economists met in 2004 to prioritise global actions who concluded that ranking health over other international goals was most urgent and that necessary action was required (Lomborg 2004). This, of course, flies in the face of the new consensus, but it reveals the danger of urgency potentially crowding out sustainability. Rather, the key is to make global health a priority, specifically underscoring the urgency of reducing HIV/AIDS infections, through measures and means that drive the systemic and institutional changes in health and critically linked sectors needed for transformative and sustainable long-run trajectories. For that, the mobilisation of actions for global health needs to be in the context of advancing the MDGs as a whole between now and 2015, rather than apart from them.

Global Action Plans

To achieve the MDGs by 2015 requires a scaling-up of domestic efforts in developing countries and in international cooperation by industrial countries sufficient to accelerate the rate of progress toward the seven MDGs related to economic, social, or environmental issues. Various studies have estimated that in terms of official development assistance (ODA) alone, achieving the MDGs would require a doubling of aid (Commission for Africa 2005). To accelerate progress over the next decade, the next step required now is to initiate multistakeholder consultations for the formulation of global action plans in the sectors crucial to the achievement of the MDG agenda. Global action plans would translate the specific objectives, targets, and indicators of the MDGs into operational programmes for achieving them.

To retain consistency with the multisectoral aspect of the MDGs as a vehicle for achieving them, three global action plans must be formulated simultaneously: one each for health, education, and the environment, with water and sanitation being a component of health, even though the indicator for it is under the environment MDG. Gender equality and poverty reduction would be cross-cutting themes within each action plan rather than treated separately. This way all eight MDGs are included in the three global action plans taken together.

Each of the three global action plans would focus on actions by all actors in the public and private sectors and the national and international actors necessary for accelerating improvements in access to health care, universal education, and sustainable, healthy environmental conditions in all countries and globally. In addition, each sectoral action plan would identify the cross-sectoral linkages in other domains that require action for each plan to be successful. Prioritisation of activities within sectoral plans would be linked to comprehensiveness rather than opposed to it.

One possibility is to integrate the prioritisation of HIV/AIDS within a global action plan for health that includes water and sanitation in compatible, mutually reinforcing ways. To achieve this balance, strengthening public health systems must be at the centre of the action as crucial for sustainability. For this centrality to become operative, ambitious investment programmes in public health systems need to be designed, prioritised, and implemented in national budgets along with external support. Investment in human resources in health care to staff the health system and in programmes for Education For All to equip individuals to manage their own health is also critical. Gender equality in education and in access to health is vital to achieving major improvements in global health, as well as battling HIV/AIDS. The HIV/AIDS crisis must be the stimulus for these investments in health systems and human resources rather than drawing health resources away from institutions and health systems to solve the crisis, only to leave societies vulnerable to the next health crisis.

Water and sanitation systems are critical components of public health systems. It is important to achieve a balance between investments in sanitation and investments in water. Too much investment in water and too little in sanitation can simply lead to another generation of diseases spawned by water contaminated by sewage. Integrated water resource management thus becomes an integral part of any global action plan for health. But water and sanitation rarely rank high in global and national priorities. They are relegated to the low politics of infrastructure and facilities management and disconnected from the human development agenda, whereas, in fact, water and good sanitation are both fundamental to the broader agenda. Without major investments in water and sanitation, the three health-related MDGs will be out of reach. Slums will mushroom and it will be impossible to halve the number of people living in poverty by 2015.

Figure 6-1 illustrates the opportunity to prioritise an assault on HIV/AIDS while maintaining the centrality of strengthening public health systems through an integrated approach for achieving the three health-related MDGs as part of a comprehensive effort to achieve all eight MDGs simultaneously. Poverty reduction (MDG No. 1) is accelerated by mobilising efforts to achieve each of the other MDGs as well as additional actions such as increased economic growth. MDG No. 8 on global partnership, in brief, means complying with commitments undertaken at Monterrey in March 2001.

The crucial question then is how to launch processes for the formulation of global action plans for health, education, and the environment in a way that catalyses

Figure 6-1 Global Action Plan for Global Health

Overall Goal: Reduce the death rate (Millennium Development Goals nos. 4, 5, and 6)

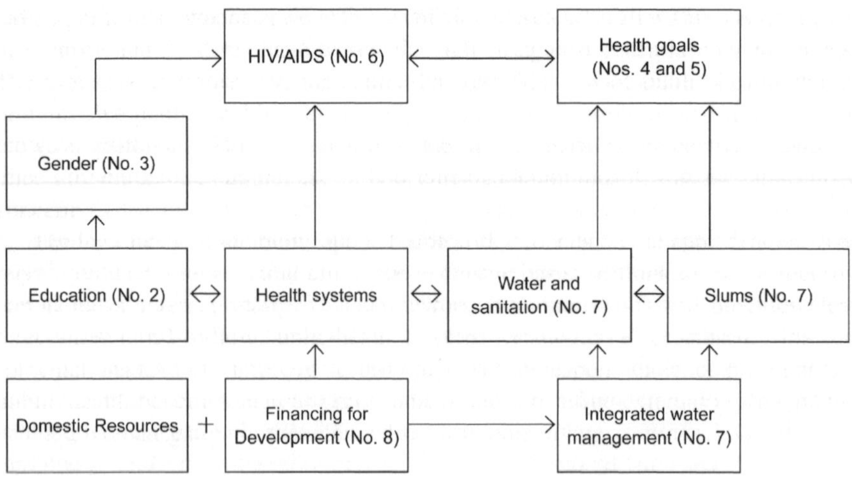

actions by all actors in innovative ways without being captured by existing interests and bureaucratic struggles that potentially stifle new interactions and interventions and revert to business as usual.

Global Governance, Global Action, and the G20

The human development agenda embodied in the MDGs is a political one. It is a political agenda because it represents a change in direction, shifts in priorities, and an ambitious effort to mobilise resources and policies for accelerated transformative change. It represents a rebalancing of the tensions between financial stability and social sustainability toward a prioritisation of interconnected investments in health, education, and the environment. These shifts have implications for all actors. International institutions do not have the authority to shift direction, reshape priorities, or raise resources; rather, they reflect those changes expressed to them by national public officials. National governments, for better or worse, are the constituted authorities precisely because they are explicitly political and accountable directly or indirectly to their national societies.

As a result, the logical locus for global governance is an intergovernmental group of national public officials, such as the G20 finance ministers and central bank governors. These kinds of *ad hoc* mechanisms have proven extremely useful in coping with a variety of global challenges. The annual G7/8 summits have existed for more than 30 years. The G20 members include the G8 as well as ten large developing countries and have been meeting at the ministerial level since 1999.[2] The proposal by former Canadian prime minister Paul Martin to elevate the G20 to a summit of heads of state and government at the leaders level (an L20) provides an opportunity to advance the global agenda embodied in the MDGs and strengthen summit processes in a new, more representative modality at the same time (English, Thakur, and Cooper 2005).

Using the G20/L20 summit mechanism to convene groups to formulate global action plans for health, education, and the environment would circumvent the problem of capture by convening national authorities and international officials. It would be done under the aegis of a global governance group accountable to more than 60 percent of the world's population. L20 heads could convene three separate consultative forums, one for health, one for education, and one for the environment, composed of G20 ministers for each of the three sectors and heads of selected international organisations with responsibility in these and adjacent domains. Working groups could be established that would be composed of senior officials below ministerial rank who would interact with civil society, the private sector, and other governments and international organisations not represented in the G20 ministerial-level sectoral groups. Working groups would report to ministerial-level sector groups, which would in turn report to leaders at the L20 level for final review, revision, and approval. Global action plans would then be fashioned in a broadly inclusive fashion and recommended to the international community by a political body consisting of the highest political authorities of most of the largest and most significant countries in the world. This is a reasonable, if not ideal, path to global action and global governance.

The advantage of building the consultative processes for the formulation of the three global action plans on the G20 base is that the G20 is fundamentally a grouping of ministers of finance. G20 ministers of health, education, and the environment would be the principal sparkplugs for these broader efforts. But there would be a need to keep their ministers of finance informed and involved because, in the end, it is the ministers of finance who have decisive influence on national priorities and national budgets. An additional step in the process might be to convene a G20 finance ministerial with each of the G20 sectoral ministers prior to referring each global action plan to the L20 for final promulgation to ensure concordance between sectoral priorities and broader fiscal constraints and national objectives.

The entire process of mobilising resources for achieving the MDGs by 2015 is one based on the understanding that stovepiped sectoral solutions are business as usual. The way to accelerate change and make qualitative leaps forward is to connect sectoral programmes continuously to intersectoral linkages in order to achieve higher yield outcomes from simultaneous cross-sectoral actions instead of isolated deepening of sectoral specialisation and parochialism. Continuously highlighting synergies and feasibility through integrated approaches building on the interconnected imperatives of the MDGs is at the core of the new global strategy. The L20/G20 is well positioned to force attention to the intersectoral linkages central to the new global agenda and to forge ambitious global action plans within feasible financial constraints. Convening consultations for global action plans would also demonstrate the need for a broadly representative leaders-level grouping as a much needed mechanism for global governance.

One of the primary reasons why a global governance summit mechanism is necessary is that the multisectoral agenda embodied in the MDGs requires an inter-institutional strategy to relate the MDGs to the international institutions responsible for different sectors. Managing issues at the interface becomes critical to implementing the MDGs. A good example of the contribution a global summit mechanism could make is to identify ways in which the WHO, the World Bank, and the regional development banks could coordinate investments with national governments in public health systems. This coordinated acceleration of institutional investment is unlikely to become prioritised without such a strategic commitment from the highest national authorities that uniquely have broader multisectoral perspectives and responsibilities. The WHO's budget is too small to significantly finance the needed investments in public health systems. In any case, the ministers of health in the WHO council only have control over half the organisation's budget. And yet, such an effort without the health expertise of the WHO makes no sense. The multilateral development banks are unlikely to prioritise investment in national public health systems without a push from higher political authorities with broader longer-term perspectives. This is a case of filling a void at the apex in global governance with a representative summit grouping that can prioritise the institutional investments necessary to manage the sequence of health crises likely to occur and the underlying health deprivation problem in poor countries at the same time.

Notes

1 This chapter builds on a project on global public health and the G20 sponsored by the Centre for International Governance Innovation (CIGI) and the Centre for Global Studies at the University of Victoria. It is based on ideas derived from an intensive interaction within the Helsinki Process sponsored by the governments of Finland and Tanzania. The author is extremely grateful to Fantu Cheru for his gracious, insightful, and intelligent intellectual leadership within the Helsinki Process and his many thoughtful contributions over the last years. He is also grateful to Henny Helmich, president of National Committee for International Cooperation and Sustainable Development (NCDO) in Amsterdam, for his excellent ideas and for bringing him together with his NCDO colleagues Nadine Beudeker and Korrie Kline as well as Ellen Verhuel of the Royal Tropical Institute, all of whom made him think hard about the role of finance ministers and the International Monetary Fund in relation to capacity building and investment in the social sectors. The author appreciates very much the contribution of David Tipping from Habitat for Humanity in Nairobi for bringing him up to speed on water and sanitation issues. He is grateful to the members of the Helsinki Process Track on the Global Economic Agenda as it was out of their intense and sometimes difficult discussions that many of the ideas herein were born. The author is most thankful to Carol Graham and Lael Brainard for supporting his work on global governance at the Brookings Institution and especially to Johannes Linn for innumerable spirited conversations about the G20 over the last two years and for his splendid colleagueship. All this said, the author alone remains responsible for the ideas and views expressed herein.

2 The G8 consists of Canada, France, Germany, Italy, Japan, Russia, United States, and the United Kingdom. The other members of the G20 are Argentina, Australia, Brazil, China, India, Indonesia, Mexico, Saudi Arabia, South Korea, and Turkey. The European Union is also a member of both the G8 and the G20. The IMF and the World Bank also participate in G20 meetings on an ex-officio basis.

References

Commission for Africa (2005). 'Our Common Interest'. Report of the Commission for Africa, London. <www.commissionforafrica.org/english/report/thereport/english/11-03-05_cr_report.pdf> (September 2006).

English, John, Ramesh Thakur, and Andrew F. Cooper (2005). *Reforming from the Top: A Leaders' 20 Summit* (Tokyo: United Nations University).

Lomborg, Bjørn, ed. (2004). *Global Crises, Global Solutions* (Cambridge: Cambridge University Press).

Chapter 7

Can the World Trade Organization Help Achieve the Health Millennium Development Goals?

Chantal Blouin

More than half a million women die every year in pregnancy or childbirth. A woman in Africa faces odds of 1 in 16 of dying in childbirth during her lifetime; in industrialised countries, the odds are only 1 out of 2800. The target of the fifth Millennium Development Goal (MDG) is to reduce the level of maternal mortality by three quarters by 2015. As of 2005, very few countries were on track to reach this target. In many poor countries, high levels of mortality are stable or even worsening. The United Nations Millennium Project recommends a number interventions to achieve this goal, including skilled attendants at birth, clean delivery and postpartum care, emergency obstetric care, antenatal care, and safe abortion services (United Nations Millennium Project 2005). The first element of this list — skilled attendants at birth (nurses, midwives, or physicians) — is key to ensure safe delivery. However, a majority of African women do not receive such services and in Asia only 60 percent of deliveries are attended by a skilled health worker (see Figure 7-1).

Can trade in health services and the trade negotiations at the World Trade Organization (WTO) improve access to health services, including access to skilled birth attendants in developing countries? Under the WTO's General Agreement on Trade in Services (GATS), countries can open their health sectors to foreign providers. The GATS sets out four basic categories of trade in health-related services. With the growth of information and communication technologies, the cross-border supply (mode 1) of health services is made increasingly feasible and convenient. For instance, telemedicine services such as diagnostic or advisory services can be offered using communications networks without the physical movement of either the patient or the provider. Currently some of the principal areas of application are e-education in health, databases of medical literature, and health information websites for physicians and the general public. However, the electronic supply of health-related services is only beginning in developing countries, beyond medical transcription, medical insurance, claim processing, and back-office services, which are becoming an increasingly large export industry in India and the Philippines.

The second form of supply (mode 2) is through the physical movement of the consumers of the service to the country of the supplier. Mode 2 includes consumers who travel abroad to receive medical care, tourists who need medical care incidentally while abroad, retirees abroad, temporary workers, cross-border commuters who may have multinational insurance coverage options, and residents of multinational areas with integrated health systems. Important here are consumers who travel to developing countries expressly to receive care. Such 'health tourism' is estimated to represent roughly 1.3 percent of total travel expenditures, amounting to approximately US$6.5 billion annually (Karsenty 2002).

Trade in health services in developing countries can also take the form of inflows of foreign investment in the establishment of a commercial presence (mode 3). Such investments can be made in hospital and management services, or in health insurance. There is still limited information on the volume of investment in this sector. Evidence shows that the level of foreign participation is relatively low, but it can be found in an increasing number of countries. In Thailand, 24 of the 302 private hospitals have received some foreign investment; the investors usually come from Japan, Singapore, China, and Europe (Buddhasri, Saithanu, and Tangcharoensathien 2003).

Finally, exports of health services can also take place through the temporary movement of health professionals (mode 4) such as physicians and nurses. The United Kingdom, the United States, Australia, Canada, Norway, and Middle Eastern countries are the main recipients. The Philippines, Bangladesh, and India are important 'exporters' of health professionals. In the Philippines, one indicator of the scale of the movement of nurses is the large number of nurses who graduate but do not register with the national professional association. More than 30 000 nurses who graduated in 2000 did not register (Lethridge 2004). A large part of the cross-border movement of health professionals consists of permanent, not temporary, migration that is not included in trade in health services. Nevertheless, there are concerns that the growth of trade through mode 4 may exacerbate current outflows of health professionals in developing countries with shortages.

Figure 7-1 Proportion of Births Attended by Skilled Health Personnel, 2005

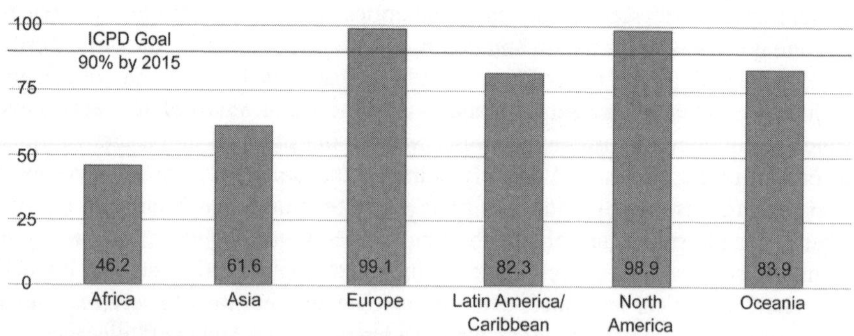

ICPD = International Conference on Population and Development

Source: *WHO (2005)*

This chapter focusses on two modes of supply of health services: health tourism and foreign investment in the health sector. It reviews existing and recent evidence on these two forms of international trade in health services and examines whether they could make a positive contribution to the achievement of MDG No. 5 by improving women's access to health services. The chapter also presents research undertaken in 2003–04 under the aegis of the World Health Organization (WHO) to document the extent and the impact of trade in health services in developing countries (see Blouin, Drager, and Smith 2005). Country studies were conducted in Argentina, Chile, China, Indonesia, Senegal, South Africa, and Thailand. Each case study was conducted by a national researcher, using a questionnaire developed by the research team. The case studies were aimed first at describing the level of international trade and foreign investment in these countries and second at examining the impact of such international transactions.

Can the Revenues from Health Tourism Improve Access to Services for Maternal Health?

Health tourism can be an important source of foreign currency for developing countries. It can provide employment and income for health workers as well as for workers in tourism sectors, as the people travelling to receive health services may also consume other services (such as hotel, transportation, and restaurants). These incomes can contribute to economic growth and poverty reduction. For example, it is estimated that health tourism could bring an additional US$2.2 billion in annual revenue to India by 2012 ('Medical Tourism in India: Get Well Away' 2004). Poverty is a key social determinant of health; if economic growth is shared equally, it can have a significant impact on poverty reduction. The additional incomes from this type of trade can also have a more direct impact on health, if they can be harnessed to benefit the health system of the country in general and the poor in particular. For instance, they can be taxed and allocated to improve the supply and quality of health services in the public sector. Indeed, financing health systems remains an important problem both in terms of the level of resources available for health care and in terms of the equity of financing arrangements.

India is a country where health tourism is growing and where additional revenues could be harnessed to improve the availability of health services, especially for maternal health. Levels of public health expenditures remain relatively low, at 3 percent of government spending, and health financing arrangements are inequitable. Indeed, a large proportion of health expenditures is made through out-of-pocket payments by patients — the most inequitable mechanism of financing (WHO 2003, 172). In 2001, private expenditures represented 82 percent of the spending on health in India and out-of-pocket payments represented 100 percent of these costs (173). Out-of-pocket payments for health services are a key factor contributing to impoverishment or dragging poor households further down into poverty (Wagstaff, Watanabe, and van Doorslaer 2001). Inequity in access to services is an obstacle to the achievement of the right to health in India. Typically, the poorest citizens have less access to services than higher income groups and patients in urban areas have much better access to services than in rural areas. For the poorest women in rural India, only 11.5 percent of deliveries are attended by a physician, a nurse, or a midwife, whereas in the richest rural quintiles of the population, almost 70 percent of the deliveries are (Gwatkin *et al.* 2005). In the urban areas, the figures stand at 26.5 percent for the poorest quintile and 81.3 percent for the richest.

A review of the literature and the case studies undertaken in this research have not documented cases where specific redistribution measures were adopted to ensure that health tourism contributed to the achievement of the health MDGs. On the contrary, some have expressed concern that the growth of large specialised hospitals that cater to foreign patients will refocus the area of specialisation of medical staff away from the local needs. Diseases such as malaria and cholera, which are major health threats for the poor in India, could be overlooked. The specialisation of the hospital itself can become an access barrier to the poor.

The growth of health tourism raises concerns regarding its impact on the health system of the recipient countries. One concern is that it can lead to a dual market structure within the healthcare system with one high-quality, expensive segment catering to wealthy nationals and foreigners and a low-quality segment with limited resources offering services to the rest of the population (Chanda 2001). For instance, the growth of health tourism in Singapore may exacerbate the existing disparity in the distribution of medical personnel and expertise between the public and the private sectors. About 48 percent of the physicians work in the public sector and admit 79 percent of all in-patients, whereas the private sector, with more physicians, admits almost four times fewer in-patients (Health Services Working Group 2003, 8). One recommendation of Singapore's expert group to remedy the problems linked to the dual structure is to facilitate the use of the private hospitals by nationals by making the government's healthcare subsidy portable, to be used in the hospital of the patient's choice.

The most pressing concern regarding the impact of health tourism on the achievement of the right to health regards the physical availability of health services given the risks of internal brain drain. Physicians and nurses from the public sector, or offering services in rural areas, move to the urban facilities offering care to foreign patients. The case of Thailand shows such a problem. The resources to service one foreign patient may be equivalent to those used to service four or five Thai patients. Thus the workload is equivalent to 3 to 4 million Thai patients. This was equivalent to approximately 3 percent of the total workload of the systems in 2001. If the growth continues at the current rate, the workload for servicing foreign patients may increase up to 12 percent of the total workload in five years. This will require an additional 3000 full-time equivalent doctors for urban private hospitals, further exacerbating the shortage of health professionals in the rural areas (Pachanee and Wibulpolprasert 2003).

In Singapore, there are also concerns that the push for making the country the regional medical hub may lead to physician shortages. Various expert groups have projected that there could be a shortage based on domestic needs alone (Health Services Working Group 2003). In addition, rapid growth of health tourism may create human resource allocation problems for the public healthcare system. Indeed, 'a booming private sector may recruit trained specialists too aggressively from the public sector and further drive up public healthcare expenditures as the public sector strives to match private sector salaries, to retain these specialists. This would put pressure on the policy objective to contain the Government's healthcare expenditure at 1% of GDP [gross domestic product]' (8). It was proposed that allowing physicians to work part time in the private sector may reduce the incentive for these professionals to leave the public sector.

In summary, there is little evidence on whether and how the additional incomes and resources from health tourism have been leveraged to improve national health system and achieve the right to health. The next section considers the difficulties of reallocating public expenditures toward the poorer patients. Moreover, there is evidence that providing health services to foreign patients strains the availability of healthcare personnel and can become a real obstacle to access to health services, especially for citizens living in rural areas. Therefore, it is hard to see how health tourism could make a positive contribution to the reduction of maternal mortality.

Can Foreign Investment Improve Maternal Health?

The inflow of foreign capital in health services provides additional resources to invest in the healthcare infrastructures and services of the country. This could mean better access to health services for the local population, including access to the services of a physician, nurse, or midwife during pregnancy (prenatal care), during delivery, and after delivery. The most direct beneficiaries of liberalisation are the households that can afford the services offered by foreign suppliers. These may be new services that were not previously offered by the domestic providers. For instance, liberalisation in the provision of health services in Chile led to the rapid growth of the supply of new high-technology services (León 2003). However, the new services may have no impact on the availability and accessibility of health services and facilities for the majority of the population, especially for low-income groups.

The Chinese experience with foreign investment in joint venture establishments also highlighted the benefits of contributing new approaches to health management and services, advanced medical technology, and good hospital environment. The country study showed that joint-venture hospitals brought competition pressures on the public hospitals (Shi Guang 2003). Even though such establishments mainly target foreigners working in China or other high-income groups, a few also provide essential healthcare services to the community. They provide basic health services to the population and have their own strategies to attract patients. They set service charges according to the market environment, taking into account the level of user fees charged by the public hospitals. Preliminary research found that public hospitals learned from the Sino-foreign joint-venture hospitals and that the quality and management of health services have improved through imitation and learning. However, the evidence from foreign-owned hospitals in China suggests that the great majority of foreign hospitals are established in urban coastal areas and not in the rural areas where the additional resources are most needed (Shi Guang 2003). The survey revealed an unbalanced distribution of the Sino-foreign health facilities in China: 78.3 percent of the Sino-foreign health facilities are located in large cities in the costal areas rather than the central and western provinces.

The key obstacle for foreign investment to make an important contribution to improving maternal health and access to health services more generally is the problem of economic accessibility. It is very likely that only patients with private or social insurance or high-income patients able to disburse a large out-of-pocket payment can gain access to the sophisticated, high-quality services offered by foreign-owned establishments. The case studies do not provide much evidence on the impact of opening the health sectors to foreign investors and providers on the economic accessibility of health services. However, there is a large literature on the impact of allowing private providers into the health sector. The literature on health financing, more specifically the well-developed literature on user fees, provides evidence on the impact of such out-of-pocket cost-recovery mechanisms on access to services.

Most of the studies are based on African examples, as most sub-Saharan African countries have introduced user fees in the health sector in order to raise revenues for the public sector. One of the early measures attempting to do so was the Bamako Initiative. It began in 1987 with support from UNICEF and the WHO as an effort to finance the expansion of access to primary care in Africa using revenues from newly introduced user charges for essential drugs. The presumption was that decentralising management and allowing for local control of locally generated revenues would provide a way to address the persistent problem of insufficient drug supplies from government sources. In some instances, it appears that the approach was successful in raising revenues and improving access and quality of care.[2]

However, in virtually all cases where user fees were increased or introduced, there has been a concurrent decrease in service utilisation. The magnitude of this drop was frequently larger, and was the effect of a longer duration, among the poor part of the population (Bennett and Gilson 2001, 11). Numerous case studies and comparative studies document this impact; in some cases the reduction in utilisation reached 50 percent (Creese 1991; Yoder 1989; McPake, Hanson, and Mills 1993; Moses *et al.* 1992; Mwabu, Mwanzia, and Liambila 1995; Haddad and Fournier 1995; Gertler and Hammer 1997; Kipp *et al.* 2001; Meuwissen 2002; Nanda 2002; Paphassarang *et al.* 2002; Ridde 2003). The impact of user fees on the utilisation of services has translated into negative health outcomes. In China, the introduction of user fees for preventive services such as immunisation and the treatment of infectious diseases led to less immunisation and higher prevalence rates for diseases such as measles and polio (Xingzhu Lui and Mills 2002).

In principle, such inequitable outcomes could be addressed by regulatory measures. However, the measures used to address this problem have proven to be difficult to implement. The literature on the introduction of user fees shows that in most cases exemptions from fees were available to the poor but the implementation of these exemptions was ineffective (Gilson 1997; Gilson *et al.* 2001; Gilson and Mills 1995; Mills 1998; Meuwissen 2002). Nevertheless, experiences in Cambodia with an earmarked fund entrusted to an independent third party show that institutional solutions can be found to the problem of access for the poor caused by cost recovery (Hardeman *et al.* 2004).

Trade in health services can also take the form of foreign investment in health insurance. Expansion of private health insurance through foreign investment offers a way to decrease the heavy reliance on out-of-pocket payment, which is the most inequitable way to finance access to services (WHO 2000). Health insurance not only shelters people from large out-of-pocket payments, but also allows for pooling, that is, spreading financial risks among the group of participants. However, it seems unlikely that the expansion of private foreign insurance will have a large-scale positive impact on improving access to services. According to the World Bank (2002, 8), 'because of cost and the pronounced market failure that occurs in private health insurance, this is not a viable option for risk pooling at the national level in low- and middle-income countries'. The evidence from Latin America shows that private insurers, be they foreign or domestic, tend to serve the higher-income and low-risk groups that can pay relatively high financial contributions to receive coverage (Baeza and Cabezas 1999; Barrientos and Lloyd-Sherlock 2000). In Chile, elderly people and women of fertile age were facing much higher premiums (Sanhueza and Ruiz-Tagle 2002). This type of age and gender discrimination based on risk level is inherent in the private insurance schemes; therefore, private foreign insurers are very unlikely to contribute to the improvement of maternal health. One way to address this discrimination is to introduce regulations to limit such behaviour by insurers. However, the creation of a strong regulatory framework is a challenge even for middle-income countries such as Argentina (see Salvador and Quiliconi 2003).

If research established that foreign investment will not make a direct contribution to improve access to health services, can it make an indirect contribution through the reallocation of resources? The inflow of foreign capital in certain parts of the health system may also reduce the burden on government resources and allow the public sector to reallocate its resources toward patients with less ability to pay. For instance, when higher income individuals receive care from a foreign-owned private hospital, the public sector does not have to provide services to them; similarly, if these individuals buy their health insurance from a foreign insurance company, the state would not have to cover the health expenses accrued by these individuals. Thus resources would be freed up and could be used for poor patients.

The need to infuse new capital in the health systems of developing countries is not disputed. To achieve MDG No. 5 and other health-related MDGs, there is a need for massive investment in health in developing countries. The WHO's Commission on Macroeconomics and Health (2001) provides estimates of how much is needed to scale up resources for health in order to achieve the MDGs. For least developed countries (LDCs), the current annual level of spending of US$11 per person must reach US$34 per person (see Table 7-1).[3] Of that US$34, US$19 will need to come from donor assistance, given the limited capacity to raise additional domestic financial resources.

For all low-income countries, external funding is required to achieve this level of financing, as mobilisation of domestic resources alone cannot deliver sufficient means. However, the current level of aid, even after being raised, is still very far from meeting the targets. The level of assistance for health is currently at US$6 billion. It should be raised to US$22 billion now and to US$31 billion in 2015 to finance the interventions that would help to achieve the health MDGs. There are — and will continue to be — mobilisations and global campaigns to persuade donors to increase the level of funding. Even with the involvement of private philanthropy, the level of commitments required from donor countries is inadequate. In these circumstances, the contribution that can be made by private capital must be seriously considered. There are two key obstacles for foreign capital to contribute to the achievement of the health MDGs and the reduction of maternal mortality. The first relates to the unattractiveness of low-income countries for foreign investors in general. The second focusses on the political economy of redistribution of public expenditures in developing countries.

First, there is a contradictory situation in which the countries in most need of additional capital and resources are the least likely to receive it. Low-income countries are generally the last recipients of foreign direct investment (FDI) among

Table 7-1 Domestic Spending and Donor Assistance on Health, 1997–1999

	Public Spending on Health (per person 1997 US$)	Total Spending on Health (per person 1997 US$)	Donor Assistance for Health (per person average annual 1997–99)	Donor Assistance for Health, Annual Average (US$ millions 1997–99)
Least developed countries	6	11	2.29	1473
Other low-income countries	13	20	0.94	1666
Lower middle-income developing countries	51	93	0.61	1300
Upper middle-income developing countries	125	241	1.08	610
High-income countries	1356	1907	0.00	2
All countries			0.75	5.052

Source: Commission on Macroeconomics and Health (2001, 56).

developing countries. Most of the capital goes to large or emerging markets that offer the foreign investor better infrastructure, stability, qualified personnel, and large domestic markets (Schmidt and Culpeper 2003; United Nations Conference on Trade and Development [UNCTAD] 1998). Moreover, when low-income countries receive FDI, it is usually in the primary sector, not in manufacturing or services. For instance, only three African LDCs (Equatorial Guinea, Angola, and Sudan) have received more than US$1 billion of FDI in 2003, and those investments focussed on petroleum exploration and extraction (UNCTAD 2004).

If low-income countries are unlikely to receive FDI in health services, middle-income countries are more likely to do so. FDI in services has been growing in the last years and tends to go to large and middle-income countries. The developing countries with the largest stock of FDI in services are Hong Kong, China, Taiwan, Thailand, Korea, Colombia, Peru, Argentina, Venezuela, and the Philippines (more than US$5 million) (UNCTAD 2004, 304–305). For now, most of this investment goes to sectors such as financial services, business services, or telecommunications, but one could expect investment in health sector to grow.

To seek such foreign investment for the health sector, a national government would need a clear strategy to reallocate public funding for services to the poor, in order to ensure that such policy contributes to reduced maternal mortality and improved access to health services more generally. Are expectations for such a reallocation of resources in developing countries realistic? Poor people generally tend to be underserved by publicly funded health services. The distribution of public health expenditures in many developing countries is skewed toward the richer groups, not the poor. 'Poor citizens have little clout with politicians' (World Bank 2004, 6). For instance, in Ghana in 1994, the poorest fifth of the population received 12 percent of public spending on health, whereas the richest fifth received 33 percent. In India in 1995–96, the poorest fifth of the population received 10 percent of public spending on health whereas the richest fifth received 32 percent (Filmer 2003). Foreign investment in health services can be expected to contribute to the health MDGs only in countries where poor citizens are in a position to hold policy makers accountable for public services in health or in countries where policy makers have already shown that the health of poor people is their priority.

Conclusions and Recommendations

This chapter raises many doubts about the capacity of trade in health services to contribute to the achievement of the health MDGs in general and the reduction of maternal mortality in particular. Health tourism seems especially problematic, given the impact it has on human resource for health. As it increases the load of patients in developing countries, it drains physicians and nurses away from the local population, especially rural patients. Hence, large growth in health tourism can lead to reduced access to health services. Therefore, national governments in developing countries should fully assess the impact of health tourism before promoting and supporting it as a key export sector. If such an assessment reveals that health tourism will worsen health personnel shortages and therefore its promotion appears incoherent with the achievement of the MDGs, national authorities should revise their strategy.

The capacity of government in developing countries to harness foreign investment in health to benefit all people is generally weak. It is very unlikely that foreign investors opening clinics or hospitals, or offering health insurance, will be improving access to health services for poor people. Very strong regulatory capacity is needed to do so. Foreign investment could benefit poor people indirectly if it would trigger a reallocation of public expenditure for health toward poor people. Such redistributive policy would run against the existing trends in funding allocation for public services, but it remains a possibility. What could be done nationally and globally to increase the chance that this scenario actually take place? Increasing policy makers' accountability to poor people, including improving the information on how money is spent, would stress the role of national and global civil society's engagement. Using human rights obligations to defend the right to health in domestic courts is one example of the strategies that have been used by some groups to hold governments accountable. At the global level, international organisations such as the WHO and the World Bank can play an advisory role to strengthen the capacity of national government to adopt such reallocative policies. For national governments in developing countries, the key message is that their main strategy to finance the achievement of MDG No. 5 and to improve access to heath services should be raising public expenditures for health or, in the case of low-income countries, increasing donor assistance for health. Foreign capital will, at best, play a complementary role, and only if clear and strong measures are adopted to ensure reallocation.

Notes

1 However, in the GATS, these health education and health data processing and storage services are classified under education and computer-related services, rather than as health services (Blouin *et al.* 2005).

2 On Mauritania see Martine Audibert and Jacky Mathonnat (2000); on Niger see François Diop, Abdo Yazbeck, and Ricardo Bitran (1995), Annemarie Wouters (1995), and Mukesh Chawla and Randall Ellis (2000); on Ecuador see John Bratt *et al.* (2002) and Santosh Mehrotra and Stephen Jarett (2002).

3 Of the annual expenditure of US$11 per person for LDCs, US$2.29 is donor assistance, US$3.71 is from government, and the rest is out of pocket.

References

Audibert, Martine and Jacky Mathonnat (2000). 'Cost Recovery in Mauritania: Initial Lessons'. *Health Policy and Planning,* vol. 15, no. 1, pp. 66–75. <heapol.oxfordjournals.org/cgi/reprint/15/1/66?ck=nck> (September 2006).

Baeza, Christian and Marcela Cabezas (1999). 'Es necesario el ajuste de riesgo el los mercados de seguros de salud en América Latina?' [Is Risk Adjustment Necessary in Health Insurance Markets in Latin America?]. Centro Latinoamericano de Investigación para Sistemas de Salud, Santiago, Chile.

Barrientos, Armando and Peter Lloyd-Sherlock (2000). 'Reforming Health Insurance in Argentina and Chile'. *Health Policy and Planning,* vol. 15, no. 4, pp. 417–423.

Bennett, Sara and Lucy Gilson (2001). 'Health Financing: Designing and Implementing Pro-Poor Policies'. DfID Health Systems Resource Centre, London. <www.dfidhealthrc.org/shared/publications/Issues_papers/Health_financing_pro-poor.pdf> (September 2006).

Blouin, Chantal, Nick Drager, and Richard Smith, eds. (2005). *International Trade in Health Services and the GATS: Current Issues and Debates* (Washington DC: World Bank and World Health Organization).

Blouin, Chantal, Jens Gobrecht, J. Lethridge, *et al.* (2005). 'Trade in Health Services under the Four Modes of Supply: Review of the Current Trends and Policy Issues'. In C. Blouin, N. Drager, and R. Smith, eds., *International Trade in Health Services and the GATS: Current Issues and Debates* (Washington DC: World Bank and World Health Organization).

Bratt, John, Mark Weaver, James Foreit, *et al.* (2002). 'The Impact of Price Changes on Demand for Family Planning and Reproductive Health Services in Ecuador'. *Health Policy and Planning*, vol. 17, no. 3, pp. 281–287.

Buddhasri, W., S. Saithanu, and V. Tangcharoensathien (2003). 'Private Hospital Industry in Thailand after the Economic Crisis, 1996–2001'. International Health Policy Programme, Nanthaburi, Thailand.

Chanda, Rupa (2001). 'Trade in Health Services'. Commission on Macroeconomics and Health Working Paper WG4:5, World Health Organization, Geneva.

Chawla, Mukesh and Randall P. Ellis (2000). 'The Impact of Financing and Quality Changes on Health Care Demand in Niger'. *Health Policy and Planning,* vol. 15, no. 1, pp. 76–84.

Commission on Macroeconomics and Health (2001). 'Macroeconomics and Health: Investing in Health for Economic Development'. World Health Organization, Geneva. <www.cid.harvard.edu/cidcmh/CMHReport.pdf> (September 2006).

Creese, Andrew (1991). 'User Charges for Health Care: A Review of Recent Experience'. *Health Policy and Planning,* vol. 6, no. 4, pp. 309–319.

Diop, François, Abdo Yazbeck, and Ricardo Bitran (1995). 'The Impact of Alternative Cost Recovery Schemes on Access and Equity in Niger'. *Health Policy and Planning,* vol. 10, no. 3, pp. 223–240.

Filmer, Deon (2003). 'The Incidence of Public Expenditures on Health and Education'. Background note for the World Development Report 2004: Making Services Work for Poor People, World Bank, Washington DC.

Gertler, Paul J. and Jeffrey S. Hammer (1997). 'Strategies for Pricing Publicly Provided Health Services'. World Bank Policy Research Working Paper No. 1762. <ssrn.com/abstract=615024> (September 2006).

Gilson, Lucy (1997). 'The Lessons of User Fee Experience in Africa'. *Health Policy and Planning,* vol. 12, no. 4, pp. 273–285.

Gilson, Lucy and Anne Mills (1995). 'Health Sector Reforms in Sub-Saharan Africa'. *Health Policy,* vol. 32, no. 1, pp. 215–243.

Gilson, Lucy, Denny Kalyalya, Felix Kuchler, *et al.* (2001). 'Strategies for Promoting Equity: Experience with Community Financing in Three African Countries'. *Health Policy,* vol. 58, no. 1, pp. 37–67.

Gwatkin, Davidson, Shea Rutstein, Kiersten Johnson, *et al.* (2005). *Socioeconomic Differences in Health, Nutrition, and Population*, 2nd ed. (Washington DC: World Bank).

Haddad, Slim and Pierre Fournier (1995). 'Quality, Cost, and Utilization of Health Services in Developing Countries: A Longitudinal Study in Zaire'. *Social Science and Medicine,* vol. 40, no. 6, pp. 743–753.

Hardeman, Wim, Wim Van Damme, Maurits Van Pelt, *et al.* (2004). 'Access to Health Care for All? User Fees plus a Health Equity Fund in Sotnikum, Cambodia'. *Health Policy and Planning,* vol. 19, no. 1, pp. 22–32.

Health Services Working Group (2003). 'Developing Singapore as the Compelling Hub for Healthcare Services in Asia: Potential Implications on Domestic Policy Objectives'. Ministry of Trade and Industry, Singapore. <app.mti.gov.sg/data/pages/507/doc/ERC_SVS_HEA_Annex2.pdf> (September 2006).

Karsenty, Guy (2002). 'Trends in International Trade in Services'. Assessment of GATS and Trade in Health Services: An International Consultation on Monitoring and Research Priorities. World Health Organization, Geneva.

Kipp, Walter, Jimmy Kamugisha, Phil Jacobs, *et al.* (2001). 'User Fees, Health Staff Incentives, and Service Utilization in Kabarole District, Uganda'. *Bulletin of the World Health Organization,* vol. 79, no. 11, pp. 1032–1037.

León, Francisco (2003). 'The Case of the Chilean Health System, 1983–2003'. Paper presented at the World Health Organization Workshop on Trade in Health Services, Ottawa.

Lethridge, J. (2004). 'Trade in Health Services under the Four Modes of Supply: Review of Current Trends and Policy Issues'. World Health Organization, Geneva.

McPake, Barbara, Kara Hanson, and Anne Mills (1993). 'Community Financing of Health Care in Africa: An Evaluation of the Bamako Initiative'. *Social Science and Medicine,* vol. 36, no. 11, pp. 1383–1395.

'Medical Tourism in India: Get Well Away' (2004). *Economist*, 7 October.

Mehrotra, Santosh and Stephen Jarett (2002). 'Improving Basic Health Service Delivery in Low-Income Countries: "Voice" to the Poor'. *Social Science and Medicine,* vol. 54, no. 11, pp. 1685–1690.

Meuwissen, Liesbeth Emm (2002). 'Problems of Cost Recovery Implementation in District Health Care: A Case Study from Niger'. *Health Policy and Planning,* vol. 17, no. 3, pp. 304–313.

Mills, Anne (1998). 'To Contract or Not to Contract? Issues for Low and Middle Income Countries'. *Health Policy and Planning,* vol. 13, no. 1, pp. 32–40.

Moses, Stephen, F. Manji, J.E. Bradley, *et al.* (1992). 'Impact of User Fees on Attendance at a Referral Centre for Sexually Transmitted Diseases in Kenya'. *Lancet*, vol. 340, no. 8817, pp. 463–466.

Mwabu, Germano, James Mwanzia, and Wilson Liambila (1995). 'User Charges in Government Health Facilities in Kenya: Effect on Attendance and Revenue'. *Health Policy and Planning,* vol. 10, no. 2, pp. 164–170.

Nanda, Priya (2002). 'Gender Dimensions of User Fees: Implications for Women's Utilization of Health Care'. *Reproductive Health Matters,* vol. 10, no. 20, pp. 127–134.

Pachanee, Cha-aim and Suwit Wibulpolprasert (2003). 'Trade in Health Services and GATS: The Case of Thailand'. Paper presented at the World Health Organization Workshop on Trade in Health Services, Ottawa.

Paphassarang, Chanthakath, Khampienne Philavong, Boungnong Boupha, *et al.* (2002). 'Equity, Privatization, and Cost Recovery in Urban Health Care: The Care of Lao PDR'. *Health Policy and Planning,* vol. 17 (Suppl. 1), pp. 72–84.

Ridde, Valéry (2003). 'Fees for Services, Cost Recovery, and Equity in a District of Burkina Faso Operating the Bamako Initiative'. *Bulletin of the World Health Organization,* vol. 81, no. 7, pp. 532–538.

Salvador, Soledad and Cintia Quiliconi (2003). 'Argentina Trade in Health Services and GATS: The Argintinean Case Study'. Paper presented at the World Health Organization Workshop on Trade in Health Services, Ottawa.

Sanhuenza, Ricardo and Jaime Ruiz-Tagle (2002). 'Choosing Health Insurance in a Dual Health Care System: The Chilean Case'. *Journal of Applied Economics*, vol. 5 (May), pp. 157–184.

Schmidt, Rodney and Roy Culpeper (2003). 'Private Foreign Investment in the Poorest Countries'. North-South Institute, Ottawa. <www.nsi-ins.ca/english/pdf/FDI_policy_brief.pdf> (September 2006).

Shi Guang (2003). 'Trade in Health Services and GATS in China: Preliminary Observation and Analysis'. Paper presented at the World Health Organization Workshop on Trade in Health Services, Ottawa.

United Nations Conference on Trade and Development (1998). 'World Investment Report 1998: Trends and Determinants'. United Nations Conference on Trade and Development, Geneva.

United Nations Conference on Trade and Development (2004). 'World Investment Report 2004: The Shift Toward Services'. United Nations Conference on Trade and Development, Geneva. <www.unctad.org/en/docs/wir2004_en.pdf> (September 2006).

United Nations Millennium Project (2005). *Preparing National Strategies to Achieve the Millennium Development Goals: A Handbook* (New York: United Nations Development Programme).

Wagstaff, Adam, Naoko Watanabe, and Eddy van Doorslaer (2001). 'Impoverishment, Insurance, and Health Care Payments'. Health, Nutrition, and Population Network, World Bank, Washington DC.

World Bank (2002). 'Health, Nutrition, and Population Sector Strategy Paper'. World Bank, Washington DC. <www.worldbank.org/html/extdr/hnp/sector_strategy/download.htm> (September 2006).

World Bank (2004). *World Development Report 2004: Making Services Work for Poor People* (Washington DC: World Bank and Oxford University Press).

World Health Organization (2000). 'World Health Report 2000 — Health Systems: Improving Performance'. World Health Organization, Geneva.

World Health Organization (2003). 'World Health Report 2003: Shaping the Future'. World Health Organization, Geneva. <www.who.int/whr/2003/en> (September 2006).

World Health Organization (2005). 'Skilled Attendant at Birth 2005 Estimates'. Geneva. <www.who.int/reproductive-health/global_monitoring/skilled_attendant_at_birth2005_estimates.pdf> (September 2006).

Wouters, Annemarie (1995). 'Improving Quality Through Cost Recovery in Niger'. *Health Policy and Planning,* vol. 10, no. 3, pp. 257–270.

Xingzhu Lui and Anne Mills (2002). 'Financing Reforms of Public Health Services in China: Lessons for Other Nations'. *Social Science and Medicine,* vol. 54, no. 11, pp. 1691–1698.

Yoder, Richard (1989). 'Are People Willing and Able to Pay for Health Services?' *Social Science and Medicine,* vol. 29, no. 1, pp. 35–42.

Chapter 8

Partnerships for Health, the Environment, and Governance

Lee-Nah Hsu and Jessica White

In September 2000, at the United Nations Millennium Summit, leaders from 189 countries jointly committed to reduce poverty and improve lives by adopting the Millennium Development Goals (MDGs) based on the United Nations Millennium Declaration (see Appendix). Specific targets, set against baselines in 1990, were set for each of the eight goals. The year 2015 was given as the target date for the world to reach the MDGs and, using 1990 as the benchmark, the mid-point milestone was set for 2005.

This chapter advocates that the achievement of the health-related goals — or any single MDG — by the target of 2015 requires a comprehensive effort to address all of the eight goals. Such a holistic and coordinated strategy would create synergies to yield much more than the sum of its parts in solving the problems faced by humanity. For example, health improvements cannot be achieved without certain levels of education or of food security. From this perspective, MDG No. 8, to develop a global partnerships for development, which has tended to be neglected by countries, takes on a crucial importance.

Health and the Millennium Development Goals

In its report 'Health in the Millennium Development Goals', the World Health Organization (WHO) emphasised that poverty and lack of development affect health. To make progress in health, it would be necessary to address these broader challenges (WHO 2005b, ch. 1). The indispensability of a global partnership for development has critical implications for health, and improved health, in turn, facilitates the achievement of the other MDGs.

Overall, the data available as reported by developing countries on the 2005 milestone for the MDGs showed progress toward achieving some goals, but showed no change or even deterioration in other goals. This information suggests that if trends observed during the 1990s continue, the majority of poor countries will not meet their MDGs by 2015 (WHO 2005b, 13). Part of the reason the anticipated halfway targets are not being reached relates to the sectoral approach to the MDGs in isolation of one another. MDG No. 8 is the one that is least addressed by many countries in their reporting. It is the goal that fell singularly short of all of its targets in all regions in 2005.

MDG No. 8 promotes North-South cooperation, as well as multisector, trade, and other partnerships. Political will, broadly informed policies, and sustained efforts are needed to meet all the MDGs. This would require each country to be the driver in implementing its own development strategies that are guided by the latest knowledge and information and transparent, accountable governance. Because developing countries generally do not have the resources required for such an effort, MDG No. 8 sets out the commitments of wealthy countries to cooperate with developing countries that are undertaking economic, political, health, and social reforms (United Nations Development Programme [UNDP] 2003, vi).

At the March 2002 United Nations Conference on Financing for Development in Monterrey, world leaders made the Millennium Development Compact to implement the Millennium Declaration. It aimed at forging a 'new partnership between developed and developing countries' (UN 2002). This compact provides a broad framework for how national development strategies and international support from donors, international agencies, and others can be both better aligned and commensurate with the scale of the challenges of the MDGs. It requires bold reforms from poor countries and urges donor countries to step forward to support these efforts.

Whereas much of the focus has been on the first seven goals, the overall success or failure of efforts to reach the MDGs may hinge on achieving the eighth goal. The targets for MDG No. 8 include a commitment to good governance, development, and poverty reduction — both nationally and internationally. This chapter suggests that good governance principles foster international partnerships and the inclusion of all stakeholders that is needed to advance people's health and well-being. Good governance principles include strategic vision, participation, consensus orientation, responsiveness, accountability, equity, efficiency, effectiveness, transparency, and rule of law (UNDP 2002, 5–6). Table 8-1 describes the good governance principles developed by the United Nations Development Programme (UNDP). This chapter considers examples of good governance in response to HIV and the highly pathogenic avian influenza. Linking the efforts toward achieving MDG No. 8 on developing global partnerships for development to the efforts made on the other MDGs could create the synergy necessary to advance the achievement of the other seven MDGs.

Development, the Environment, and Health

Poverty and hunger (MDG No. 1) and women's educational levels (MDG No. 3) affect maternal health (MDG No. 5) and influence infant mortality (MDG No. 4). More than one in five deaths among children under five years old occur during the first week of life, mostly due to malnutrition of the mother and of the foetus, which leads to low birthweight (WHO 2005b, 16). Nearly 11 million children die each year before reaching the age of five, mostly from preventable causes (Annan 2001, 4). The majority of high child mortality rates are found in developing countries. Child survival is influenced by multiple social factors. Of all the social factors associated with reducing child mortality, maternal education — especially literacy — has been singled out as one of the key factors (Findley *et al.* 1997).

Poverty and hunger prevent children from entering into primary education and cause children who are enrolled to drop out (MDG No. 2) (UN 2005a, 11). School drop-out rates for girls are higher than those for boys and are a manifestation of gender inequality (MDG No. 3).

HIV, malaria, and other diseases are associated with poverty and hunger, gender inequality, and primary school enrolment (MDG No. 6). The UN's Food and Agriculture Organization (FAO) has estimated that in the 27 most affected countries in Africa, 7 million agricultural workers died from AIDS between 1985 and 2000 and 16 million more deaths will likely occur in the next two decades (FAO 2001). In the ten most affected African countries, the agricultural labour force will decline between 11 percent and 26 percent by 2020. The loss of labour from AIDS-related illnesses and deaths reduces the amount of land that can be cultivated, resulting in lower food production and food insecurity (FAO 1997). For instance, a survey in

Table 8-1 Good Governance Principles

Participation
All men and women have a voice in decision making, either directly or through legitimate intermediate institutions that represent their interests. Such broad participation is built on freedom of association and speech, as well as capacities to participate constructively.

Rule of Law
Legal frameworks are fair and enforced impartially, particularly the laws on human rights.

Transparency
Transparency is built on the free flow of information. Processes, institutions, and information are directly accessible to those concerned with them, and enough information is provided to understand and monitor them.

Responsiveness
Institutions and processes try to serve all stakeholders.

Consensus Orientation
Good governance mediates among differing interests to reach a broad consensus on what is in the best interest of the group and, where possible, on policies and procedures.

Equity
All men and women have opportunities to improve or maintain their well-being.

Effectiveness and Efficiency
Processes and institutions produce results that meet needs while making the best use of resources.

Accountability
Decision makers in government, the private sector, and civil society organisations are accountable to the public, as well as to institutional stakeholders. This accountability differs depending on the organisation and whether the decision is internal or external to an organisation.

Strategic Vision
Leaders and the public have a broad and long-term perspective on good governance and human development, along with a sense of what is needed for such development. There is also an understanding of the historical, cultural, and social complexities in which that perspective is grounded.

Source: Adapted from UNDP (1999).

Zimbabwe showed that agricultural output in communal areas had declined by nearly 50 percent among households affected by AIDS (Kwaramba 1997; UN 2005b).

The proportion of women and girls infected by HIV is growing globally. Overall, approximately half of the people living with HIV are females, but in some countries, the number of female infections has surpassed that of males. In some sub-Saharan countries there are three young women living with HIV for every young man (UN 2005a, 25). Pregnant women with HIV are more vulnerable to malaria, resulting in higher perinatal mortality, low birthweight of newborns, and maternal anaemia (WHO 2005b, 22). In addition, many children must drop out of school to care for sick family members, and an increasing number of children are orphaned as a consequence of HIV and AIDS. On average, in sub-Saharan Africa, children who are orphans are 17 percent less likely to attend school than children with at least one parent living (22). Even prior to the death of their parents, these children begin to shoulder the burden of care and support of the remaining members of the households, thus mortgaging their own futures.

The Link between Health and the Environment

Many causes of disease lie outside the purview of healthcare systems. The link between health and environmental sustainability is critical and requires strengthened partnerships between the health and non-health sectors (MDG No. 7).

Approximately 25 percent of the world's burden of disease is attributable to eco-environmental factors (WHO 1997). For example, the emergence and re-emergence of diseases that are particularly lethal and debilitating, such as severe acute respiratory syndrome (SARS), avian influenza, dengue, malaria, and Nipah virus, are linked to human interactions with their ecosystems. These emerging diseases relate to changes in habitat conditions leading, in turn, to changes in vector breeding sites and host reservoir distributions. The invasion of new species or inter-species host transfers, such as between animal and human hosts, also contributes further to emerging diseases such as SARS, avian influenza, and Nipah virus. Changes in biodiversity, such as the reduction of biodiversity due to mono-cropping or loss of predator species and changes in host population densities, further influence the re-emergence of diseases. Human technologies also contribute to genetic modifications of pathogens or disease vectors such as insect resistance to pesticides or the emergence of antibiotic-resistant bacteria (WHO 2005a, 22).

Water-associated infectious diseases claim up to 3.2 million lives each year, amounting to nearly 6 percent of all deaths globally and a loss of 75 million healthy life years (WHO 2005a, 2). More than 900 million people live in absolute poverty in rural areas (UNDP 2003, 123). Their livelihoods and food security depend directly on the goods and services of ecosystems. However, they often lack the access to adequate information on markets and on how to protect the environment that is the source of their livelihoods. Furthermore, much environmental degradation relates to poor governance in environmental management. The failures in environmental management include, for example, deforestation, overgrazing, and over-fishing, which also link to user rights. The situation is often compounded by insufficient information and opportunities for local stakeholders to participate in decision making that affects the use of ecosystem resources and services (127).

Achieving the health-related MDGs requires the generation of knowledge and the design of interventions that situate human health within its broad ecological context. One such approach is the ecosystem approach to human health framework. This trans-disciplinary framework promotes positive action on the environment that improves community well-being and health (Lebel 2003). Participation of multiple stakeholders and the analysis of social and gender equality are both fundamental to the approach. Stakeholder participation allows diverse inputs from experts of different disciplines, women and men from affected communities, and policy makers. In other words, it is an application of good governance principles for health and development. Local, national, regional, and global partnerships, built on models for good governance such as an ecosystem approach to health, could facilitate the achievement of the health and other MDGs.

Current Status in Reaching 2005 Millennium Development Goal Targets

Most of the information used to assess the 2005 milestones of the MDGs comes from national data and international surveys conducted in 2002 and 2003. The UN's 2005 report on the progress on MDGs provides the basis for the summary in this section (UN 2005a). Table 8-2 provides an aggregation, by region, of information for the eight MDGs on improvements, regression, or lack of change between 1990 and 2005. Brief descriptions for the status for each of the eight MDGs in the regional aggregates are listed below. For the purposes of this discussion, countries

Table 8-2 Score Card for the Millennium Development Goals by Region, 2005

	Africa	Asia	Commonwealth of Independent States	Latin America/ Caribbean	Oceania
MDG No. 1	–	+	–	+	0
MDG No. 2	+	+	0	+	+
MDG No. 3	+	+	+	+	+
MDG No. 4	+	+	+/–	+	0
MDG No. 5	H	M	L	M	H
MDG No. 6	0	+	–	+	–
MDG No. 7	0	+	+	+	–
MDG No. 8	0	–	–	–	–

Notes: + = met, on track, or in progress; 0 = no change; – = negative change; H = remains high for maternal mortality and considerable efforts are needed; M= moderate level; L= low level.

Source: Adapted from UN (2005a) with data from the United Nations Statistics Division.

are aggregated into five regions: Africa, Asia, Commonwealth of Independent States (CIS), Latin America/Caribbean, and Oceania.

MDG No. 1: Eradicate extreme poverty and hunger. Extreme poverty remains a daily reality for more than 1 billion people who subsist on less than US$1 per day. More than 800 million people have too little to eat to meet their daily energy needs. However, most of Asia, with the exception of the west, leads the way in reducing poverty. Latin America has slowly reduced its poverty, whereas little has changed in North Africa and western Asia. Although the countries in transition are starting to see their situation improve, in sub-Saharan Africa, with the highest poverty rates in the world, the numbers of poor continue to increase: the extremely poor are getting poorer. Conflicts, diseases, and disasters continued to fuel poverty and hunger.

MDG No. 2: Achieve universal primary education. Countries in all five regions are making progress in primary school enrolment. However, eight of every ten children who are out of school live in sub-Saharan Africa or southern Asia. It should be noted that AIDS is one of the factors contributing to the low education level of children who are not enrolled in schools.

MDG No. 3: Promote gender equality and empower women. Most countries are making progress in increasing girls' school enrolment in primary schools, although gaps still exist in sub-Saharan Africa and in southern and western Asia. Gender disparity continues to be wider at higher levels of education. Furthermore, women still have a far smaller share of paid jobs than men and men continue to dominate decision making at the highest levels in most fields, particularly in politics.

MDG No. 4: Reduce child mortality. Countries in all regions are making progress in reducing child mortality. However, countries with high levels of AIDS in the population are starting to see a reversal of the progress gained and, instead of a reduction, are seeing an increase in mortality for children under five years of age.

MDG No. 5: Improve maternal health. Improvements have been made in reaching this goal. Skilled healthcare personnel attend more deliveries and fewer women die during childbirth. There were, however, no observable improvements on this goal in sub-Saharan Africa.

MDG No. 6: Combat HIV/AIDS, malaria, and other diseases. The prevalence of HIV has increased in all regions. The number of women and girls infected with HIV is rising. The reduced immunity associated with HIV has made people more vulnerable to malaria, tuberculosis, and other infectious diseases.

MDG No. 7: Ensure environmental sustainability. Forests provide valuable ecosystem services, including the production of food, fuel, and building materials, as well as water filtration and climate regulation. However, the amount of the world's forested areas is decreasing rapidly. Many of the forested areas have been reduced due to logging and clearing the land to make way for large-scale plantations or for small farms. Biological diversity is declining and marine ecosystems and coastal marsh habitats are disappearing rapidly. Access to safe drinking water has improved in all regions of the world, but the world is facing the threat of reduced freshwater reserves. Population movements are unprecedented compared to previous decades. Ever more people move from rural to urban areas. The expansion of urban and industrial development has reduced the amount of prime agricultural land available for production.

MDG No. 8: Develop a global partnership for development. Trade, youth employment, pharmaceuticals, agricultural development, and information and communication technologies are some of the many sectors that could facilitate health and sustainable ecosystem management for development. In order to ensure the sustainability of ecosystems while advancing technologies that can improve human security, it is necessary to strengthen trans-disciplinary collaboration in responding to the challenges of reaching the MDGs.

Overall, each region has shown some progress in some of the MDGs at the aggregate level. Yet, despite the fact that global partnership is an essential component for achieving the rest of the MDGs, the eighth goal is the only one where no progress was observable in all the regions of the world. Increased attention to enhance global partnership is necessary if all the MDGs are to be reached by 2015.

Applying Good Governance Principles for Health and the Millennium Development Goals

What additional efforts could be made to support countries in achieving the MDGs by 2015? Development is an inter-sectoral and interdependent process. The eight MDGs are synergistic, and no single goal can be achieved without improvements in the others. The achievements of the health-related MDGs are determined by political, social, and economic factors (WHO 2005b, ch. 3). The interdependency among the MDGs reflects the necessary inter-sectoral collaboration as well as participation by diverse stakeholders. The principles of good governance facilitate the participation and collaboration of sectors and stakeholders.

HIV/AIDS and Governance

The 2005 status report by countries reflects the fact that progress on many of the MDGs was set back as HIV and AIDS prevalence continued to rise. This situation is particularly evident in sub-Saharan Africa. HIV is now widely understood to be a development issue closely intertwined with poverty, hunger, maternal and child mortality, gender inequality, and rural-to-urban migration.

Rule of Law and Participation

By applying good governance principles, it is possible to build people's resilience to HIV and AIDS, thus improving the chance of reaching the MDGs. The rule-of-law principle of good governance contains the protection of human rights. For HIV and AIDS, the right of access to antiretroviral treatment (ART) has been a turning point in improving the survival of people living with HIV and AIDS. It has also helped to reduce the maternal to newborn transmission of HIV as well as facilitated the prolongation of maternal life span, which, in turn, improves the survival of children born to HIV-infected mothers.

The participation of people living with HIV and AIDS in research, planning, policy, and programme decisions that affect them has contributed significantly to HIV prevention efforts in communities and to improved care and support services to patients, widows, and orphans.

The Gini index was used as a proxy of equity in a study conducted on HIV and governance in 2003 (Hsu 2004, 7–9). At the time of the 2003 study, global governance indicators were being developed; therefore there was no specific governance index that could be used to correlate global governance to HIV prevalence. The Gini index measures the extent to which the distribution of income (or consumption) among individuals or households within a country deviates from a perfectly equal distribution. Figure 8-1 shows the correlation of the Gini index with that of HIV prevalence. The lower the equity in wealth distribution, the higher the HIV prevalence. However, the Gini index is an imperfect index to estimate governance. Since that study was conducted in 2003, the UNDP, in collaboration with the European Commission, has developed a governance index, which became available in 2005. But due to the newness of this index, there has not been sufficient data collected in countries to provide a global trend. It is hoped that future research will provide country-specific data to allow for better investigations on the correlation between governance and HIV.

Figure 8-1 Correlation between the Gini Index and HIV Prevalence

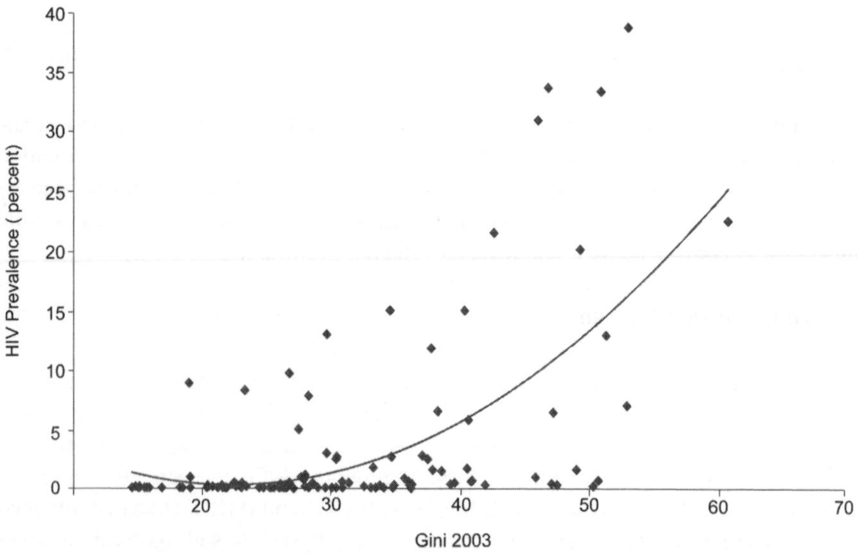

Highly Pathogenic Avian Influenza Preparedness: Responsiveness, Effectiveness, and Efficiency

Global health today is influenced by multiple factors, and effective responses to this new complexity require partnerships that transcend borders, sectors, and disciplines. The emergence of highly pathogenic avian influenza has revealed the influence of behavioural, biological, ecological, economic, and social factors in the re-emergence of pandemics, and has stimulated an unprecedented global partnership in preparing for and implementing timely responses.

The Canadian government hosted an international consultation among ministers of health in Ottawa in October 2005. This was followed a month later in Geneva by a strategic planning consultation coordinated among the WHO, the FAO, and the World Organisation for Animal Health (OIE), with the participation of the World Bank. Following these consultations, countries in Southeast Asia jointly organised a donor pledging consultation hosted by the China in Beijing in January 2006. This international multisectoral collaboration is addressing the links among agricultural practices, animal health, human health and behaviour, economics, and trade. It is a comprehensive effort that will be critical to improving the effectiveness and efficiency of a pandemic preparedness system and policies at community, national, regional, and global levels.

However, in order to be ultimately effective, this partnership must expand to include other regions. With migratory birds moving to the southern hemisphere during the northern winter, the transport of poultry products, and the movement of people, highly pathogenic avian influenza is spreading to the other regions, including the African continent. The combination of avian influenza with multiple diseases that have already devastated the social and economic progress in Africa could have disastrous consequences.

This is where a trans-disciplinary and participatory ecosystem approach to health could make a significant contribution to preventing a health and development crisis. The necessary consideration of social, environmental, economic, cultural, behavioural, and logistic aspects, in addition to the medical dimensions (vaccines, treatment drugs, and so on) would be critical to respond effectively to a potential spread of highly pathogenic avian influenza. From a global perspective, such a collaborative response could build upon and strengthen the effectiveness of the prevention network being developed in Southeast Asia and in other countries and with African countries. The value of a global partnership in this effort is critical to health and development outcomes because it is essential in dealing with the challenges faced in controlling an emerging avian influenza pandemic.

Conclusion

Global health is interdependent with development, environmental sustainability, and medical technological advances. To achieve the MDGs — and global health — it is necessary to have trans-disciplinary collaboration to address the multitude of linkages and make effective use of resources. It is also necessary to have the participation of people affected, the researchers, the policy makers, the business sector, and service providers. Transparency is needed to ensure access to pertinent knowledge and information for those who require it to formulate policy or to determine their practice or daily behaviour. Accountability, equity, and responsiveness are essential in breaking a vicious chain of disease transmissions. These good governance principles, when applied, could facilitate the achievement of MDGs. In turn, improved education and strengthened economies could also facilitate good governance. This reflects the inter-relatedness of the MDGs (UN Millennium Project 2005).

The time is now to promote cross-sectoral policies that address the underlying driving forces for each of the MDGs. There are many uncertainties with the current knowledge base for the impact of today's decisions over the long term. The implications for the potential outcomes of specific policies and programme decisions are multiple. To reduce these uncertainties and ensure sustainable management of ecosystems while advancing human health and development, it is no longer practical to tackle such challenges with a single-sector approach. To achieve the MDG goals, it is necessary to form global partnerships to further trans-disciplinary programmes and policies built upon the participation of multiple stakeholders and engaging multiple sectors for effective and timely action. Responsive strategies and action need to account for specific social and environmental contexts while also ensuring social and gender equality. Together in partnership for good governance, the MDGs could become a reality.

References

Annan, Kofi (2001). 'We the Children: Meeting the Promises of the World Summit for Children'. United Nations, New York. <www.unicef.org/specialsession/about/sg-report.htm> (September 2006).

Findley, Sally, Ahmed Zayan, Maria Kere, *et al.* (1997). 'Stretching the Limits of Health Interventions in Burkina Faso'. *Health Transition Review,* vol. 7, no. 1, pp. 95–107.

Food and Agriculture Organization (1997). 'The Rural Population of Africa Confronted with AIDS: A Challenge to Development'. Summary of FAO Studies on AIDS, Rome.

Food and Agriculture Organization (2001). 'The Impact of HIV/AIDS on Food Security'. Paper prepared for the 27th Session of the Committee on World Food Security, 28 May–1 June, Rome.

Hsu, Lee-Nah (2004). 'Building Dynamic Democratic Governance and HIV-Resilient Societies'. Paper presented at the Oslo Governance Centre, 3 November 2003, United Nations Development Programme.

Kwaramba, P. (1997). 'The Socio-Economic Impact of HIV/AIDS on Communal Agricultural Production Systems in Zimbabwe'. Working Paper 19, Economic Advisory Project, Friedrich Ebert Stiftung Foundation.

Lebel, Jean (2003). *Health: An Ecosystem Approach* (Ottawa: International Development Research Centre).

United Nations (2002). 'Final Outcome of the International Conference on Financing for Development'. A/CONF/198. 1 March. Monterrey. <www.un.org/esa/ffd/0302finalMonterreyConsensus.pdf> (September 2006).

United Nations (2005a). 'The Millennium Development Goals Report 2005'. New York. <millenniumindicators.un.org/unsd/mi/pdf/MDG%20Book.pdf> (September 2006).

United Nations (2005b). 'Population, Development, and HIV/AIDS with Particular Emphasis on Poverty: The Concise Report'. ST/ESA/SER.A/247. <www.un.org/esa/population/publications/concise2005/PopdevHIVAIDS.pdf> (September 2006).

United Nations Development Programme (1999). 'Governance for Sustainable Development'. Policy document, New York.

United Nations Development Programme (2002). 'Introducing Governance into HIV/AIDS Programmes: People's Republic of China, Lao PDR, and Viet Nam'. <www.undp.org/hiv/docs/alldocs/Asia %20-%20Introducing%20Governance%20into%20HIV-AIDS%20Programmes%20(2002).pdf> (September 2006).

United Nations Development Programme (2003). *Human Development Report 2003 Millennium Development Goals: A Compact among Nations to End Human Poverty* (New York: Oxford University Press) <hdr.undp.org/reports/global/2003/?CFID=2670336&CFTOKEN=65436232> (September 2006).

United Nations Millennium Project (2005). 'Investing in Development: A Practical Plan to Achieve the Millennium Development Goals'. United Nations Development Programme, New York. <www.unmillenniumproject.org/reports/fullreport.htm> (September 2006).

World Health Organization (1997). 'Health and Environment in Sustainable Development 1997: Five Years after the Earth Summit'. WHO/EHG/97.8. Geneva.

World Health Organization (2005a). 'Ecosystems and Human Well-Being: Health Synthesis'. Geneva. <www.who.int/entity/globalchange/ecosystems/ecosys.pdf> (September 2006).

World Health Organization (2005b). 'Health in the Millennium Development Goals'. Geneva. <www.who.int/entity/mdg/publications/MDG_Report_revised.pdf> (September 2006).

PART IV
The Central Institutions: The G8 System

Chapter 9

The G8 and Global Health Governance

John J. Kirton and Jenevieve Mannell[1]

Since 1975, global health governance has been transformed by new physical challenges and by the behaviour of old multilateral global health organisations in response. During this time the dominant conception for global health governance and its prevailing policy paradigm has moved from the medical absence of disease to socioeconomic well-being, resource availability, poverty reduction, and ecological integrity (Pannenborg 1979). This shift was driven by the World Health Organization (WHO), at the apex of its strength in the 1970s, through its ambitious human rights initiative of Health For All. The WHO also drove the world from a concept of health as a national issue, which had prevailed during previous centuries, toward a more internationally focussed global approach to health governance (Cooper 1989).

Yet three decades later, the WHO has proven inadequate in addressing the major health challenges and crises of a rapidly globalising, post–Cold War, post–September 11 world. The rapid spread of HIV/AIDS through the West and then the rest of the world was the first sign of the failure of the old multilateral and regional health organisations. Compounding the failure have been other factors: the cumulative body count from the continuing chronic afflictions of malaria and tuberculosis (TB), the re-emergence of old diseases once on the verge of extinction such as polio, the eruption of bioterrorism with the anthrax attacks on America after 11 September 2001, the assault from severe acute respiratory syndrome (SARS) in 2002–03, and the subsequent threat of an avian influenza pandemic.

This failure has fuelled the search for a new generation of global health governance for the 21st-century world. In response, the G8 major market democracies, created in 1975 as part of a new generation of global institutions, has taken up the challenge. Starting narrowly with health research on diseases within the G8 countries, the G8's agenda soon broadened to address the major illnesses afflicting the world as a whole. At first the G8 worked to support the WHO and broader United Nations system in raising the money they needed but were unable to attract on their own. However, as the 21st century began, the G8 found it necessary to launch its own initiatives to deliver global health more directly. This phase started with the creation of the Global Fund to Fight AIDS, Tuberculosis, and Malaria in 2001. It continued with the 2001–02 development of the G8 Africa Action Plan and new attention and institutions to combat bioterrorism following the shock the September 11 and subsequent American anthrax attacks. At the 2003 Evian Summit, the G8's Health Action Plan directly tackled some of the world's most terrible diseases. By the 2004 Sea Island Summit, the G8 was focussed on specific interventions such as developing an HIV/AIDS vaccine and the eradication of polio. Gleneagles in 2005 continued this thrust. St. Petersburg in 2006 took infectious disease as one of its three priority themes and had the G8 health ministers meet for the first time.

How effective has this ever more active and ambitious G8 been as an emerging centre of global health governance, and why has it worked when the old multilateral organisations have failed? Only on the empirical and explanatory foundation provided by answers to these questions can reliable innovations be designed to improve global health governance in the years ahead. Yet there remains a great debate among scholars and other observers over the G8's record and the contribution the G8 can and should make. This debate ranges widely from the critics who think the G8 has done too little, done too much of the wrong thing, or failed to deliver the good promises it has made through to supporters who claim the G8 has already filled some gaps, has the potential to do much more, and is already delivering a new generation of health governance for a globalising world.

The first school of critics sees the G8 as a great fundraising failure (Drohan 2005; Lewis 2005). It views the G8's proper role as narrowly confined to raising massive amounts of new money to pass on, with few conditions attached, to the old organisations of the UN system that have been unable to induce their own members to provide the necessary sums. Acknowledging the failure of the old international organisations to deal adequately with the HIV/AIDS pandemic and arguing for a human right to health, these critics highlight the low level of financial commitments made to provide antiretroviral therapy (ART) for HIV/AIDS in developing countries. They also note the political lobbying of the United States government for the protection of the intellectual property rights of the world's most powerful pharmaceutical companies and the G8's easy acceptance of a dominant America's approach.

(2005), an advocate employed by the United Nations as Special Envoy on HIV/AIDS in Africa, has referred to this placement of intellectual property rights and international trade law above the alleged human right to health as 'mass murder by complacency'. A second cause he regularly alludes to is the common attitude of racism shared by G8 members and others in a largely wealthy white West. His third cause is the 'thinly disguised neo-colonial manipulation' that maintained the G8's 'unbroken record of betraying their promises' through to Gleneagles in 2005 (31, 149).

A second school sees the G8 as having a much broader role, but failing to deliver the promising new directions now required (Labonté and Schrecker 2004; Labonté *et al.* 2004). Here the G8's failure to improve health outcomes in the face of a new generation of disease flows from the collateral damage caused by its members' attachment to neo-liberal principles in the economic and social policy areas that are vital in generating health. As Ronald Labonté, Ted Schrecker, David Sanders, and Wilma Mieeus (2004, 228) put it: 'With respect to such an agenda that begins seriously to redress the human health and development catastrophes arising in the wake of contemporary globalization, the G8's response can best, if disturbingly, be described as fatal indifference.'

A third school locates the cause in institutional rather than ideological factors, notably the G8's search as an informal, summit-level institution for short-term public relations success ('G8 Failed to Tackle the Toxic Politics of Drug Making and Selling' 2003; Foster 2002, 2003). This view of the G8 as an informal institutional failure asserts that the G8's proper role goes beyond merely supporting the UN. But the G8's focus on other issues and its narrow audience lead it to fail. Thus, in the lead-up to the 2002 Kananaskis Summit, John Foster (2002) concluded that 'other priorities and photo opportunities may transcend the issue of follow-up and fulfillment' on the G8's global health file.

A fourth school argues, in contrast, that the G8 is emerging as the global health governor of last resort, as a consequence of the poor performance of the old multilateral organisations and the high technical and economic capacity of G8 members (Price-Smith 2001, 2002). This school sees the UN organisations as having failed in addressing the world's new health needs. It thus perceives the G8 as a useful supplement, gap filler, and insurance policy for an inadequate WHO. Andrew Price-Smith (2001, 178–179) concludes that the G8's recent involvement in health stems from this weakening of the WHO, and from the G8's ability to pick up the pieces from the failed global health institutions. He argues that the technical and economic capacity of the G8 will make it the most appropriate leader for the development of a badly needed 'global disease containment regime'.

A fifth school sees the G8 as the potential governor of globalisation in the health field as a whole (Savona and Oldani 2003). It argues that the G8 has already forged the new path for global health governance for an era where globalised markets threaten to overwhelm states. Paolo Savona and Chiara Oldani (2003, 100) claim that the G8 began by providing leadership as a consultative forum in the oil crisis of the 1970s and has since become a global decision centre. The G8 is suited for global health governance because it adheres to the proper role of international institutions: 'not to plunder nations' residual sovereignty but to recover some shares of it from the market on behalf of national authorities.'

A sixth school views the G8 as the emerging centre of 21st-century global health governance, due to the inclusive, multi-stakeholder model on which it is now based (Bayne 2000, 2001; Aginam 2004, 2005). Nicholas Bayne (2001, 34) attributes the G8's success in dealing with global health to its mobilisation of 'intellectual, human and financial resources from all available quarters — government, business, and NGOs [nongovernmental organisations] active in the field'. According to Bayne, the 'most promising advance' of the Okinawa Summit in 2000 came in health, with the summit's call for a partnership to reduce the prevalence of AIDS, TB, and malaria. This call was answered the following year at Genoa with the establishment of the Global Fund — a landmark initiative in its integration of governmental and non-state actors. Its task-oriented collaboration between the private and public sectors represents the model for the future of global health governance (Orbinski 2002).

Despite the growing diversity and dynamism of the debate, there has as yet been no full-scale analysis of the G8's actual performance in global health governance or of the forces that have propelled it to act in particular ways. Activists and analysts such as Lewis, Foster, and Labonté *et al.* focus on the many problems that remain rather than on the efforts made or actions taken to provide solutions. They often ignore the G8 members' high compliance with the health commitments the G8 has made. Those such as Price-Smith who emphasise the mismanagement of funds by the WHO and the capacities of the G8 in disease containment do not explain how the high-profile, crisis-oriented G8 can adequately address broader global health needs. Nor do they examine the actual performance of the G8 in global health governance to see if its members' capacities can handle the requirements of a multifaceted disease containment regime. Savona, Oldani, and Bayne highlight the G8's integration of private and public actors, but do not show how this produces global health. Nor has Bayne provided a detailed tracing of the process by which G8-centred multi-stakeholder networks produce the G8's many health deliberations, principles, commitments, and compliance.

This chapter presents the first systematic analysis of the G8's performance in global health governance. Part 1 defines health as a policy area within the G8, examines the G8's domestic political, deliberative, directional, decisional, delivery, and development of global governance performance in health, and identifies the overall patterns of performance that arise. Part 2 addresses the major causes of these patterns, exploring in turn the six factors highlighted by the concert equality model that has proven to explain G8 governance in other policy areas and overall (Kirton 2004, 2005a).

This analysis shows that since the onset of rapid globalisation in 1996, the G8 has emerged through several stages as an effective, high-performing centre of global health governance across the board. In 1996 and 1997, under French and American leadership, the G8 summits started discussing and deciding on global health issues in a substantial way. In 2000–01, under Japanese and Italian leadership, the G8 more than doubled its health deliberations and decisions, delivered its decisions to a very high degree, and mobilised new money to this end. In 2002–03, under Canadian and French leadership, the G8 began to articulate new directions and produce new peaks in its deliberative, directional, decisional, and development of G8-led global governance performance. In 2005, it took a step-level jump in the new money it mobilised for global public health.

This rapidly rising G8 performance in global health governance has been led by almost all G8 countries, especially when each has served as host. Effective action by this concert of equals has been driven by the deeper forces highlighted by the concert equality model of G8 governance. The most powerful cause has been the increasingly equal vulnerability of each G8 member to a new generation of infectious diseases, as the early AIDS assault on America spread rapidly to all G8 members, made the G8's newest member of Russia most infected member of the G8, and then proliferated across an Africa that secured major attention and attendance at G8 summits since 2001. In response, the old organisations of the UN system, led by the WHO, have proven increasingly ineffective in raising their own members' resources on the scale required or in meeting the targets and timetables they themselves have set. In contrast, the G8 countries possess the globally predominant and internally equal capabilities needed to combat the new diseases on a global scale. Their core common principles of open democracy and social advance bring them close to their newly democratic African partners and make them comfortable with the multi-stakeholder approaches most appropriate to combat the new generation of disease. From 2001 to 2005 the high degree of domestic political control of the popularly elected G8 leaders allowed the same seven individuals to come to an unprecedented five summits in a row, to meet the same four core democratic African partners in the still constricted and cosy leaders-dominated G8 club, and to discuss global health in the inclusive, interlinked, innovative way the world needs.

Part 1: The G8's Growing Health Governance

The new health paradigm that emerged in the 1970s expanded the dominant conception of health beyond disease or health care to include the social and economic determinants of health. In keeping with this broader conception, health is defined in this study as the human condition of being sound in body, mind, and spirit, and free from physical disease, infirmity, or pain. But health is also considered in its relationship with economy and society, and in its connections with the environment, security, and human rights.

In the G8 context, health can be divided into two categories: core health, where health is the ultimate welfare objective, and health-related issues, where health is an instrument affecting other welfare outcomes. Core health encompasses the human condition of health, the presence or absence of life, disease, or pain, and the efforts made toward maintaining a healthy human condition. Core health issues thus include infectious diseases (such as HIV/AIDS, malaria, TB, polio), medical research, the healthcare system, improved health as a function of development (development for health), health promotion, medicine and treatment, global collaboration and resource mobilisation for health, the current global health organisations (notably the WHO, the Joint United Nations Programme on HIV/AIDS [UNAIDS], and the multilateral development banks), and bioterrorism. Core health also embraces the use of health-generating instruments, where health is specified as the welfare objective to be obtained, as in debt relief (for the benefit of health systems in developing countries), information and communications technology to improve healthcare facilities, or environmental issues (which affect human health). Health-related issues deal with the specified ways in which health instruments affect outcomes on other policy areas, such as economic development or education.

The G8's performance on both core health and health-related issues is assessed across the six basic functions of international institutions: managing domestic politics in member countries; deliberating on specific global issues and thus setting the global agenda; directing particular principles and norms to prevail; deciding on clear, concrete, future-oriented, collective commitments or rules, with at least minimal levels of precision and obligation; delivering on these commitments through subsequent implementing action that constitutes compliance; and developing global governance through creating or guiding international institutions to which future tasks can be delegated.

Domestic Political Management

On the first function of domestic political management, the G8's health performance has been mixed. G8 leaders have not heralded their G8 health accomplishments in their annual national policy addresses to their voters at home. But they have increasingly received attention and approval for their G8 health achievements in their national media news and editorial coverage. This progress culminated in 2005, when the virtually unanimous domestic media approval received by British prime minister Tony Blair for the 2005 Gleneagles Summit was fuelled in part by its prominent attention to and action on African health (Kirton 2005b).

Civil society actions have been largely negative. Most campaign groups have highlighted remaining needs rather than the existing progress, and criticised the G8 as the new focal point, rather than the UN bodies, for not doing nearly enough. Indeed, one reason why the leaders gave relatively little attention to health in 2002 was the strong criticism they received from nongovernmental organisations (NGOs) for what the leaders regarded as their major breakthrough on health at the Genoa Summit in 2001. The violent protests that erupted and the death of a protestor at that summit dominated the media coverage and drowned out any attention and approval for the leaders' advances on health at Genoa.

Deliberation

On the second function of deliberation, the G8's health performance has become high. Since the subject first appeared on the G8's core agenda in 1982, there has been increasing interest in health, both in the documentation released by the leaders and in their private deliberations among themselves (see Appendix 9-1). This increase has been punctuated by seven peaks, generally reflecting the sudden emergence of new diseases such as AIDS, SARS, and bioterrorism in 1991 and 2002.

The first peak occurred with the introduction of health to the agenda at the French-hosted Versailles Summit in 1982. The issue arose in relation to the use of biotechnologies to reduce disease as well as famine and overpopulation in developing countries (G7 1982). This reference to the role the G8 could play in improving health facilities represented a large percentage of the overall agenda because of the relatively short length of the communiqué. It was followed by an oral statement on cancer made by the chair at London in 1984.

The second peak occurred with the Venice Summit in 1987. Here the Italian host released the Chairman's Statement on AIDS, a four-paragraph separate statement calling for greater support of the WHO's programmes (G7 1987). This was the first separate publicly released document pertaining entirely to health.

The third peak came in 1990 and 1991 with the emphasis on bioweapons. The threat of disease outbreaks from bioterrorism was highlighted as a result of the war with Iraq and concerns over Iraq's biological weapons programme. Another driver was the review of the Biological Weapons Convention in September 1991.

The fourth peak arose in 1996 and 1997 as the summits changed their focus from G8-centred health to global health. The 1996 Lyon Summit produced substantially more paragraphs on health than any previous summit — 9 of the total 296. This text focussed on the need for restructuring the WHO to cope with HIV/AIDS and other infectious diseases. By Denver in 1997, infectious diseases in the developing world took centre stage (WHO 1997). Although there was a subsequent slide, health commitments remained strong in 1998 with the Roll Back Malaria Partnership taking the spotlight at Birmingham.

The fifth peak came in Okinawa in 2000 with the greatest percentage of paragraphs on core health for any summit in G8 history. Okinawa concentrated on health in developing countries, committing to a 'new global partnership' to reduce the prevalence of HIV, TB, and malaria. This became the Global Fund that was created at Genoa in 2001 (Zupi 2001). Despite the significance of the health issue at Okinawa, attention subsequently slipped until Evian 2003.

The sixth peak arose at Evian in 2003. It was pushed by the implication of the SARS outbreak of 2002–03 and a renewed initiative to eradicate polio. The summit saw the release of an entire collective document devoted to health, out of 15 in total. Health had become a major component of the G8's social agenda, comprising a significant portion of the leaders' deliberations.

The health peak of 2003 was, like the others, short lived and driven by the year's health preoccupation of SARS. Although the number of paragraphs devoted to health and health-related issues in 2004 was higher than the peak of 2000, the percentage of health in the overall agenda, at only 5.4 percent, was the lowest it had been since 1998, and well below the peak in 2000 of over 14 percent and 2003's 11.6 percent. Moreover, the fight against AIDS showed a dramatic turn toward the role of medical research and pharmaceutical companies in finding a vaccine and away from the more urgent needs of treatment and prevention required by individuals in sub-Saharan Africa and other high-prevalence areas. In addition, following the 2003 Iraq war's focus on weapons inspections and terrorism, bioweapons once again became a major component of the health-related agenda.

A seventh peak soon came at St. Petersburg in 2006, when infectious diseases served as one of the summit's three priority themes. The summit's 5717-word document on the Fight Against Infectious Disease was the longest of the total 15 documents and constituted more than 18 percent of the summit's output. For the first time it featured avian influenza, emergency responses to natural and human-made disasters, measles, HIV/AIDS in Eurasia, and the migration of healthcare workers from poor countries, while maintaining attention on HIV/AIDS, TB, malaria, and polio as well as the importance of financing.

Direction Setting

The third function, direction setting, has seen the G8 do much to define new principles, norms, priorities, and epistemes in global health. The 2000 Okinawa

Summit acknowledged for the first time the link between health and poverty. It declared:

> Health is key to prosperity. Good health contributes directly to economic growth whilst poor health drives poverty. Infectious and parasitic diseases, most notably HIV/AIDS, TB and malaria, as well as childhood diseases and common infections, threaten to reverse decades of development and to rob an entire generation of hope for a better future. Only through sustained action and coherent international co-operation to fully mobilise new and existing medical, technical and financial resources, can we strengthen health delivery systems and reach beyond traditional approaches to break the vicious cycle of disease and poverty (G8 2000).

Subsequently, health became a priority principle with the G8's move in 2002 to issue a chair's statement as the summit's defining capstone document that would reflect only what the leaders actually discussed. This process culminated at the 2005 Gleneagles Summit, where health, in relation to Africa, was given a prominent place. The 21st-century priority principles centred on the need for more funding, research, international cooperation, and accessible, affordable medicines for Africa in the fight against HIV/AIDS, polio, malaria, TB, and SARS, and healthcare reform within the G8. While there was a hint that health for the poor would trump trade values, there was no recognition of health for security or health as a human right (Labonté and Schrecker 2004, 226). St. Petersburg in 2006 stood out for its affirmation of the centrality of democratic values such as openness, transparency, information exchange, monitoring, surveillance, reporting, ethics, and civil society participation as vital in promoting health in the new era of fast-moving globalised infectious diseases.

Decision Making

On its fourth function of decision making, the G8's health performance has been increasingly strong, as measured by the number, appropriateness, and ambition of the collective commitments its leaders publicly make at their annual summit. Commitments are defined as discrete, specific, future-oriented, measurable, publicly encoded commitments, often with specified instruments, outcome targets, and timetables or deadlines attached. Health commitments represent 5.5 percent of the total commitments made at the summits from 1975 to 2005. The G8 has been a consistent producer of health commitments since 1996 at Lyon, when the G8 moved beyond merely discussing the issue to making clear commitments aimed at change in the global health system.

Prior to 1996, the single commitments on health — in 1983, 1986, 1991, and 1993 — accounted for a very small portion of the total output. Since the Lyon Summit, there has been sustained and growing G8 decisional action on health. The summits of 2002 and 2003 produced the highest ratio of health commitments during the summit's first 30 years.

This progression was a slow development, both in the number of commitments made and in the significance of the commitments themselves. In the period building up to Kananaskis and Evian, Nicholas Bayne (2002, 147) noted the low ambition of the commitments. He judged that 'in general, the Genoa documents set out clear diagnoses of the problems addressed. But often the G7/G8 response is not to take new policy measures or to provide new resources, but only to intensify exiting actions and coordinate them better.'

However, at Evian, both the number and the significance of the health commitments expanded, with a standalone health action plan included in the summit documents. Evian produced an all-time high of 21 commitments on health. While the G8 Health Action Plan focussed on 'welcoming' and 'supporting' other initiatives pertaining to HIV/AIDS, it also made a strong pledge to policy change or resource commitments in providing developing countries with access to essential medicines, vaccine development, and fighting polio (G8 2003). A total of US$500 million was mobilised for polio at the summit, representing the first financial commitment on health to come since the establishment of the Global Fund.

At Sea Island in 2004, the number of health commitments dropped from 21 (10 percent of the total commitments) to 12 (5 percent). They focussed on two issues: eradicating polio and developing an HIV/AIDS vaccine. Moreover, Sea Island was the first summit since 1996 where all the commitments either instructed the existing international organisations or represented an independent initiative by the G8. No commitments called for the direct support of other initiatives or institutions. The twelve commitments made at Sea Island therefore represent more direct concentration on health issues and a desire to take control of these specific issues. They reflect a desire by the G8 to fill the gaps, whether technical or financial, in the specific areas it saw as lagging in development and to provide leadership when the older institutions were found lacking.

At Gleneagles in 2005, the number of health commitments rose to 18, or more than 8 percent of the total. A new high of US$24 billion was raised for health purposes, broadly defined. St. Petersburg in 2006 continued the rising cadence. It generated 64 health commitments, representing 20 percent of the summit's 317 total. This was far the highest number and portion of health commitments in the G8's 31-year history.

Delivery

On the fifth function, delivery, the summit has also performed well in health, as G8 members have largely fulfilled their collective commitments through a broad range of behaviour in the year after they were made. Since 1998, G8 members' compliance with their health commitments has been quite high. On the 20 measured health commitments between 1988 and 2004, the average compliance level was +60 percent. From levels close to the overall summit compliance average in 1998 and 1999, compliance with health commitments soared to a nearly perfect +95 percent in 2000. They have since stayed at above-average levels, even with a noticeable dip in 2002. Yet there was some slippage in delivering the 2005 priority health commitments, as that on HIV/AIDS fell to +33 percent and that on polio to only +11 percent, compared to an overall summit compliance average of +65 percent (G8 Research Group 2006).

One form of commitment for which compliance is important is that of new money mobilised. In the field of health, the centrepiece has been the Global Fund. In the years immediately following its establishment, there was significant criticism of the lack of financial support provided by the G8. Bayne (2003, 237) observed that at Kananaskis 'the leaders ignored the funding pressures on the Global Fund to Fight AIDS, Malaria, and Tuberculosis, which they had launched only the year before … the fund already needed replenishment but the leaders made no move to do this.'

Yet compliance with significant, non-financial commitments made to the fund has been high, such as the promise made at Evian to participate actively in donor and support conferences. Every G8 country complied, and this specifically resulted in increased pledges to the Global Fund by France and the United Kingdom (G8 Research Group 2004a, 2004b). Moreover, although the summit commitments made to the Global Fund have not included concrete financial targets, and although G8 donations have not always lived up to some NGOs' assertions of what constitutes an equitable contribution, the G8 members have improved their contributions significantly since 2002 (France, Ooms, and Rivers 2002). Indeed, by 2004, the U.S. was now at 117 percent of its recommended 'equitable' contribution for 2004, the UK had reached 140 percent, and Italy led the way with 430 percent. Showing some improvement since 2002, Canada and Japan had 51 percent and 33 percent respectively. More recently, at a pledging conference on 6 September 2005, US$3.7 billion was pledged to the Global Fund for 2006–07. The donors were led by G8 members, with France at US$600 million, Japan at US$500 million, and Britain at US$375 million. The G8's total donations to the Global Fund had more than doubled from US$1.3 billion in 2001 to more than US$2.8 billion in 2005. At St. Petersburg the leaders made a major effort to get the funds already promised actually delivered and reported, if inadequately, on their own record in delivering at the end of their health declaration.

The Development of Global Governance

The sixth performance dimension is the development of institutions for ongoing global governance in new ways. From 2002 onward, the G8 has moved from supporting or directing the UN system to taking initiatives to build G8-centred instruments and institutions on its own. It started G8-centred institution building with AIDS, creating the International Ethics Committee on AIDS in 1987 (consistent with the agenda focus on HIV/AIDS the same year) and the Group of Experts on the Prevention and Treatment of AIDS in 1992.

With the establishment of the Global Fund to Fight AIDS, Tuberculosis, and Malaria in 2000, the G8 began a period of increased institutionalisation, establishing four other institutions in the years following. Late in 2001, the G7 members together with Mexico also began a ministerial meeting not linked to the G7, the Global Health Security Initiative (GHSI). Together these G7 and G7-parallel bodies have focussed on health security and infectious diseases. However, three distinct areas of sustained institutionalisation appear. First, in 2002 and 2003, immediately following SARS, three institutions were created that concentrated specifically on containing disease outbreaks and establishing better international cooperation. Second, HIV/AIDS has seen substantial G8 governance both through the establishment of the Global Fund in 2000 and the creation of the Global HIV Vaccine Enterprise in 2004. Third, the ministerial meetings were established with the intention of dealing with the issue of biological warfare and security, yet the post-SARS agenda has shifted its attention to the containment of potential naturally occurring disease outbreaks.

At the ministerial level, the British considered holding a meeting in the fall of 2005 as part of their presidency. The Russians, as hosts in 2006, held the first G8 health ministers meeting, in Moscow in April 2006, to develop the St. Petersburg Summit's priority theme on infectious diseases. The St. Petersburg leaders further committed themselves in their communiqué to conduct a regular review of their work in tackling pandemics.

The Pattern of G8 Performance

The overall pattern of performance of the G8 in health that emerges across these six functions is consistent with that from other analyses. In Bayne's (2005) annual assessments of the G8, the health issue area received the highest grade for the establishment of the Global Fund at Genoa in 2001. The University of Toronto's G8 Research Group gave A grades to both Denver and Okinawa on health. It awarded an A to St. Petersburg for its performance on avian influenza and a B+ for that on HIV/AIDS.

Together these analyses show that the G8's health performance passed through five stages. First, the G8 became a global health governor at an early stage across a broad array of governance functions. In the mid 1980s, the rising awareness of HIV led to the Chairman's Statement on AIDS in 1987 and to the formation of the International Ethics Committee on AIDS. The Iraq wars of 1990–91 and 2003– led to increased agenda attention on bioterrorism and bioweapons.

Second, starting in 1996 the G8 moved to a more global focus and a more fully international health agenda, with the introduction of diseases such as Ebola and cholera, which primarily affect the developing world. This period brought a dramatic improvement in the summit's performance, beginning with the arrival of global health at Lyon. The 1996 Lyon Summit saw four commitments, when previously only single health commitments had been made at a time. However, the pattern of health performance did not consistently improve from one summit to the next. Few summits stand out during this time of high health performance.

The third major leap forward, inaugurating the 21st-century takeoff, came with Okinawa in 2000. It was awarded a grade of A+ by the G8 Research Group for its performance in health (G8 Research Group 2000). Okinawa was very strong in its health deliberations (with 30 mentions of health), decision making (11 health commitments), and compliance (an almost perfect score by all members). Okinawa also brought to the G8's agenda guinea worm and onchocerciasis (river blindness), diseases virtually unheard of in G8 countries.

The fourth jump came at Evian in 2003. Evian saw sweeping success in almost all functions, with historic highs in deliberation, direction setting, decision making, and the development of global governance and the second strongest performance in delivery. Infectious diseases and treatment (specifically AIDS in the developing world) formed the major focus of the core health agenda, backed up by clean water and sanitation in the health-related agenda. Sea Island in 2004 and Gleneagles in 2005 maintained this momentum and brought new highs for money mobilised.

The fifth advance came at St. Petersburg in 2006. It took infectious diseases as one of its three priority themes and produced the longest dedicated document and most extensive deliberation on health. It strongly emphasised a democratic approach to global health governance, with the highest number of health commitments ever. Its strong emphasis on monitoring compliance suggests that these decisions are likely to be delivered in the years ahead. The first ever G8 health ministers meeting took the development of G8-centred global health governance to a new high.

Part 2: Causes of the G8's Growing Health Governance

The G8's increasingly high performance in health has been achieved through the leadership of virtually all G8 countries as host, with each adding important components to the cumulative edifice. Behind this leadership of the individual agents lie the six forces highlighted by the concert equality model of G8 governance: the shared health vulnerability of G8 members, the diminishing health performance of older international organisations, the equalising capability of the G8 members, the social democratic principles common to G8 members, the G8 leaders' high political control and capital, and the constricted membership and participation in the G8.

The Intensifying Equal Health Vulnerabilities of the G8 and the World

The first and most powerful force is the increasingly equal vulnerability of each G8 member to a new generation of infectious diseases. This came as the early AIDS assault on America rapidly spread to all G8 members, made the recently recruited Russia the leading source of new infections within the club, proliferated throughout an Africa that became the dominant agenda priority and attending partner of the G8 summits since 2001, and threatened a new pandemic in an India and China that attended in 2003, 2005, and 2006.

This intensifying vulnerability to health threats, and thus common incentive to act, is seen first in the number of new infections of HIV/AIDS — the most deadly of the 'new generation' diseases — in each of the G8 countries (see Appendix 9-2). These data show that the G8's growing health governance was a direct, rational response by G8 members to the physical vulnerability of proliferating new infections within and throughout their societies. Yet it was also punctuated by a psychological vulnerability, as the governors and publics in G8 countries were shocked into greater action when important physical thresholds were crossed (Picard 2001). It was also the provision of a global public good in response to a pandemic of global scope and scale (the magnitude of which is illustrated in Appendix 9-3).

The physical assault from AIDS began first in the United States, Canada, and France in the early 1980s. By 1985, for the first time, all the G7 countries had recorded new incidents of HIV/AIDS. By 1987 the number of cases was quickly mounting in almost all G7 countries. At the time, the U.S. was taking the brunt of the disease burden, with the number of newly infected individuals in America skyrocketing to 28 599 in 1987. Compounding the physical assault was a psychological one, for AIDS had begun to cause widespread panic in the American public as the disease itself was still largely mysterious to medical researchers.

Driven by this rise in AIDS cases and public anxiety, the 1997 Denver Summit introduced AIDS and infectious diseases to the leaders' collective documents. The chair's statement highlighted the vulnerability the G7 felt by speaking to the severity of the disease, addressing the panic it was causing in the public by calling for increases in public education and asking the medical community for more studies on prevention and treatment. In 1987 HIV/AIDS was perceived as an issue requiring immediate G7 attention, as until Denver in 1997 it was the only infectious disease the G7/8 leaders would discuss. And it was the shock of this initial vulnerability, rapidly spreading equally among all G7 members, that brought AIDS to the G8 agenda.

During the 1990s the physical assault on all G7 countries from HIV/AIDS continued. The peak number of new cases a year came for the U.S. in 1993, France in 1994, Italy and Canada in 1995, and Germany in 1996. With a majority of G7 members now so severely afflicted, HIV/AIDS returned to the summit agenda in a major way and never left again. In 1996 the G7 summit added the equally mysterious diseases of Ebola, as well as the merely exotic ones in G7 countries of malaria, TB, cholera, and pneumonia. This broadening was consistent with a new fear that intensifying demographic globalisation was bringing the old diseases still prevalent in poorer countries into a long secure G8. At the same time, where fact and familiarity were high and fear was low, the G8 left the diseases alone. Persistent diseases such as cancer and cardiovascular disease, which account for significant numbers of deaths in G8 nations, received almost no attention at the summits.

By 2001, the G8 crossed three new physical thresholds — a new peak in the average number of new infections across all G8 countries, in Japan, and in the G8's newest member, Russia. In the U.S., the decline in the incidence of new cases stopped in 2000 and a slow rise started again. In 2001, the number of new cases in Russia jumped up to 88 253, the highest number ever recorded in any year for any G8 country, including the U.S. itself at its 1993 peak.

The years 2002–03 brought a second vulnerability from a new source, this time coming through the shock of SARS (see Appendix 9-4). Although the Asian-born disease did not reach the U.S., it struck hard in its deadly form in its two other G8

Pacific partners, Canada and Japan, while infecting Russia as well. It drove home the deadly lesson that even advanced G8 countries with world-class and well-funded healthcare systems were vulnerable to diseases that developed in very poor countries and were half a world — but only one plane ride — away. While SARS saw rather low levels of morbidity and mortality, its unknown cause and cure created a compounded sense of shock and panic, and a relatively high level of agenda attention after the first outbreak in 2002. The impact of the awareness SARS created for global collaboration was clearly felt at the summit.

In 2003, the year following the 2002 SARS outbreak, the G8 at Evian produced the highest summit on record in both health deliberation and commitments; two institutions were established, money was mobilised, and compliance was higher than average. It can be concluded from this pattern that emerging health threats and the public concern surrounding them have been largely responsible for introducing new health issues to the G8 agenda during this initial period. The shock of SARS thus drove home a further recognition of reality: the vulnerability of the global health system itself in an age when national defence at the border by sovereign territorial Westphalian major powers was virtually irrelevant.

In 2005, this lesson was driven home by a second shock — the attack of avian influenza, originating in Asia, on the homelands of G8 members themselves (see Appendix 9-5). Starting in the first quarter of 2004 in Japan, the disease spread steadily to all G8 regions by the end of 2005. Although no human cases or fatalities were reported in G8 countries, the rising human death toll in neighbouring Asia, and in systemically important countries that were G20 members and 21st-century G8 attendees, inspired the G8 to act quickly and preventively to this second shock. By the summer of 2006, avian influenza had touched all G8 countries. It acquired a new epicentre in Indonesia, where the first extended cluster of cases of human-to-human transmission took place.

The Poor Performance of the Old International Health Organisations

The second cause of growing health governance is the poor performance of the old organisations of the UN system, led by the WHO, in the face of this rapid proliferation of vulnerability from the new diseases on a G8-wide and global scale (Cooper 1989; Howard 1989; Zacher 1999).

The G8's initial lack of concern with health had flowed from its deference to the WHO, as the official formal and presumably functionally effective body for global health governance. All G8 summits with major health commitments thus included calls for support of the WHO's activities and references to the important role of the organisation in combating the world's diseases.

However, growing global vulnerability in the 21st century called for much stronger international collaboration than the WHO, with its deference to national sovereignty and regional pillars, proved able to provide (Fidler 2002, 2004; Kickbusch 2003; Price-Smith 2001). Ilona Kickbusch (2000, 983) has emphasised how the old system has been overwhelmed by 'the increasing number of actors in the international health arena; the increasing privatization of medical care and the growing global health care market; increased importance of health intelligence, data and surveillance for economic development and trade; increased feeling of threat through new and reemerging diseases; and increased awareness of health as a human rights'. This constellation led to conflicts between global governance institutions and private industry, such as the debate over access to essential medicines for HIV/AIDS in Africa. There emerged an inherent instability as the number of actors on the global health stage increased without the mechanisms necessary for increased collaboration. The result is that emerging diseases go unnoticed or there is not the necessary cross-sector collaboration between national health systems and the pharmaceutical companies responsible for vaccine or antidote development, as has been the case with river blindness.

The G8's adoption of issues such as river blindness sought to fill the gap in collaboration. At Kananaskis, the G8's Africa Action Plan endorsed 'supporting relevant public-private partnerships for the immunization of children and the elimination of micro-nutrient deficiencies in Africa' (G8 2002). The deliberation on public health at the summits has focussed on building these types of public-private partnerships and attempting to build trust among the actors in global health.

Such gap-filling efforts have been propelled by the failure of the old international health organisations, notably the WHO and the UN, to retain sufficient confidence from their members to lead these countries to provide the required resources. As the financial reports contained in the WHO World Health Assembly documents show, from 1996 to 2001, as the HIV/AIDS pandemic proliferated throughout the G8 and the globe, the budget of the WHO did not undergo its usual biannual increase. In sharp contrast, during this time G8 health performance grew strongly, culminating in the 2000–01 launch of the Global Fund.

With current infection rates of HIV/AIDS now exceeding 40 million worldwide and threatening a new pandemic across Eurasia, it is clear that no international institution has been doing enough of the right things in response.

Yet, as the first line of defence, the WHO in particular has received widespread criticism both from within the organisation and from the larger international community. Moreover, those within the UN system have also recognised that its own internal failures in handling the crisis have contributed in part to its severity: 'We have to admit that the way global targets were set is not conducive to success simply because the HIV pandemic was acknowledged but not internalised' (Vandemoortele 2003; see also Foster 2003). In an overt display of its lack of confidence in the WHO's handling of the AIDS crisis as early as 1993, the UN itself had taken the Global Programme for AIDS, which was the WHO's largest programme, out of the WHO's sole control (Godlee 1994, 7). It created UNAIDS instead. Yet the UN itself also failed (Lewis 2005, 155).

Responding to the WHO's perceived inadequacies, the G8 first focussed on making commitments that supported the organisation. Yet by 2001, the G8 concluded that support for a failing UN system was in vain. An Italian presidency document released at the Okinawa Summit stated:

> The experience matured in the past twenty years demonstrates that aid provided by the international community has contributed to a significant improvement in the health conditions of millions of people. However, at the beginning of the third millennium, 'Health for All' targets agreed upon in 1978 have yet to be reached; today, 880 million people are excluded from the most basic access to care and public services (Italy [G8 Host] 2001).

This failure of WHO governance continued. The WHO's '3 by 5' initiative, under which the WHO promised to have three million patients in treatment for AIDS by the end of 2005, was a striking failure, as only one third of the targeted 3 million were receiving treatment at this time (Lewis 2005, 154). Thus it was left to the G8 at Gleneagles to promise not just partial but virtually 'universal access to treatment for AIDS by 2010' (G8 2005). Moreover, when the SARS crisis erupted in 2003, the WHO, with its deference to the sovereign prerogatives of closed countries such as China, was slow to respond to protect the global community against this fast-moving new disease.

High G8 Health Capability

The third cause is the globally predominant and internally equalising capability of the countries in the G8. In sharp contrast to the limited capacity and poor performance of the old multilateral organisations, the G8 countries increasingly possess the globally dominant share of the overall and specialised capabilities required to combat the new diseases, and share these among G8 members in a way that enables and requires all to contribute in a materially meaningful way.

The G8's global predominance is highlighted by a comparison of G8 healthcare spending and the healthcare capacity of the developing world. The G8 average for 2001 was an expenditure on health care of US$1492 per capita. In sharp contrast, the average health expenditure per capita for developing countries is US$73.4, and for the poorest of the poor in sub-Saharan Africa is US$31.9.[2] The Commission on Macroeconomics and Health (2001) predicts the financial need for health services in developing countries will reach US$27 billion by 2007. The disease burden of these countries has profound impacts on their economic capacity and therefore their ability to improve the situation. According to the WHO, 'analysis of data from thirty-one African countries during the period 1980 to 1995 showed that the annual loss of economic growth due to malaria has been as high as 1.3 percent per year' (Brundtland 2000). For G8 nations — the primary development donors — this presents an economic as well as a healthcare burden.

This disparity in healthcare budgets and the economic strain that has resulted from the proliferation of disease in the developing world can partly explain the G8's focus on international health since 1996. This is where the greatest need meets a great capacity. The need itself has become more apparent in recent years as AIDS has taken hold of Africa and other developing areas. The G8, through the Global Fund, is now providing more money to meet this global public need than the WHO itself. By

2004 the money committed to health at the summits combined was US$4.9 billion. Promises for official development assistance (ODA) on health outside the G8 structure accounted for US$6 billion (Commission on Macroeconomics and Health 2001). At Gleneagles the G8 promised to double ODA within five years, and inspired the additional US$3.1 billion raised in the autumn replenishment of the Global Fund.

The equality among G8 members in health is evident in the way each has taken the leadership on a disease in which it has developed a specialised capacity. France has been active on AIDS, a disease first discovered by a French scientist, closely followed by an American one. Britain, with historical strengths in tropical medicine, has led in putting TB and malaria on the agenda. Canada has been in the lead on polio and SARS. Italy accepted stewardship in 2005 for developing a financial facility to ensure the development of vaccines. And in 2006 Russia made health a prioirty and established a regional coordination mechanism to involve Eastern European and Central Asian countries in the Global HIV Vaccine Enterprise.

The G8's Common Principles of Open Democratic Health

The fourth cause is the G8's shared common principles of open democracy and social advance. These core values bring the G8 members ideologically closer to their new African and most outreach partners now embracing democratic development. Together they have made it easy for the G8 to move beyond national sovereignty into the openness and transparency needed to protect human security. These common values have also fuelled the functionally appropriate, multi-stakeholder approaches most appropriate to combat the new generation of disease.

Providing high-quality health care is a principle shared by all G8 members. This shared social purpose leads to higher performance in deliberation and decision making, as all members see the value of handling health concerns at the summits. As shown by the World Bank's statistics for the percentage of gross domestic product (GDP) spent on health care by the G8, health represents a relatively equal preference in country budgets with an average of 9.15 percent (2001).[3] The World Bank thus recognises how public heath is vital to the G8's seminal mission of social advance. The shock of SARS in 2003 has shown how deadly disease can proliferate because of inadequate transparency in countries that lack open democracy. Far less relevant as a unifying force is the G8's seminal value of individual liberty, as not all G8 members have accepted at home a human right to health.

G8 Leaders High Political Control and Capital at Home

The fifth cause of growing health governance is leadership continuity. From 2001 to 2005, high political control at home by the popularly elected G8 leaders allowed the same seven individuals to come to an unprecedented five summits in a row. This encouraged a sustained, iterative, and expanding treatment of the issue of health over half a decade, as continuity generated experience and self-confidence and a determination to get the job done (Bayne 1999).

In 1998, the newly elected Tony Blair, as G8 host, brought the Roll Back Malaria Partnership to the summit. But the Birmingham Summit did little to further G8 health governance as a whole. In general, the peaks in G8 health performance have come during the secure years between elections or at the end of a leader's final term. In 2000 a particularly significant peak in health performance came as U.S. president Bill Clinton attended his last summit, and the unelected host Japanese prime minister Yoshiro Mori hosted his first.[4] Clinton was looking for a legacy and an all-encompassing effort domestically and internationally to push forward the agenda items he had previously been holding off on for the sake of popular support; this desire drove the summit's progress, even if the launch of the Global Fund had to wait until Genoa the next year. The 2002 Kananaskis Summit's high deliberation and decision-making performance coincided with the leadership of Canadian prime minister Jean Chrétien, attending the summit for the tenth time and hosting it for the second. The 2004 Sea Island Summit's focussed deliberation and decreased decision making came as host U.S. president George W. Bush was entering a very tight race for his second term later that same year and needed to be seen as conservative as well as effective in his commitments.

In 2005, with Blair hosting his second summit, after eight years of summit experience and having just received his third majority mandate at home, many gains on African health were made. In 2006, while there were several new leaders around the summit table, domestic publics across the G8 picked infectious diseases as the second most popular issue they wanted the summit to address, with those in the U.S. and Canada putting it in first place and those in Russia, France, and Britain in second spot (Global Markets Institute 2006).

The Constricted Participation of the G8 Leaders' Club

The sixth cause is the constricted membership and participation in the G8 summit. This has allowed the same G8 leaders to meet face to face, annually, and increasingly as equals, with the same four core African partners in the still constricted G8 club, and to reach out to other stakeholders at the ministerial and official levels below (Hajnal 1999).

Constricted participation, and the spontaneous innovation among leaders it allowed, was responsible for placing health on the G8's agenda in the early years. In the 1980s it was Margaret Thatcher's informal, personal conversation with Ronald Reagan at the summit that led the leaders to take up the issue of drugs, which led directly to the G7's attention to HIV/AIDS. The move to a more restricted format in 1998, when only the leaders started to meet at the summit, helped Blair as host have the summit broaden the G8's attention from AIDS to malaria and TB.

Yet the G8's highly selected and targeted expansion of participation has also fuelled the increase in its health governance performance in both breadth and depth. The inclusion of Russia as a full and then permanent member starting in 1997 has coincided with the G8's rapidly growing governance of health since that time. The dramatic increase in the number of HIV/AIDS cases in Russia during this time, together with Russia's growing inclusion and experience as a full member, has sustained the G8's growing attention to health, even if Russia had long been reluctant or unable to highlight the problem in its national agenda at home. The peak of G8 health performance at the Okinawa Summit in 2000 coincided with actions by the Japanese chair to consult informally southern countries over the course of the summit. Most directly, the presence at the summit every year from 2001 to 2005 of the same four leaders of Africa's major democratic powers has fuelled the '21st century' takeoff in G8 health governance, particularly in its concentration on those diseases that are destroying Africa most.

A third consequential component of constricted participation has been the G8's mobilisation of the multi-stakeholder model in the health field. At Birmingham in 1998 and Cologne 1999, NGO pressure from the Jubilee 2000 coalition pushed G8 leaders to do more for debt relief to free up resources to devote to health and education in developing countries. At Genoa, the G8 pioneered the use of public-private partnerships in a major form with the creation of the Global Fund, which included G8 and other governments, international institutions, and civil society actors from many spheres. By Genoa, in regard to health and other issues, the G8 had demonstrated its progress in 'involving both private firms and non-profit bodies in summit preparation and follow-up' (Bayne 2002).

Driving the importance of multi-stakeholder participation in G8 health governance are increasing numbers of actors participating in global health governance; NGOs have made their voices heard in the international arena and have shown considerable power of persuasion in influencing public opinion and public policy. Most notably, the Médecins Sans Frontières (MSF) Campaign for Access to Essential Medicines has played a significant role in altering policy on drug access and the International Baby Food Action Network's global campaign in the 1980s led to the International Code of Marketing on Breastmilk Substitutes (Fidler 2004, 54). Multinational corporations (MNCs) have also demonstrated their influence as non-state actors in affecting public policy. For example, the lobbying of the U.S. government on the part of pharmaceutical companies has been a major impediment to progress in providing access to ART for developing countries. Private foundations, led by the Bill and Melinda Gates Foundation, have become major financial sponsors of the new initiatives on global health.

Conclusion

Past Performance

Since the onset of rapid globalisation in 1996, the G8 has emerged through several stages as an effective, high-performing centre of global health governance across the board. In 1996 and 1997, under French and American leadership, the G8 summits moved to deliberate and decide on global health issues in a substantial way. In 2000–01, under Japanese and Italian leadership, the G8 became a permanent high-performing centre of global health governance, more than doubling its health deliberations and decisions, delivering its decisions to a very high degree, and starting to mobilise new money to this end. In 2002–03, under Canadian and French leadership, the G8 began to articulate new directions and produce new peaks in its deliberative, directional, decisional, and development of G8-led global governance performance. In 2005, it took a step-level jump in the new money mobilised for global public health and in 2006 adopted health as one of its three priority themes.

This rapidly rising performance has been led by almost all G8 countries, with each adding important components to the cumulative edifice when serving as summit host. Such effective action by this group of equals has been driven by those deeper causes that the concert equality model of G8 governance highlights. The most powerful cause has been the increasingly equal vulnerability of each G8 member to a new generation of infectious diseases. The early AIDS assault on America rapidly spread to all G8 members, made the recently recruited Russia the most infected member, proliferated across an Africa that has secured major attention and attendance at G8 summits since 2001, threatened Eurasia and the G8's new 'Plus Five' partners of India and China, and was joined in 2006 by the threat of avian influenza.[5] In response, the old organisations of the UN system, led by the WHO, have proven increasingly ineffective, while the G8 countries alone possess the globally predominant and internally equal overall and specialised capabilities needed to combat the new diseases on a global scale. Their common principles of open democracy and social advance have brought them close to their newly democratic African and Plus Five partners and made them comfortable with the multi-stakeholder approaches most appropriate to combat the new generation of disease. From 2001 to 2005 the high political control at home of the popularly elected G8 leaders has allowed the same seven individuals to come to an unprecedented five summits in a row. Here they have met face to face each year with the same four core African partners, and been joined by four other outreach partners, in the still constricted and cosy leaders-dominated G8 club.

Driving this 21st-century takeoff in G8 health governance have been the complexities that globalisation has brought to the health field. The paradigm of health has changed, moving toward a conception that includes a breadth of socioeconomic, ecological, political security, and human rights factors as causes, consequences, and targets of health. There are more players on the field, with health NGOs and MNCs looking to have their say in the decision-making process. In this era of frequent air travel, the stakes are higher than ever because an infectious disease can travel from one continent to another in hours. And it can spread in an even more pervasive and uncontrollable way as migratory birds move around the world. The G8 is an informal international institution led by an annual summit where the world's most powerful leaders can comprehensively and swiftly address all policy areas across international and domestic domains, and make the complex connections among them in policy that map those in the physical world. It is thus uniquely well designed to generate the desired global health governance for this new world.

At their annual summits, the G8 leaders have brought health issues to the table to discuss the new realities presented by globalisation and assist the WHO in its efforts to contain the world's diseases. The rising panic over HIV/AIDS and the apparent threat it posed to the U.S. and Europe first drove the G8's concern. Other health concerns subsequently came onto the G8's agenda out of public panic over infectious diseases, such as SARS, bioterrorism, and avian influenza. The seven peaks in agenda attention reflect the contribution that health crises have made in stimulating and steering the G8's focus. At the Denver Summit in 1997 the G8 moved away from dealing with health sporadically whenever there was a crisis and began more sustained governance, with a growing performance in the deliberative, decision-making, and delivery domains. Up to 2003, Evian was the highest performer in all these functions and produced an entire collective document devoted to health.

This sustained period of attention and activity on diseases that do not primarily affect the G8 countries themselves has been driven by the weakness of the WHO. Its manifest failures in the face of the new fast-moving global pandemics have opened the door for other global organisations, especially those that can facilitate collaboration between the many participants now consequentially involved in the global health system. The flexibility of the G8 to expand the participants in its deliberations to include NGOs, MNCs, and the existing health organisations has been a great asset in its ability to achieve its health goals. This has been seen most clearly in the G8's effective leadership in creating the Global Fund to Fight AIDS, Tuberculosis, and Malaria, which now enjoys substantial financial and political support worldwide.

Future Challenges

This impressive past performance by the G8 confronts the stark and deadly realities of the growing global body count from preventable infectious diseases, the huge gaps in healthcare funding, systems, and practices in developing countries, and the large capacity the G8 possesses for closing these gaps. The need for even greater G8 leadership was underscored by the striking contrast between the world's two major summits that took place within a few months of each other in 2005.

On 6–8 July 2005, the G8 leaders met at their annual summit with their African and systemically significant partners at Gleneagles. There they issued a document that put health in a prominent place. Two months later, on 14–15 September, more than a hundred world leaders met at the UN in New York for their first summit in half a decade. They issued a document that in its priority passages (the first 16 paragraphs) noted the value or existence of health not at all (UN General Assembly 2005). In their overall documentary output, the Gleneagles G8 devoted 15 paragraphs to health, and the New York UN leaders only 10. Polio made the G8 but not the UN list. While the World Summit documents made more commitments on health than the Gleneagles G8 did, the UN leaders mobilised no new money to meet them. Indeed, the Gleneagles G8 leaders raised more money for global health than ever before.

There were thus good grounds for looking to the G8 as the primary global health governance platform on which to innovate in the years ahead. The 2006 St. Petersburg Summit, hosted for the first time by Russia, responded to the need, driven by Russia's position as the most vulnerable G8 partner to the infectious disease threat.

The rapid spread of avian influenza globally and into Russia and other G8 countries, constituting a second shock after SARS, helped lead Russia to select infectious diseases as one of its three summit priorities (Panova 2005; Savostiyanov 2005). In preparing for the summit, the Russians began with a wide-ranging and ambitious comprehensive programme for the control of infectious diseases, including AIDS, TB, malaria, polio, emerging diseases, and avian influenza. It embraced G8 measures to strengthen global information and analysis-monitoring networks for infectious diseases, a G8 plan of action to control avian influenza and prevent a pandemic, the prevention and mitigation of the epidemiological consequences of natural disasters (such as the shocks of the hurricanes that ravaged a vulnerable America in the summer of 2005, as well as the Asian tsunami and Pakistani earthquake), and scientific exchanges to study infectious disease agents, including those involved in bioterrorism. Largely absent from their agenda were their acute domestic health problems relating to alcoholism and poor diet, thus confirming the G8's evolution as an outward-looking centre of global health governance, rather than an inward-looking club focussed on its own citizens' health.

Proposals for Progress

To further the G8's growing performance as the centre of global health governance, there are several steps that the G8 at subsequent summits would be well advised to act upon (Kirton 2006). The first is to complete and expand the US$7 billion funding package required by the Global Fund for 2006–07, by doubling the funds committed at the pledging session held immediately after the Gleneagles Summit. The second is to devote resources to ensure that the WHO's failed '3 by 5' initiative is achieved within the next few years. The third is to commit to the resources and actions to ensure that the G8's commitment to eliminate polio is fulfilled within the next few years. The third is to ensure that the first ever meeting of G8 health ministers, called by the Russians, becomes a permanent, annual, G8 ministerial-centred institution, and that it quickly embraces a broad range of other relevant stakeholders as well. And the fifth is to endure that the G8's work on bioterrorism takes place in a way that is fully integrated with that of the highly effective Global Health Security Initiative.

Notes

1 The authors gratefully acknowledge the support of the Social Sciences and Humanities Research Council of Canada and the research assistance of Laura Sunderland and members of the G8 Research Group.
2 Data taken from the World Bank (2006).
3 Data taken from the World Bank (2006).
4 Mori, who was the secretary general of Japan's Liberal Democratic Party, became prime minister in April 2000 after his predecessor, Keizo Obuchi, suffered a fatal stroke.
5 The 'Plus Five' are the five countries whose leaders were invited to the outreach session on climate change at Gleneagles in 2005: Brazil, China, India, Mexico, and South Africa.

References

Aginam, Obijifor (2004). 'Salvaging Our Global Neighbourhood: Critical Reflections on the G8 Summit and Global Health Governance in an Interdependent World'. *Law, Social Justice, and Global Development,* vol. 1. <www2.warwick.ac.uk/fac/soc/law/elj/lgd/2004_1/aginam> (September 2006).

Aginam, Obijifor (2005). *Global Health Governance: International Law and Public Health in a Divided World* (Toronto: University of Toronto Press).

AVERT (2006a). 'HIV and AIDS: History, Pictures, and Posters'. <www.avert.org/historyi.htm> (September 2006).

AVERT (2006b). 'United States AIDS Cases and Deaths by Year'. <www.avert.org/usastaty.htm> (September 2006).

AVERT (2006c). 'United Kingdom Statistics by Year'. <www.avert.org/statsyr.htm> (September 2006).

AVERT (2006d). 'Canada Statistics by Year and Age'. <www.avert.org/canstatr.htm> (September 2006).

Bayne, Nicholas (1999). 'Continuity and Leadership in an Age of Globalisation'. In M.R. Hodges, J.J. Kirton, and J.P. Daniels, eds., *The G8's Role in the New Millennium,* pp. 21–44 (Aldershot: Ashgate).

Bayne, Nicholas (2000). *Hanging In There: The G7 and G8 Summit in Maturity and Renewal* (Aldershot: Ashgate).

Bayne, Nicholas (2001). 'Managing Globalisation and the New Economy: The Contribution of the G8 Summit'. In J.J. Kirton and G.M. von Furstenberg, eds., *New Directions in Global Economic Governance: Managing Globalisation in the Twenty-First Century,* pp. 171–188 (Aldershot: Ashgate).

Bayne, Nicholas (2002). 'Impressions of the Genoa Summit, 20–22 July, 2001'. In M. Fratianni, P. Savona, and J.J. Kirton, eds., *Governing Global Finance: New Challenges, G7 and IMF Contributions,* pp. 199–210 (Aldershot: Ashgate).

Bayne, Nicholas (2003). 'Impressions of the Kananaskis Summit'. In M. Fratianni, P. Savona, and J.J. Kirton, eds., *Sustaining Global Growth and Development: G7 and IMF Governance,* pp. 229–240 (Aldershot: Ashgate).

Bayne, Nicholas (2005). *Staying Together: The G8 Summit Confronts the 21st Century* (Aldershot: Ashgate).

Brundtland, Gro Harlem (2000). 'Address at the Opening Dinner of the Massive Effort Advocacy Meeting'. 3 October, Winterthur. <www.who.int/director-general/speeches/2000/english/20001003_massive_effort.html> (September 2006).

Commission on Macroeconomics and Health (2001). 'Macroeconomics and Health: Investing in Health for Economic Development'. World Health Organization, Geneva. <www.cid.harvard.edu/cidcmh/CMHReport.pdf> (September 2006).

Cooper, Richard N. (1989). 'International Cooperation in Public Health as a Prologue to Macroeconomic Cooperation'. In R.N. Cooper, ed., *Can Nations Agree? Issues in International Economic Cooperation,* pp. 183–190 (Washington DC: Brookings Institution).

Drohan, Madelaine (2005). 'Broken Promises'. *Literary Review of Canada,* vol. 13, no. 10, pp. 11–12.

European Centre for the Epidemiological Monitoring of AIDS (1998). 'HIV/AIDS Surveillance in Europe'. Quarterly Report No. 60, Saint-Maurice, France. <www-aids.med.unibo.it/eustat> (September 2006).

Fidler, David P. (2002). 'Global Health Governance: Overview of the Role of International Law in Protecting and Promoting Global Public Health'. Discussion Paper No. 3, World Health Organization and London School of Hygiene and Tropical Medicine, Geneva.

Fidler, David P. (2004). *SARS: Governance and the Globalization of Disease* (New York: Palgrave Macmillan).

Foster, John W. (2002). 'Canada and International Health: A Time of Testing on AIDS'. In N. Hillmer and M.A. Molot, eds., *Canada among Nations 2002: A Fading Power,* pp. 191–208 (Toronto: Oxford University Press).

Foster, John W. (2003). 'Canada's Foreign Policy in Health: Signs and Signals from HIV/AIDS'. Paper presented at the workshop on Canadian Foreign Policy and Global Health, Institut québécois des hautes études internationales and the North-South Institute, 5 December, Quebec City. <www.nsi-ins.ca/english/pdf/Cdn_policy_global_health.pdf> (September 2006).

France, Tim, Gorik Ooms, and Bernard Rivers (2002). 'The Global Fund: Which Countries Owe How Much?' Aidspan. <www.aidspan.org/Papers/GlobalFundContributions21April2002.htm> (September 2006).

G7 (1982). 'Report by François Mitterrand, President of the French Republic at the Summit of the Industrialized Nations' [Rapport de M. le Président de la République au Sommet des pays industrielles: technologie, emploi et croissance]. 10 June, Versailles. <www.g8.utoronto.ca/summit/1982versailles/report_english> (September 2006).

G7 (1987). 'Chairman's Statement on AIDS'. 10 June, Venice. <www.g8.utoronto.ca/summit/1987venice/aids.html> (September 2006).

G8 (2000). 'G8 Communiqué Okinawa 2000'. 23 July, Okinawa. <www.g8.utoronto.ca/summit/2000okinawa/finalcom.htm> (September 2006).

G8 (2002). 'G8 Africa Action Plan'. 27 June, Kananaskis. <www.g8.utoronto.ca/summit/2002kananaskis/africaplan.html> (September 2006).

G8 (2003). 'Health: A G8 Action Plan'. 2 June, Evian. <www.g8.utoronto.ca/summit/2003evian/health_en.html> (September 2006).

G8 (2005). 'Chair's Summary'. 8 July, Gleneagles. <www.g8.utoronto.ca/summit/2005gleneagles/summary.html> (September 2006).

'G8 Failed to Tackle the Toxic Politics of Drug Making and Selling'. (2003). *East African,* 10 June.

G8 Research Group (2000). '2000 Okinawa Summit Performance Assessments'. <www.g8.utoronto.ca/evaluations/2000okinawa/country.htm#issues> (September 2006).

G8 Research Group (2004a). '2003 Evian Final Compliance Report'. <www.g8.utoronto.ca/evaluations/2003evian_comp_final> (September 2006).

G8 Research Group (2004b). '2003 Evian Interim Compliance Report'. <www.g8.utoronto.ca/evaluations/2003evian_comp_interim> (September 2006).

G8 Research Group (2006). '2005 Gleneagles Final Compliance Report'. <www.g8.utoronto.ca/evaluations/2005compliance_final> (September 2006).

Gagel, Sabine and Elodie Niederlaender (2004). 'VIH et SIDA dans l'Union europeénne' [HIV and AIDS in the European Union]. Eurostat. <epp.eurostat.cec.eu.int/cache/ITY_OFFPUB/KS-NK-04-018/FR/KS-NK-04-018-FR.PDF> (September 2006).

Global Markets Institute (2006). 'G8 Summit in St. Petersburg'. Poll conducted for the 2006 St. Petersburg Summit, Goldman Sachs, New York.

Godlee, Fiona (1994). 'WHO in Retreat: Is It Losing Its Influence?' *British Medical Journal,* vol. 309, no. 6967, pp. 1491–1495.

Hajnal, Peter I. (1999). *The G7/G8 System: Evolution, Role, and Documentation* (Aldershot: Ashgate).

Health Canada (2000). 'HIV and AIDS in Canada: Surveillance Report to December 31, 1999'. Ottawa. <www.phac-aspc.gc.ca/publicat/aids-sida/aic04-00/pdf/aic0400e.pdf> (September 2006).

Howard, Lee (1989). 'The Evolution of Bilateral and Multilateral Cooperation for Health in Developing Countries'. In M.R. Reich and E. Marui, eds., *International Cooperation for Health: Problems, Prospects, and Priorities* (Dover MA: Auburn House).

Infectious Disease Surveillance Center (Japan) (2006). 'Index of IASR Topics'. <idsc.nih.go.jp/iasr/iasr-ge1.html> (September 2006).

International Labour Organization (2003). 'The HIV/AIDS Epidemic in the Russian Federation'. <www.ilo.ru/aids/docs/dec02/cis/Russia-eng.pdf> (September 2006).

Italy [G8 Host] (2001). 'Beyond Debt Relief'. Genoa. <www.g8.utoronto.ca/summit/2001genoa/pres_docs/pres_doc2.html> (September 2006).

Kickbusch, Ilona (2000). 'The Development of International Health Policies — Accountability Intact?' *Social Science and Medicine,* vol. 51, no. 6, pp. 979–989.

Kickbusch, Ilona (2003). 'The Contribution of the World Health Organization to a New Public Health and Health Promotion'. *American Journal of Public Health,* vol. 93, no. 3, pp. 383–388. <www.ajph.org/cgi/content/full/93/3/383> (September 2006).

Kirton, John J. (2004). 'Explaining G8 Effectiveness: A Concert of Vulnerable Equals in a Globalizing World'. Paper prepared for the International Studies Association conference, 17–20 March, Montreal. <www.g8.utoronto.ca/scholar/kirton2004/kirton_isa_040304.pdf> (September 2006).

Kirton, John J. (2005a). 'America at the G8: From Vulnerability to Victory at the Sea Island Summit'. In M. Fratianni, J.J. Kirton, A.M. Rugman, *et al.*, eds., *New Perspectives on Global Governance: Why America Needs the G8,* pp. 31–50 (Aldershot: Ashgate).

Kirton, John J. (2005b). 'Gleneagles G8 Boosts Blair at Home'. 1 August, G8 Research Group, Toronto. <www.g8.utoronto.ca/evaluations/2005gleneagles/coverage.html> (September 2006).

Kirton, John J. (2006). 'The G8 and Global Health Governance: The Case for a 2006 Eurasian HIV/AIDS Initiative'. Paper prepared for the International Parliamentary Conference in Conjunction with Russia's G8 Presidency on HIV/AIDS in Eurasia and the Role of the G8, sponsored by the Transatlantic Partners Against AIDS, 8 June, Moscow. <www.g8.utoronto.ca/scholar/kirton2006/kirton_health_060609.pdf> (September 2006).

Labonté, Ronald and Ted Schrecker (2004). 'Committed to Health for All? How the G7/8 Rate'. *Social Science and Medicine,* vol. 59, no. 8, pp. 1661–1676.

Labonté, Ronald, Ted Schrecker, David Sanders, *et al.* (2004). *Fatal Indifference: The G8, Africa, and Global Health* (Cape Town: University of Cape Town Press).

Lewis, Stephen (2005). *Race against Time: Searching for Hope in AIDS-Ravaged Africa* (Toronto: House of Anansi).

Orbinski, James (2002). 'AIDS, Médecins Sans Frontières, and Access to Essential Medicines'. In P.I. Hajnal, ed., *Civil Society in the Information Age,* pp. 127–135 (Aldershot: Ashgate).

Pannenborg, Charles O. (1979). *A New International Health Order: An Inquiry into the International Relations of World Health and Medical Care* (Alphen aan den Rijn, Netherlands: Sijthoff and Noordhoff).

Panova, Victoria (2005). 'Impressions of the 2005 Gleneagles Summit'. 18 July, G8 Research Group. <www.g8.utoronto.ca/evaluations/2005gleneagles/panova2005-0718.html> (September 2006).

Picard, André (2001). 'Malaria Cases Soar in Canada'. *Globe and Mail,* 6 March.

Price-Smith, Andrew (2001). *Plagues and Politics: Infectious Disease and International Policy* (New York: Palgrave).

Price-Smith, Andrew (2002). *The Health of Nations: Infectious Disease, Environmental Change, and Their Effects on National Security and Development* (Cambridge MA: MIT Press).

Savona, Paolo and Chiara Oldani (2003). 'Globalisation: The Private Sector Perspective'. In M. Fratianni, P. Savona, and J.J. Kirton, eds., *Sustaining Global Growth and Development: G7 and IMF Governance,* pp. 99–112 (Aldershot: Ashgate).

Savostiyanov, Mikhail (2005). 'Presentation at the Pre-G8 Summit Academic Conference'. Paper presented at the conference on Development, Sustainability and Finance: The Role of the G8 and the Gleneagles Summit, University of Glasgow, 29–30 June, Glasgow. <www.g8.utoronto.ca/conferences/2005/conf/savostiyanov.html> (September 2006).

UNAIDS (2005). 'AIDS Epidemic Update: December 2005'. <www.unaids.org/epi/2005/doc/EPIupdate2005_html_en/epi05_00_en.htm> (September 2006).

UNAIDS (2006). '2006 Report on the Global AIDS Epidemic'. Geneva. <www.unaids.org/en/HIV_data/2006GlobalReport/default.asp> (September 2006).

United Nations General Assembly (2005). '2005 World Summit Outcome'. 15 September. <www.un.org/summit2005/documents.html> (September 2006).

Vandemoortele, Jan (2003). 'The MDGs and Pro-Poor Policies: Can External Partners Make a Difference?' Paper prepared for the annual Global Development Conference of the Global Development Network on Understanding Reform, 28–30 January, New Delhi. <www.gdnet.org/pdf2/gdn_library/annual_conferences/fifth_annual_conference/vandemoortele_paper.pdf> (September 2006).

World Bank (2006). 'HNP Comparative Data' [Database]. <devdata.worldbank.org/hnpstats/cd3.asp> (September 2006).

World Health Organization (1997). 'The Denver G8 Summit Highlights Infectious Disease'. Press release WHO/50, 24 June, Geneva.

World Health Organization (2005). 'World Health Assembly Official Records'. <policy.who.int/cgi-bin/om_isapi.dll?infobase=wharec-e&softpage=Browse_Frame_Pg42> (September 2006).

World Health Organization (2006a). 'Situation Updates — Avian Influenza'. Geneva. <www.who.int/csr/disease/avian_influenza/updates/en> (September 2006).

World Health Organization (2006b). 'Cumulative Number of Reported Probably Cases of Severe Acute Respiratory Syndrome (SARS)'. Geneva. <www.who.int/csr/sars/country/en> (September 2006).

World Health Organization (2006c). 'Reports on Global HIV/AIDS Situation'. Geneva. <www.who.int/hiv/epiupdates/en> (September 2006).

Zacher, Mark W. (1999). 'Global Epidemiological Surveillance: International Cooperation to Monitor Infectious Diseases'. In I. Kaul, I. Grunberg, and M.A. Stern, eds., *Global Public Goods: International Cooperation in the 21st Century,* pp. 266–283 (New York: Oxford University Press for the United Nations Development Programme).

Zupi, Marco (2001). 'The Genoa G8 Summit: Great Expectations, Disappointing Results'. *International Spectator,* vol. 36, no. 3, p. 59.

Appendix 9-1
Pattern of G8 Health Performance

	Deliberative	Directional	Decisional: commitments	Decisional: money	Delivery	Development of Global Governance	Score
1975	0	0	0	0	–	0	–
1976	0	0	0	0	–	0	–
1977	0	0	0	0	–	0	–
1978	0	0	0	0	–	0	–
1979	1	0	0	0	–	0	–
1980	1	0	0	0	–	0	–
1981	0	0	0	0	–	0	–
1982	4	0	0	0	–	0	–
1983	1	0	1	0	–	0	N/A
1984	1	0	0	0	–	0	–
1985	2	0	0	0	–	0	–
1986	2	0	1	0	–	0	N/A
1987	7	0	0	0	–	1	–
1988	2	0	0	0	–	0	–
1989	3	0	0	0	–	0	–
1990	7	0	0	0	–	0	–
1991	9	0	1	0	–	0	N/A
1992	3	0	0	0	–	1	–
1993	3	0	1	0	–	0	N/A
1994	2	0	0	0	–	0	–
1995	2	0	0	0	–	0	–
1996	14	0	4	0	–	0	N/A
1997	17	0	7	0	–	0	A
1998	6	0	4	0	+26%	0	B+
1999	11	0	3	0	+32%	0	N/A
2000	30	0	11	0	+87%[a]	0	**A+**
2001	15	0	3	$1.3 billion	+75%[a]	1	N/A
2002	19	2	19	0	+38%[b]	1	B–
2003	50	6	**21**	$500 million	**+89%**[c]	**2**	N/A
2004	36	5	12	$3.3 billion	+50%	1	N/A
2005	22	1	18	$24 billion	+22%	0	–
2006	**84**	**8**	52	**$4.4 billion**	N/A	1	A–

Notes: If no figure is indicated, no significant references to health were made by the G8 in that year. N/A = No data available. Note that the Global Fund to Fight AIDS, Tuberculosis, and Malaria was established in 2001. Peak scores are in bold. Deliberative = references in annual documentation, unit is paragraph, includes chair's summary. Directional = references in summit chapeau or chair's summary, unit is paragraph. Development of global governance = the number of G8-centred health institutions created at the official or ministerial level during the summit hosting year; includes G8 health ministers meeting in 2006. N/A = not available.

Sources: Compliance reports completed by the University of Toronto G8 Research Group available at <www.g8.utoronto.ca/compliance>.

Appendix 9-2
New Cases of AIDS per Year in G8 Countries

	G7 average[a]	U.S.	Japan	Germany	France	UK	Italy	Canada	Russia[b]
1979								1	
1980				0	4		0	5	0
1981		339		1	8		0	9	0
1982		1201		9	31		1	26	0
1983		3153		40	92		8	68	0
1984		6368		116	236		37	167	0
1985	2254	12 044	6	311	583	–	198	381	1
1986	3726	19 414	5	573	1259	–	458	647	–
1987	5736	29 105	14	1038	2252	–	1030	977	–
1988	7238	36 126	14	1268	3054	–	1775	1190	–
1989	8803	43 499	21	1589	3809	–	2482	1420	–
1990	8758	49 546	31	1553	4320	1241	3134	1478	103
1991	10 553	60 573	35	1767	4657	1393	3827	1622	81
1992	13 480	79 657	51	1811	5183	1579	4261	1817	87
1993	**13 688**	**79 879**	85	1900	5514	1788	4818	**1889**	106
1994	12 875	73 086	135	**1913**	**5737**	**1851**	5522	1882	156
1995	11 653	69 984	169	1695	5253	1771	**5659**	1773	198
1996	10 618	61 124	234	1358	3941	1443	4997	1230	1526
1997	8251	49 379	250	773	2168	1078	3292	815	1804
1998	6959	43 225	231	442	1335	792	1926	762	8067
1999	8024	41 356	300	–	1808	756	3220	701	19 846
2000	6376	39 513	327	736	1717	830	2026	481	59 340
2001	6404	39 206	332	693	1679	728	1797	395	**88 422**
2002	7373	40 267	308	655	–	877	1753	380	
2003	6602	41 831	336	353	686	908	1759	349	39 699[c]
2004	9169	42 514	**385**	–	2697	813	–	237	–
Number of people living with HIV (G8 total = 2 497 000)									
2005	312 125	1 200 000	17 000	49 000	13 000	68 000	150 000	60 000	94 000

Notes: This table does not include HIV statistics. In most G8 countries HIV prevalence is currently rising rapidly (the epidemic is unclear in France and Italy) (see UNAIDS 2005). Peak scores are in bold.

[a] Does not include Russia, for which data were available only on HIV, not AIDS.

[b] Russian statistics are based on HIV-positive testing, not AIDS cases.

[c] The apparent decline in HIV prevalence in Russia 'appears not to have represented an actual slowing of the epidemic; it reflected changes in HIV testing policy, the smaller number of tests carried out in population groups with high-risk behaviour (especially drug injectors and prisoners), and shortages of test kits' (UNAIDS 2005, 46).

Sources: AVERT (2006b; 2006c; 2006d) Health Canada (2000), European Centre for the Epidemiological Monitoring of AIDS (1998), Gagel and Niederlaender (2004), Infectious Disease Surveillance Center (2006), International Labour Organization (2003).

Appendix 9-3
Global HIV/AIDS Cases

Year	New Infections	Cumulative Infections (AIDS)	Cumulative No. people living with HIV/AIDS	Annual Deaths	Cumulative Deaths	Number in Treatment
1970–80	*100 000–300 000*					
1983[a]	3064			1292		
1984[b]		8569			3711	
1985		20 303				
1986		38 401				
1987		71 751				
1988						
1989		142 000[c]	5 000 000–10 000 000			
1990		307 000[d]	8 000 000–10 000 000			
1991		450 000[e]	9 000 000–11 000 000			
1992						
1993						
1994		985 119				
1995	*4 700 000*	1 291 810				
1996[g]	*3 000 000*		*23 000 000*		*6 400 000*	
1997				*2 300 000*		
1998	*5 800 000*					
1999			*33 000 000*	*2 600 000*		
2000	5 300 000		36 100 000	3 000 000	21 800 000	
2001	5 000 000	35 000 000	40 000 000	3 000 000		
2002	5 000 000		42 000 000	3 100 000		
2003	5 000 000	38 000 000	40 000 000	3 000 000		
2004						
2005	4 900 000	40 300 000	*38 600 000*	3 100 000	25 000 000+	1 000 000

Notes: Italics indicates the figure is an estimate.

[a] Data for United States only.

[b] Data for United States and Europe only.

[c] Number of reported AIDS cases; World Health Organization (WHO) estimated that actual number (beyond those reported) was more than 400 000.

[d] Number of reported AIDS cases; WHO estimated that actual number (beyond those reported) was closer to 1 million.

[e] Number of reported AIDS cases; WHO estimated that actual number (beyond those reported) was 1.5 million.

[f] UNAIDS became operational on 1 January 1996, bringing new methodologies for reporting and estimating cases.

Sources: AVERT (2006a), UNAIDS (2006), WHO (2006c).

Appendix 9-4
Cumulative (Probable) Cases of Severe Acute Respiratory Syndrome World-Wide, 2003

Country	February	March	April	May	June	July	Final (December)
Asia (excluding G8)							
Vietnam	1:0	54:4	63:5	63:5	63:5	63:5	63:5
Hong Kong		530:13	1589:157	1739:278	1755:298	1755:298	1755:299
Singapore		91:2	201:24	206:31	206:32	206:32	238:33
Thailand		5:1	7:2	8:2	9:2	9:2	9:2
Taiwan		10:0	78:1	676:81	678:84	671:84	346:37
Macao			1:0	1:0	1:0	1:0	1:0
Malaysia			6:2	5:2	5:2	5:2	5:2
Mongolia			6:0	9:0	9:0	9:0	9:0
Philippines			4:2	12:2	14:2	14:2	14:2
Korea			1:0	3:0	3:0	3:0	3:0
G8							
Canada		44:4	148:20	188:30	252:37	250:38	251:43
Germany		5:0	7:0	10:0	10:0	10:0	9:0
UK		3:0	6:0	4:0	4:0	4:0	4:0
Ireland		2:0	1:0	1:0	1:0	1:0	1:0
U.S.		59:0	52:0	66:0	73:0	75:0	27:0
Italy		2:0	9:0	9:0	5:0	4:0	4:0
France		1:0	5:0	7:0	7:0	7:1	7:1
Japan			2:0				
Russia				1:0	1:0	1:0	1:0
European Union							
Spain			1:0	1:0	1:0	1:0	1:0
Sweden			3:0	3:0	3:0	3:0	5:0
Finland				1:0	1:0	1:0	
G20							
Australia			4:0	6:0	5:0	5:0	6:0
Brazil			2:0	2:0	3:0	1:0	
China		806:34	3460:159	5328:332	5327:348	5327:348	5327:349
India				3:0	3:0	–	3:0
Indonesia			2:0	2:0	2:0	2:0	2:0
South Africa			1:0	1:1	1:1	1:1	1:1
Other European Countries							
Romania		3:0	1:0	1:0	1:0	1:0	1:0
Switzerland		3:0	1:0	1:0	1:0	1:0	1:0
Bulgaria			1:0				
Other Countries							
Kuwait			1:0	1:0	1:0	1:0	1:0
Colombia				1:0	1:0	1:0	
New Zealand				1:0	1:0	1:0	1:0
TOTAL	/	1622:58	5663:372	8360:764	8447:811	8437:813	8098:774

Note: Reported cases : reported deaths.

Source: WHO (2006b).

Appendix 9-5
Confirmed Cases (Cumulative) of Avian Influenza

Country	1996–2003	2003–2004	2004 (Jan.–June)	2004 (July–Dec.)	2005 (Jan.–June)	2005 (July–Dec.)	2006 (Jan.–June)	July 2006	Total human cases: deaths[a]
Asia (excluding G8 and G12)									
Thailand		P:0:0	P:12:8	P:17:12[b]	P:0:0	P:22:14		P:23:25	23:25
Vietnam			P:23:16	P:27:20	P:33:20	P:66:22			66:22
Cambodia			P:0:0	P:0:0	P:4:4		P:6:6		6:6
Lao PDR			P:0:0	P:0:0					0
Malaysia				P:0:0					0
Mongolia						P:0:0			0
Europe (excluding European Union)									
Kazakhstan						P:0:0			0
Romania						P:0:0			0
Croatia						P:0:0			0
Turkey						P:0:0	P:21:4		21:4
Azerbaijan							P:8:5		8:5
Bulgaria							P:0:0		0
Slovenia							P:0:0		0
G12									
Hong Kong	P:18:6	0:20:7							20:7
China	P:0:0		P:0:0	P:0:0	P:0:0	P:7:3	P:19:12		19:12
Korea		P:0:0							0
Indonesia			P:0:0	P:0:0		P:16:11	P:51:39	P:54:42	54:42
India							P:0:0		0
G8									
Japan			P:0:0						0
Russia						P:0:0			0
UK						P0:0			0
Canada						P:0:0			0
Italy							P:0:0		0
Germany							P:0:0		0
France							P:0:0		0
European Union									
Belgium				P:0:0					0
Greece							P:0:0		0
Austria							P:0:0		0
Sweden							P:0:0		0
Middle East									
Iraq							P:2:2		2:2
Iran							P:0:0		0
Egypt							P:14:6		14:6
Afghanistan							P:0:0		0
Africa									
Nigeria							P:0:0		0
Niger							P:0:0		0
Djibouti							P:1:0		1:0
TOTAL									234:126

Notes: Mortality rate from cases of avian influenza in humans is approximately 54 percent. Ratio used is birds infected : human cases : human deaths. P = Poultry outbreak.

[a] All cases confirmed by laboratory tests, not accounting for all suspected or probable human infections.

[b] First case of human-to-human transmission.

Source: WHO (2006a).

Chapter 10

Diplomatic Rhetoric or Rhetorical Diplomacy: The G8 and Global Health Governance

Obijiofor Aginam

Health is a state of complete physical, mental and social well-being and not merely the absence of disease or infirmity. The enjoyment of the highest attainable standard of health is one of the fundamental rights of every human being without distinction of race, religion, political belief, economic or social condition.

— Preamble to the Constitution of the World Health Organization

It follows that unequal development in the promotion of health in different countries, and particularly in the control of disease, is a common danger. This is well demonstrated not only by past epidemics but currently by the pervasive threat of HIV/AIDS which has not been successfully contained in any one jurisdiction, and which has also destabilized several nations.

— Frank Grad

In the past two decades, public health has emerged as a foreign policy issue. In the global context, the transnational menace of infectious and non-communicable diseases in a globalising world has immersed all of humanity in a single microbial sea. Both the dominant traditional international governance actors in the Westphalian system — nation-states and multilateral institutions — and emerging actors in global governance — nongovernmental organisations (NGOs) and civil society, philanthropic and charitable organisations, foundations, businesses, and corporations — agree that inherited models of global health governance have become ineffective in the face of the global crisis of emerging and re-emerging infectious and non-communicable diseases. The vulnerability of humans to microbial threats in a globalising world calls for a reassessment of the traditional Westphalian model of global health governance (Fidler 1999, 2001; Aginam 2005; Nakajima 1997; Price-Smith 2001; Foster 2002).

This chapter offers a critical assessment of the actual and potential contributions of an emergent powerful actor in global health governance, the G8. Successive G8 summits, at least since 2000, have made global health more conspicuous in the annual summit of the world's major industrial democracies. Yet a critical assessment of G8 commitments to global health manifests an appalling disconnect with other normative and multilateral mechanisms on global health (Labonté *et al.* 2004; Aginam 2004). This chapter focusses on three G8 summits: Okinawa, Japan (2000), Genoa, Italy (2001), and Kananaskis, Canada (2002). Although Okinawa and Genoa catalysed the establishment of the Geneva-based Global Fund to Fight AIDS, Tuberculosis, and Malaria as a public-private partnership, the G8's commitment to global health governance must nonetheless align with existing global health mechanisms in mutually reinforcing ways to diminish human vulnerability to disease globally. The key question therefore is not whether the G8 is a relevant actor in global health governance, but rather whether the G8 could fill or has already filled the vacuum in global health governance created by the inadequacy of the Westphalian model. To do this, there has to be convincing evidence that G8 commitments to global health correspond to and engage with existing multilateral normative and policy frameworks to boost the effectiveness of the Westphalian model. Is the G8 summit a forum for incubating humane global health governance norms, or is it a diplomatic forum for rhetoric with little concrete action and few results in the underdeveloped countries where vulnerable populations live their daily lives with the heaviest mortality and morbidity burdens of infectious and non-communicable diseases? In answering these questions, this chapter explores the relationship between the G8 and the emerging trends at the World Trade Organization (WTO) to enable developing countries to use the flexibility of the WTO's Trade-Related Aspects of Intellectual Property Rights (TRIPS) to maximise access to essential medicines for prevailing diseases such as HIV/AIDS, malaria, and tuberculosis (TB).

There are two reasons why the G8 commitments to global health governance must be assessed in terms of their alignment and engagement or, otherwise, with existing multilateral health governance mechanisms. First, the G8 countries should not contribute something to global health governance in one way, for instance through the establishment of the Global Fund, and then denigrate global health in another forum, for example, by not facilitating the process of making TRIPS flexibilities on essential medicines available to developing countries at the WTO. Second, Westphalian and emerging post-Westphalian global health governance mechanisms within and outside the United Nations system must be coherent and sustainable. All relevant actors of global health governance, both the traditional actors in the Westphalian system and the emerging actors in a post-Westphalian architecture, must assess the policy coherence, commonalities, and tensions across their respective mandates. Within the UN system, as observed by Christopher Weeramantry, former vice-president of the International Court of Justice,

> the United Nations family of organizations today is widely expanded, closely knit, and works together, in developing areas of international activity, within the framework of the international rule of law. While each of these organizations has its specific functions, they all interlock in the common service of the ideals of the United Nations and they all operate under the common aegis of international law. Though each of them is given a particular sphere of activity, they do not necessarily function in closed compartments, for the complex nature of United Nations activities may often result in overlapping areas of

interest. The work of one organization may interweave with that of other organizations, and hence would have repercussions on the work of other members of the United Nations family (International Court of Justice 1996).

This persuasive judicial opinion, although limited to multilateralism within the UN system, provides a framework for fresh thinking on effective policy coherence at the global level involving a multiplicity of global health governance actors within and outside the UN system: the World Health Organization (WHO), the WTO, the World Bank, the G8, and the emerging non-state actors.

The G8 as an Emerging Actor in Global Health Governance

The G8 countries, as the major industrial democracies, control a considerable percentage of global capital in trade, finance, and foreign direct investment (FDI). The summit gives direction to the international community by setting priorities and delivering guidance to established international organisations (G8 Research Group 2006). Michael Hodges (1999, 69) refers to the G8 summit as a think tank that includes 'the individuals who matter most in the world'. Successive G8 summits have discussed international trade, migration, debt, the global digital divide, the environment, crime and drugs, transnational security issues and arms control, terrorism, hunger and food safety, poverty reduction, and global infectious disease challenges. The 2000 Okinawa Summit focussed on the global and multilateral governance of leading infectious d-iseases. The G8 leaders committed to address the global challenges posed by leading infectious and parasitic diseases — HIV/AIDS, TB, and malaria. The summit recognised health as the key to economic posterity by linking health to development (see Chapter 9). At Okinawa, the G8 committed to working in strengthened partnerships with governments, the WHO and other multilateral institutions, industry (especially pharmaceutical companies), academic institutions, NGOs, and other civil society actors to deliver three critical UN targets: reducing the number of HIV/AIDS-infected young people by 25 percent in 2010 pursuant to UN Secretary General's Report to the General Assembly in March 2000, reducing TB mortality rates and prevalence burdens by 50 percent in 2010 pursuant to the WHO's Stop TB Partnership, and reducing the burden of disease associated with malaria by 50 percent in 2010 pursuant to the Roll Back Malaria Partnership, launched in 1998 by the WHO, the United Nations Children's Fund (UNICEF), the United Nations Development Programme (UNDP), and the World Bank (G8 2000). To achieve these targets, the G8 committed to support innovative partnerships, including NGOs and private sector and multilateral organisations, and to explore the evolution of an innovative governance strategy to accomplish these commitments. The Okinawa International Conference on Infectious Diseases held in December 2000 paved the way for the commitments made by the 2001 Genoa Summit to reduce the burdens of HIV/AIDS, TB, and malaria through the establishment of the Global Fund.

In 2001, the Genoa Summit pledged US$1.3 billion to the Global Fund. As a public-private partnership, the fund aimed at promoting an integrated approach to these three killer diseases by emphasising prevention, treatment, and care (see Chapter 11). While pledging its support, the G8 also promised to work with the pharmaceutical industry together with the affected countries to facilitate the broadest possible provision of drugs in an affordable and medically effective manner. The summit reaffirmed the commitment of the G8 toward balancing the intellectual property and public health imperatives of the TRIPS Agreement (G8 2001). In the context of this specific G8 commitment, it is imperative to inquire whether the balance of intellectual property and public health imperatives of TRIPS is being achieved. If indeed it is, did the G8 countries individually or collectively facilitate it?

The World Trade Organization, Access to Essential Medicines, and G8 Responses

The tension between intellectual property rights driven by economic globalisation and the promotion of public health as a global public good is exemplified by the norms of the free trade architecture enforced by the WTO.[1] The TRIPS Agreement is the embodiment of the tension between the right to life and essential medicines on the one hand, and profit maximisation and incentives for drug discovery by pharmaceutical corporations on the other. TRIPS, which was part of the Marrakesh Agreement that established the WTO in 1995, covers both aspects of intellectual property rights: literary and artistic property (copyrights and neighbouring rights) and industrial property (trademarks, patents, geographical indications, industrial designs, and trade secrets). The TRIPS Agreement seeks to harmonise certain aspects of intellectual property rights at the global level. It sets a minimum standard of intellectual property protection for all WTO member states' national legislation. Patent protection for pharmaceuticals is set for a minimum of 20 years.[2] Although the TRIPS Agreement has flexibilities, subject to certain conditions, that allow parallel importation and compulsory licensing, legitimate efforts by a few developing countries to make use of these flexibilities, even in the face of very high prevalence of HIV/AIDS in South Africa and Brazil, were rebuffed by a few industrialised states led by the United States (Thomas 2002; Bass 2002; t'Hoen 2002).

On 14 November 2001, after prolonged agitation by developing countries and sustained advocacy by a coalition of civil society groups, the WTO ministerial conference in Doha adopted the Declaration on the TRIPS Agreement and Public Health (WTO 2001b; see also Gathii 2002). The declaration affirmed that TRIPS can and should be interpreted and implemented in a manner supportive of WTO members' right to protect public health and, in particular, to promote access to medicines for all (WTO 2001a, para. 4). It recognised that WTO members with insufficient or no manufacturing capacities in the pharmaceutical sector could face difficulties in making effective use of compulsory licensing under the TRIPS Agreement (para. 6). On 30 August 2003, the WTO's General Council adopted a decision on the Implementation of Paragraph 6 of the Declaration on the TRIPS Agreement and Public Health (WTO 2003). The decision provides for the criteria aimed at facilitating access to essential medicines, including antiretroviral treatment (ART) for HIV/AIDS, by vulnerable populations in the least developed and developing countries.

Despite the General Council's decision in 2003, difficult questions remain on the best ways to maximise access to essential medicines, especially ART. While the decision imposes certain key obligations on exporting and importing countries for these medicines, only two industrialised countries — Canada and Norway — have initiated legislative changes to patent laws to allow domestic production of generic drugs for export to poor countries hit by HIV/AIDS and other diseases. The decision imposes an obligation on developing countries to notify the WTO of an intention to become an eligible importing member and to notify the WTO specifically about the products and quantities (see Correa 2004).

While the General Council decision is promising, the fact remains that more than 90 percent of developing country members of the WTO lack a functional and thriving pharmaceutical sector with the capacity for domestic production of ART and essential medicines for other killer diseases such as malaria. These countries cannot issue compulsory licences for domestic production of generic HIV/AIDS drugs because they lack the functional pharmaceutical and technological capacity to do so. But the WTO decision offered another opportunity for such countries that involves importing generics from an industrialised country willing to amend its patent legislation to allow the export of generics. This would largely depend on whether such industrialised countries could withstand the corporate lobby by powerful pharmaceutical giants that have patent rights on essential HIV/AIDS drugs. If the experience of the TRIPS negotiations in the 1990s is anything to go by, the industry lobby remains very influential and powerful in international economic relations. The entire gamut of international trade and global economic relations is now shaped by the 'neo-liberal dogma of minimizing intrusions on the market, and "downsizing" the role of government in relation to the provision of public goods that compose the social agenda' (Falk 1998b, 15). The establishment of the WTO has challenged the actors in global governance (both states and non-states) to take the task of balancing neo-liberal ideology with the promotion of global public goods seriously.

To date, Canada has remained, in the context of the WTO's General Council decision, the only G8 member ever to initiate a legislative process aimed at reconciling its WTO-TRIPS obligations with facilitating access to essential medicines in developing countries. In May 2004, the Canadian Parliament passed Bill C-9, which amended the *Patent Act* and the *Food and Drugs Act*. The amendments affirmed Canada's intention to respond to the WTO decision by initiating practical steps that would allow Canadian generic drug companies to negotiate contracts for the production and export of patented drugs to developing countries based on need (see Orbinski 2004; Elliott 2006). Bill C-9 has many restrictions and preconditions, for instance, by maintaining a list of drugs subject to the legislation, a list of countries eligible to use flexibilities in the legislation, and approvals by the Canadian Commission of Patents and other relevant governmental agencies. Nonetheless, other G8 countries should individually and collectively follow and possibly improve on the Canadian initiative. It follows that the pledge by the 2001 Genoa Summit to balance the intellectual property and public health imperatives of the TRIPS Agreement, which has resonated in somewhat different language in successive G8 summit statements, amounts to rhetorical diplomacy or diplomatic rhetoric if these powerful industrialised countries cannot take concrete and practical steps either within the WTO or individually, as Canada has done, to work toward achieving this commitment to global health.

Conclusion: From Diplomatic Rhetoric to Humane Diplomacy

The conspiracy between disease and the conditions of chronic underdevelopment, especially in most underdeveloped and developing countries, poses a serious challenge to emerging norms of global health governance. The embedded orthodoxy of drawing a distinction between diseases of the global economic South and those of the global economic North has been shattered by the globalisation of public health (Lee and Dodgson 2000; Yach and Bettcher 1998a, 1998b). Since infallible evidence now links socioeconomic underdevelopment in developing countries with the mortality and morbidity burdens of leading killer diseases — HIV/AIDS, TB, and malaria — the global health and developmental communities must strive to redistribute the dividends of health as a public good across societies in the emerging global village. The G8 summit's commitments on debt and other aspects of socioeconomic development in the developing world would remain lopsided if public health remains at the peripheries of these global initiatives. The report of the WHO's Commission on Macroeconomics and Health (2001, 1) offers convincing evidence of the links among poverty, development, and disease, and how the endless cycle of poverty, disease, and underdevelopment could be addressed in multilateral health governance. The commission argued that health is inexorably linked to poverty reduction as well as to long-term economic growth. The mortality and morbidity burdens of disease in some low-income regions, especially Africa, impede economic growth and therefore must be addressed centrally in any comprehensive development strategy (1). The challenges posed by HIV/AIDS undoubtedly requires a global policy universe and humane governance framework involving a multiplicity of actors — international organisations, private and corporate actors, and civil society. An indispensable part of this governance architecture, in an era of globalised public health, lies within the normative boundaries of Richard Falk's (1998a, 33) 'law of humanity'. An imperative for humane governance is further compelled by the fact that normatively, there is a preponderance of opinion that contemporary global governance is distorted in so far as it promotes the interests of the most powerful states and global social forces and restricts the realisation of greater global social justice and human security, thereby propelling the dynamics of inequalities of power between states and the structural privileging of the interests and agenda of global capital (Held and McGrew 2002, 13). Evolving governance structures must focus on the 'world' as its primary constituency, and humanity (human life) as the endangered species that it seeks to conserve. While the G8 and the WTO must be commended for their Okinawa initiative to establish the Global Fund and the Doha declaration respectively, they both must be reminded constantly that they have a duty to millions of vulnerable populations globally whose lives are viciously threatened by the mortality and morbidity burdens of HIV/AIDS and other opportunistic infections as well as by chronic conditions of underdevelopment. The G8 has a prominent role to play in addressing global health problems in the context of socioeconomic development. While these eight powerful countries have done well to elevate global health as an important foreign policy issue in recent years, they need to do more individually and collectively toward policy coherence and sustainability of their commitments in the context of other multilateral health commitments in other forums: the WHO, the WTO, and the Global Fund. Genuine pursuit of this coherence and sustainability in global health governance will likely transform the G8 summit commitments from rhetorical to humane diplomacy.

Notes

1 For a history of international trade and the evolution of the WTO, including the agreements under its mandate, see John Jackson (1997) and Michael Trebilcock and Robert Howse (2001). On the tension between trade liberalisation and the promotion of human rights in the global economy, see Robert Howse and Makao wa Matua (2000).

2 For an insightful discussion of TRIPS in the context of global health and access to drugs, see Susan Sell (2003, 2004).

References

Aginam, Obijifor (2004). 'Salvaging Our Global Neighbourhood: Critical Reflections on the G8 Summit and Global Health Governance in an Interdependent World'. *Law, Social Justice, and Global Development,* vol. 1. <www2.warwick.ac.uk/fac/soc/law/elj/lgd/2004_1/aginam> (September 2006).

Aginam, Obijifor (2005). *Global Health Governance: International Law and Public Health in a Divided World* (Toronto: University of Toronto Press).

Bass, Naomi A. (2002). 'Implications of the TRIPS Agreement for Developing Countries: Pharmaceutical Patent Laws in Brazil and South Africa in the 21st Century'. *George Washington International Law Review,* vol. 34, no. 1, pp. 191–223.

Commission on Macroeconomics and Health (2001). 'Macroeconomics and Health: Investing in Health for Economic Development'. World Health Organization, Geneva. <www.cid.harvard.edu/cidcmh/CMHReport.pdf> (September 2006).

Correa, Carlos (2004). 'Implementation of the WTO General Council Decision on Paragraph 6 of the Doha Declaration on the TRIPS Agreement and Public Health'. World Health Organization, Geneva. <www.eldis.org/static/DOC17336.htm> (September 2006).

Elliott, Richard (2006). 'Global Access to Medicines: Canada's Law on Compulsory Licensing for Export'. Canadian HIV/AIDS Legal Network. <www.aidslaw.ca/publications/publicationsdocEN.php?ref=552> (September 2006).

Falk, Richard A. (1998a). *Law in an Emerging Global Village: A Post-Westphalian Perspective* (Ardsley NY: Transnational Publishers).

Falk, Richard A. (1998b). 'The Coming Global Civilization: Neo-Liberal or Humanist'. In A. Anghie and G. Sturgess, eds., *Legal Visions of the 21st Century: Essays in Honour of Judge Christopher Weeramantry* (The Hague: Kluwer Law International).

Fidler, David P. (1999). *International Law and Infectious Diseases* (Oxford: Oxford University Press).

Fidler, David P. (2001). 'The Globalization of Public Health: The First 100 Years of International Health Diplomacy'. *Bulletin of the World Health Organization,* vol. 79, no. 9, pp. 842–849.

Foster, John W. (2002). 'Canada and International Health: A Time of Testing on AIDS'. In N. Hillmer and M.A. Molot, eds., *Canada among Nations 2002: A Fading Power,* pp. 191–208 (Toronto: Oxford University Press).

G8 (2000). 'G8 Communiqué Okinawa 2000'. 23 July, Okinawa. <www.g8.utoronto.ca/summit/2000okinawa/finalcom.htm> (September 2006).

G8 (2001). 'Communiqué'. 22 July, Genoa. <www.g8.utoronto.ca/summit/2001genoa/finalcommunique.html> (September 2006).

G8 Research Group (2006). 'What Is the G8'. <www.g8.utoronto.ca/what_is_g8.html> (September 2006).

Gathii, James Thuo (2002). 'The Legal Status of the Doha Declaration on TRIPS and Public Health under the Vienna Convention on the Law of Treaties'. *Harvard Journal of Law and Technology,* vol. 15, no. 2, pp. 291–317.

Held, David and Anthony McGrew (2002). 'Introduction'. In D. Held and A. McGrew, eds., *Governing Globalization: Power, Authority, and Global Governance* (Cambridge: Polity Press).

Hodges, Michael (1999). 'The G8 and the New Political Economy'. In M.R. Hodges, J.J. Kirton, and J.P. Daniels, eds., *The G8's Role in the New Millennium,* pp. 69–74 (Aldershot: Ashgate).

Howse, Robert and Makau Mutua (2000). 'Protecting Human Rights in a Global Economy: Challenges for the World Trade Organization'. International Centre for Human Rights and Democratic Development, Montreal.

International Court of Justice (1996). 'Legality of the Use by a State of Nuclear Weapons in Armed Conflict'. Advisory Opinion of 8 July 1996: Dissenting Opinion of Judge Weeramantry. <www.icj-cij.org/icjwww/icases/ianw/ianwframe.htm> (September 2006).

Jackson, John (1998). *The World Trade Organization: Constitution and Jurisprudence* (London: Royal Institute of International Affairs).

Labonté, Ronald, Ted Schrecker, David Sanders, *et al.* (2004). *Fatal Indifference: The G8, Africa, and Global Health* (Cape Town: University of Cape Town Press).

Lee, Kelley and Richard Dodgson (2000). 'Globalization and Cholera: Implications for Global Governance'. *Global Goverance,* vol. 6, no. 2, pp. 213–236.

Nakajima, Hiroshi (1997). 'Global Disease Threats and Foreign Policy'. *Brown Journal of World Affairs,* vol. 4, no. 1, pp. 319–332.

Orbinski, James (2004). 'Access to Medicines and Global Health: Will Canada Lead or Flounder?'. *Canadian Medical Association Journal,* vol. 170, no. 2, pp. 224–226. <www.cmaj.ca/cgi/content/full/170/2/224> (September 2006).

Price-Smith, Andrew (2001). *Plagues and Politics: Infectious Disease and International Policy* (New York: Palgrave).

Sell, Susan K. (2003). *Private Power, Public Law: The Globalization of Intellectual Property Rights* (Cambridge: Cambridge University Press).

Sell, Susan K. (2004). 'The Quest for Global Governance in Intellectual Property and Public Health: Structural, Discursive, and Institutional Dimensions'. *Temple Law Review,* vol. 77, no. 2, pp. 363–400.

t'Hoen, Ellen (2002). 'TRIPS, Pharmaceutical Patents, and Access to Essential Medicines: A Long Way from Seattle to Doha'. *Chicago Journal of International Law,* vol. 3, no. 1, pp. 27–46.

Thomas, Caroline (2002). 'Trade Policy and the Politics of Access to Drugs'. *Third World Quarterly,* vol. 23, no. 2, pp. 251–264.

Trebilcock, Michael J. and Robert Howse (1999). *The Regulation of International Trade*, 2nd ed. (New York: Routledge).

World Trade Organization (2001a). 'Ministerial Declaration'. 14 November, Doha. <www.wto.org/english/thewto_e/minist_e/min01_e/mindecl_e.htm> (September 2006).

World Trade Organization (2001b). 'Declaration on the TRIPS Agreement and Public Health'. WT/MIN(01)/DEC/2. 14 November. <www.wto.org/English/thewto_e/minist_e/min01_e/mindecl_trips_e.htm> (September 2006).

World Trade Organization (2003). 'Implementation of Paragraph 6 of the Doha Declaration of the TRIPS Agreement and Public Health'. Decision of the General Council of 30 August. <www.wto.org/english/tratop_e/trips_e/implem_para6_e.htm> (September 2006).

Yach, Derek and Douglas Bettcher (1998a). 'The Globalization of Public Health I: Threats and Opportunities'. *American Journal of Public Health,* vol. 88, no. 5, pp. 735–738.

Yach, Derek and Douglas Bettcher (1998b). 'The Globalization of Public Health II: The Convergence of Self-Interest and Altruism'. *American Journal of Public Health*, vol. 88, no. 5, pp. 738–741.

Chapter 11

Keeping Faith with Africa's Health: Catalysing G8 Compliance

John Kirton and Ella Kokotsis[1]

On many dimensions of performance, the G8 summit held at Gleneagles from 6 to 8 July 2005 was the most successful in the G8's 31-year history. Despite the potential distractions from the London terrorist bombings of 7 July, the leaders of the world's most powerful democracies mobilised the largest amount of new money ever amassed at a G8 summit for global public goods. They also produced 212 specific commitments, the third highest in summit history. Most of these commitments focussed on host Tony Blair's twin priorities of African development and climate change.

What happens, however, once the lights of the world's media elite dim at summit's end and the leaders return home to their respective national constituencies with the difficult task of delivering on the promises they so boldly made? There has long been much scepticism that G8 promises made will be transformed into G8 promises kept (Labonté *et al.* 2004; Lewis 2005). And history has shown that promises made at the annual summits do not always translate into promises kept and have never done so in full (von Furstenberg and Daniels 1991; Kokotsis 1999; Kokotsis and Daniels 1999; Kirton and Kokotsis 2005; Hodges 1999). Indeed, compliance has varied markedly by year, issue area, and member country, for reasons that scholars have yet to understand adequately (Kokotsis 1999; Li 2001; Kirton 2004). What causes these variations in compliance? Which of these causes are under the leaders' and the G8 system's own control? Can leaders, as they craft their commitments at the summit itself, ground those commitments in compliance-inducing catalysts that push compliance higher than it otherwise would be?

To help establish a theoretically informed, empirically supported, and policy-relevant explanation of members' compliance with G8 commitments, this chapter examines the available evidence on compliance with overall and health-related G7/8 summit commitments and whether compliance improves when G8 leaders embed particular 'compliance catalysts' within the commitment itself. This chapter first reviews the G8's treatment of heath issues over its three-decade history from 1975 to 2005. Second, it looks more closely at the G8's health-related commitment and compliance performance from 1996 to 2005. Third, it examines the G8's overall compliance from 1996 to 2004 to see if compliance is improved when commitments contain one or more of eight compliance catalysts: priority placement, targets, timetables, specified agents, money mobilised, remit mandates, other institutions instructed, and G8 institutions instructed. Fourth, it assesses which of these compliance catalysts appear to have worked in improving compliance with G7/8 health commitments in particular. It concludes by assessing compliance with the 2005 Gleneagles G8 commitments on Africa and health.

This chapter argues that the G8 has had a steadily rising performance in health over its 31 years. This has been particularly true in its expanding commitments and high compliance since 1996. Since that year, higher compliance with overall G8 commitments has tended to come when the G8 leaders have endowed a commitment with a priority placement in the summit communiqué's opening chapeau or chair's summary and injected into a commitment a large number of different compliance catalysts. The importance of priority placement also appears to have become important in inducing compliance with the G8's commitments on health, although instructions to other international organisations and, above all, precise timetables have a stronger effect. The prospects for compliance with the many African-related and health-related commitments made at the 2005 Gleneagles Summit were promising, for several contained those compliance catalysts of proven potency in the past. Yet the relatively poor compliance with the Gleneagles health commitments suggests more effort is required on the G8's part. The scepticism surrounding prospects for the delivery of the G8's often ambitious health commitments may thus be excessive, for G8 leaders have available to them, and are using, compliance catalysts of proven performance in converting promises made into promises kept. At the same time both G8 governors and outside analysts have more work to do.

The G7/8's African-Related Health Agenda, 1975–2005

Health emerged early on the G7's agenda. At the 1979 Tokyo Summit the leaders affirmed that they 'place more emphasis on cooperation with developing countries in overcoming hunger and malnutrition' (G7 1979).[2] From 1979 to 1996, health appeared in the leaders' final declarations in most years, on issues such as health research, famine, bioethics, and improved healthcare systems.[3]

The 1996 Lyon Summit began a dramatic shift. The final communiqué produced the highest number of paragraphs on health to that time (9 of 296) (G7 1996). The G8 health agenda expanded to a much more global perspective, as leaders gave explicit priority to the alleviation of poverty, including adequate official development assistance (ODA) for essential sectors such as health. There were references to increasing prevalence of epidemics and infectious diseases including HIV/AIDS, malaria, cholera, Ebola, and tuberculosis (TB). The communiqué dealt presciently with the threat of bioweapons. The merits of the World Health Organization (WHO) were brought to the fore, as reform issues and resource management were recognised as limits to the organisation's ability to deal with global health policy effectively. At Lyon, the G8 began to lose faith in the WHO, and started to govern global health on its own. The summits from 1997 to 1999 saw increased attention, expanding to active aging, microbiology and safe drinking water, environmental threats to children's health, human cloning, illicit drugs, healthcare costs, and food safety.

At the 2000 Okinawa Summit, the idea of a new global partnership was introduced. It focussed on international efforts by the G8, the WHO, nongovernmental organisations (NGOs), civil society, and pharmaceutical companies to fight infectious and parasitic diseases. The goal was to reduce the number of HIV/AIDS-infected people by 25 percent and the number of TB and malaria deaths by 50 percent by 2010. At the 2001 Genoa Summit, the G8 created the Global Fund to Fight AIDS, Tuberculosis, and Malaria, with an initial commitment of US$1.3 billion by the G8 leaders.

At the 2002 Kananaskis Summit, through the launch of the G8 Africa Action Plan, the G8 produced the greatest attention and highest number of collective commitments to Africa in summit history. The Africa Action Plan's 132 commitments were extraordinarily comprehensive. The leaders recognised the importance of supporting African efforts to build sustainable health systems in order to deliver effective disease intervention. To this end, the action plan devoted 26 paragraphs to core health and health-related initiatives. These included enhancing polio immunisation efforts and promoting the availability of an adequate supply of life-saving medicines, as well as assisting African producers in meeting product and health standards in export markets and supporting the development and adoption of HIV/AIDS programmes for prevention, care, and treatment. African health-related issues penetrated the areas of education and information technology as the action plan highlighted the impact of HIV/AIDS on Africa's educational systems and the importance of access to relevant and timely information in reversing downward health trends.

At the 2003 Evian Summit the leaders reaffirmed their commitment in the chair's summary to improved access to health care and more affordable drug treatments, as well as famine prevention and food security. They also issued, for the first time, four standalone documents dealing with health issues: Health: A G8 Action Plan; Water: A G8 Action Plan; Action Against Famine Especially in Africa: A G8 Action Plan; and Science and Technology for Sustainable Development: A G8 Action Plan. Collectively, these documents reflected the extent to which global health issues had emerged at the forefront of the G8's social agenda. Moreover, with the announcement of US$500 million toward the eradication of polio, Evian represented the first financial contribution to health since the launch of the Global Fund.

At Sea Island in 2004, the G8 leaders issued a record 16 documents (spanning ten different issue areas) and generating a record 253 commitments (Kirton 2005a). Although the Broader Middle East and North Africa (BMENA) Initiative was a primary concern, Africa emerged second, with the issuance of six declarations and actions plans covering debt relief, famine, and health. On health, attention focussed on the eradication of polio and the development of an HIV/AIDS vaccine. Here the G8 became a major fundraiser, with targets and timetables attached. On polio, the leaders agreed to bridge the WHO's funding gap in the Polio Eradication Initiative by up to US$200 million, concentrating particularly on those regions still affected, notably Afghanistan, Egypt, India, Niger, Nigeria, and Pakistan. The goal here was to 'take all necessary steps to eradicate polio by 2005 and close the funding gap by our next Summit' (G8 2004). On HIV/AIDS, the G8 agreed to a US$375 million plan to develop and disseminate a vaccine. They added a remit mandate to report back by the time of the 2005 summit. They also endorsed the establishment of the Global HIV Vaccine Enterprise to 'accelerate HIV vaccine development'.

At Gleneagles in 2005, global health issues arose under both of the summit's two main themes of African development and climate change. Extensive references were made to basic health care, universal access to AIDS treatment, and the reduction in pollution as a means of protecting public health. Along with the participating African leaders, the G8 agreed to a comprehensive plan that would boost investment in health and 'take action to combat HIV/AIDS, malaria, TB and other killer diseases' (G8 2005b). The leaders agreed that measures in the plan would 'deliver free basic health care and primary education for all' and 'provide as close as possible to universal access to treatment for AIDS by 2010'. The leaders also noted the importance of reducing pollution as a means of protecting public health. Here they emphasised the 'need to improve air and water quality in order to alleviate suffering from respiratory disease, reduce public health costs and prolong lives' (G8 2005c). Moreover, the US$50 billion increase in aid represented not only the 'signal for a new deal on trade, the cancellation of the debt of the poorest nations and universal access to Aids treatment', but also the G8's 'definitive expression of [their] collective will to act in the face of death and disease' (G8 2005d).

G8 Health Commitment and Compliance: 1996–2005

Since 1996, the G8 has moved steadily to translate its growing attention to health into concrete, future-oriented, and often ambitious commitments, and to comply with them within a year to an increasing and high degree (G8 Research Group 2006b).[4]

Commitment

Since its 1975 inception as the G7, the G8 has made 165 core health commitments. Only four came from the summits between 1975 and 1995. A full 161 have arisen since 1996. Starting at the French-hosted Lyon Summit in 1996, the G8 have made health commitments every year, made multiple heath commitments, and made a rising number of health commitments. The annual number moved into double digits in the 21st century, reached a new peak of 21 commitments at the next French-hosted summit at Evian in 2003, and soared to an all-time high of 64 at St. Petersburg in 2006. The significance of these commitments also rose during this period. Since 1996, there have emerged seven standalone summit documents on health. Several G8 health institutions, and the mobilisation of US$9.5 billion on health-related initiatives.[5]

The Canadian-hosted Kananaskis Summit in 2002 marked a second turning point. During the 2002–05 period, a total of 136 concrete, measurable, and identifiable commitments on African-related health issues were produced. Given that more than

850 commitments were generated across all issue areas during this time, the ratio of African health-related issues to overall issues averages 16 percent. In those four years, the G8 produced more commitments on African-related health issues (136) than on core health from every summit since its inception (101). This serves as compelling testament to the weight and consideration paid by the G8 to health issues within the African context.

Compliance

Since 1996, G8 members have complied with these commitments to an increasing and now generally high degree (see Appendix 11-1).[6] From 1998 to 2004, final compliance (that is, within one year after the summit) with health commitments averaged +58 percent when each individual final compliance score is weighted equally, and +57 percent when the average annual scores of the seven years from 1998 to 2004 are equally weighted. Health compliance has thus been well above the summit's historic 1975–99 overall average of +31 percent, and above the rising overall average for more recent and comparable years. Almost perfect compliance scores on core health commitments have come with the +87 percent in 2000 and the +89 percent in 2003. Only the +38 percent in 2002 broke the trend, as the intra-G8 divisions generated by the spring 2003 invasion of Iraq reduced compliance with G8 commitments in health and overall.

All G8 members have a positive record in complying with their core health commitments for the period from 1998 to 2005 (see Appendix 11-1). The highest score has come from the European Union, with a perfect +100 percent compliance with the 22 commitments assessed. Also complying well and above average have been the UK with +80 percent, Canada with +77 percent, and the U.S. with +73 percent. Only Russia at 0 percent has put in a notably below average performance.

The strength of this final compliance record is seen in the experience of the centrepiece health commitments each summit has made. The 2001 Genoa Summit brought the largest initiative to date on global health policy. Here the leaders pledged 'to make a quantum leap in the fight against infectious diseases and to break the vicious cycle between disease and poverty' (G8 2001). To this end, they launched, together with the UN, the Global Fund to Fight AIDS, Tuberculosis, and Malaria.[7] Leaders committed US$1.3 billion and set a goal of making the fund operational by the end of 2001. Both of these commitments were met as the Global Fund announced the first round of grants totalling US$378 million to be allocated in 30 countries, across 40 projects over a two-year period ('The AIDS Fund Gets Going' 2002). In terms of financial resources, by May 2002, the fund had amassed more than US$2 billion, of which US$1.4 billion came directly from G8 member states.

In 2002 at Kananaskis, the leaders pledged to support the Global Fund and to increase the overall effectiveness of its operations. Within the framework of the G8 Africa Action Plan and the New Partnership for Africa's Development (NEPAD), the G8 vowed to increase Africa's access to the fund as well as its participation in it. Additional financial allocations were not committed. What did materialise was a broader approach on global health, however, with Africa at its core. The leaders recognised that any comprehensive plan on African development would have to address the crippling impact of infectious diseases with more than just the allocation of financial resources. An effective strategy would also require the recognition that research, prevention, treatment, education, partnership programmes, and capacity building for health infrastructure were inextricably linked to the root causes of infectious diseases. Kananaskis thus served to reinforce the point that addressing the root causes of health problems and developing viable health systems on the African continent were both critical and necessary development goals. To this end, one of the strongest pushes by the leaders at Kananaskis came with their commitment to work with the pharmaceutical industry and civil society to promote the availability of life-saving medicines in affected African countries. In 2002 the leaders fared modestly, delivering a compliance score of 38 percent on health, or just above the average +34 percent for the summit overall.

At the 2003 Evian Summit, the 2002 SARS outbreak helped generate a record 21 commitments. The G8 Action Plan on Health committed the leaders to work in partnership with developing countries, the private sector, multilateral organisations, and NGOs to help achieve their health goals. These promises included a donors conference in Paris that July to secure sustainable long-term financing for the Global Fund and pledges to strengthen healthcare systems in the developing world, to increase global access to medicines, to further research on health technologies for the prevention, control, treatment, and cure for infectious diseases, and to increase global disease surveillance and laboratory, diagnostic, and research efforts for SARS. Moreover, in keeping with their pledge at Kananaskis to provide sufficient resources to eradicate polio by 2005, the leaders raised an additional US$500 million 'to ensure that the remaining funding gap is closed' (G8 2003).

Although the U.S. did not offer any concrete financial pledges to the fund at Evian, deferring instead to the forthcoming donors conference in Paris, it took the lead by announcing it would pledge US$1 billion annually to the Global Fund until 2008.[8] The EU followed suit, indicating its readiness to pledge another US$1 billion, subject to confirmation at the next European Council meeting (Bayne 2003). Apart from Germany, which blocked EU legislation that would have allocated an additional €170 million, all other G8 countries allocated money to the fund in 2003, including Russia, which increased its contribution by US$5 million a year for 2004–06 (G8 Research Group 2004, 51–57). By producing the highest number of health commitments and delivering one of the highest compliance scores (88 percent), Evian became the pivotal summit on global health.

Compliance with African-related health issues continued at the 2004 Sea Island Summit. The G8 recognised that challenges, including 'HIV/AIDS, famine and poverty, represent[ed] a compelling call for international cooperation to support [Africa's] efforts to achieve lasting progress' (G8 2004). Despite a slight drop in the number of commitments at Evian the year before, the leaders at Sea Island did commit to eradicating polio by 2005 by closing the funding gap by the time of the 2005 Gleneagles Summit, and by taking all necessary steps to accelerate the development of an HIV vaccine. To this end, the G8 endorsed the establishment of the Global HIV Vaccine Enterprise and mobilised, together with partners from public and private sectors, more than US$3.3 billion to fund polio immunisation campaigns around the world.

The commitment to establish the enterprise was realised in January 2005 through the release of the Scientific Strategic Plan, which detailed the enterprise's ten-year roadmap for research and development (R&D) to combat the HIV/AIDS pandemic. Yet some critics argued that the G8 would have to strengthen its political leadership if an HIV vaccine was to be possible. Either way, the G8 delivered a compliance score of 56 percent by committing to its goal of establishing the enterprise and, through it, not only allocate financial contributions but also support efforts to upgrade research laboratories in Africa to international standards, train African scientists, and ensure measures for equitable vaccine access (G8 Research Group 2005).

Regarding their commitment to closing the financing gap on polio eradication by the time of the 2005 G8 summit, the leaders scored 44 percent. They fell short by US$50 million in funding required to end polio transmission by year's end. Despite the positive progress achieved until that point, in April 2005 polio was imported into Indonesia and Yemen, two countries previously thought to have eliminated the disease. Both these polio strains were traced back to Nigeria, where immunisation campaigns had been stalled for longer than a year after northern Muslim provinces blocked WHO efforts. Without the US$200 million required for 2006, the Global Polio Eradication Initiative would not be able to implement its 2004–08 goal, which included 'certifying the elimination of the disease, developing products for the international termination of the oral polio vaccine, and using the infrastructure and information to assist in other health initiatives' (G8 Research Group 2005, 172).

At the 2005 Gleneagles Summit, the G8 agreed to boost investment and take action to combat HIV/AIDS, malaria, TB, and other killer diseases through the delivery of 18 health-related African commitments. The G8 and African leaders agreed that, if implemented, measures set out in their comprehensive plan could deliver free basic health care for all and could provide nearly universal access to AIDS treatment by 2010. The US$50 billion in aid to Africa that was committed at Gleneagles signalled not only a new deal on trade and the cancellation of debt of the poorest, but also a commitment to provide universal access to AIDS treatment (see G8 2005b). In this regard, the leaders committed to 'work to meet the financing needs for HIV/AIDS, including through the replenishment this year of the Global Fund to Fight AIDS, TB and Malaria; and actively working with local stakeholders to implement the "3 Ones" principles in all countries' (G8 2005a). A second major commitment was 'supporting the Polio Eradication Initiative for the post eradication period in 2006–8 through continuing or increasing our own contributions toward the US$829 million target and mobilising the support of others'.

One year later, compliance with both of these health commitments was very low, with the Global Fund replenishment at +33 percent and polio eradication at +11 percent, for an average of +22 percent (G8 Research Group 2006b). Full compliance with the Global Fund commitment came only from the U.S., the EU,

Japan, and Russia; that with polio came from the U.S., the EU, Britain, Canada, and Germany. Concerned NGOs understandably expressed disappointment with the results (DATA 2006).

Catalysing Compliance, 1996–2004

In making commitments, the G8 leaders regularly seek to enhance the likelihood of subsequent compliance by including within the individual commitment itself components they judge to be catalysts of compliance action (see Appendix 11-2).[9] Outside critics have also urged upon them particular formulae for crafting commitments in an effort to engender compliance, often by easing the task of outside monitoring that is thought to be important in inducing compliant behaviour by G8 governments (Lewis 2005).

Over the years, the G8 leaders have relied primarily on eight such compliance catalysts: priority placement in the chair's statement or the introductory chapeau of the main summit communiqué; the inclusion of a specified, often numerical welfare target or objective; the inclusion of a similarly specific numerical timetable for action or accomplishment; a remit mandate committing the leaders to re-examine the commitment, its implementing action, or an accomplishment at a subsequent summit; mobilised money that dedicates specific or additional monetary resources or the equivalent to the commitment; a specified agent or agency as the individual, country, group, or other actor to do, take charge of, or otherwise be responsible for compliance or implementing action; a G8-centred body at the ministerial, official, or multi-stakeholder level to be responsible for implementing actions; and another international institution, of plurilateral or multilateral membership, similarly responsible for ensuring compliance.

Catalysing Compliance Overall

From 1996 to 2004, in the commitments for which compliance information is available, all of these eight compliance catalysts have been used by G8 leaders every year. The most frequent every year and overall are, in order, priority placement, other international institutions, specified agency, timetables, and G8-centred bodies. Yet only some of these compliance catalysts have actually worked. By far the most potent has been priority placement. It is followed in turn by specified agency and, less clearly, timetables, targets, and remit mandates. There is no suggestion that G8 bodies and other international institutions make any difference at all. Indeed, priority placement and specified agency appear to be the only compliance catalysts that contemporary G8 leaders can really count on to have their collective will realised in the real world.

A correlation and regression analysis of the 164 final commitments and 56 interim commitments for which compliance data were available from 1996 to 2004 confirms the importance of priority placement. But this analysis suggests that specified agency is not the more potent supplement. For the 164 final compliance scores, the mean final compliance score was 0.41 and the mean number of catalysts 1.49. For the 56 interim compliance scores since 2002 (measured six months after the summit), the mean compliance score was 0.42 and the mean number of catalysts 1.49 as well. Both these compliance scores are significantly higher than the 0.31 for the 1975–89 period found by George von Furstenberg and Joseph Daniels (1991). G8 members' compliance with their overall G8 commitments is rising over time, especially since the advent of intense post–Cold War globalisation and Russia's incorporation as a full member into the expanded G8.

Some compliance catalysts, when used alone or in particular combinations, do raise compliance scores, and do so more quickly than would otherwise be the case. Most notably, priority placement caused higher levels of final compliance and much higher levels of interim or quick compliance. The total number of catalysts strongly increased interim compliance, perhaps because the sheer number and diversity of catalysts in a commitment signals to a broad range of relevant implementing actors that the G8 leaders really do want action taken now. In contrast, money mobilised harmed interim compliance. In contrast to the easy assumptions of many critics (see, for example, Lewis 2005), the G8 should thus not be viewed primarily as a great global fundraiser. Promises of quick cash from the summit leaders actually diminish the prospects of a fast start on compliance.

A few particular combinations of catalysts have a potent effect. Priority placement, when combined with targets and other international institutions in a regression model, had a weak effect on raising final compliance and a strong effect on raising interim compliance. But when priority placement, targets, and other international institutions are combined with the total number of catalysts in a regression model, priority replacement raises final compliance but other international institutions diminishes it. This suggests that when the G8 is determined to act, by including many of the compliance catalysts it controls, final compliance increases. In contrast, when it relies on other international institutions for implementation, final compliance is reduced. This combination of priority placement, targets, other international institutions, and the total number of catalysts in a regression model also generates greater interim compliance. A G8 reliance on other international institutions may create a quick start on implementation, but reduce compliance over the longer term.

A further analysis divides the commitments into the 104 made prior to the 2002 Kananaskis Summit and the 60 made at and after it. Before Kananaskis, the mean and average final compliance score was +39 percent and the mean number of catalysts 1.26. Since Kananaskis, the mean and average final compliance score has risen to +45 percent and the mean number of catalysts has also risen noticeably to 1.9. The two trends in rising catalysts and compliance are statistically related. From Kananaskis onward there was a highly significant correlation between final compliance and priority placement ($r = 0.51, p = 0$).[10] A linear regression of all eight catalysts yielded a highly significant effect on final compliance ($F [8,59] = 4.10, p = 0.001, r2 = 0.36$), with priority placement having the main effect. A regression of priority placement, target, other international institutions, and total catalysts was highly significant in explaining final compliance ($F [4,59] = 7.00$, $P < .001$); as before, priority placement had a main positive effect and other international institutions a main negative effect. This model without total catalysts was almost as significant, with the negative effect of other international institutions gone. Regressions of priority placement alone and total catalysts alone again showed each had a significant effect in explaining final compliance.

These findings strongly suggest that the new Kananaskis format, the fully equal inclusion of the Russians, and the regular attendance of the powerful democratic African leaders produced a new 21st-century summit where the leaders sought to bind themselves more, found more effective ways to do so, and produced higher compliance as a result. Their most powerful and reliable tools to do so were the priority placements of their commitments and the use of a higher total number of catalysts in each commitment. Reliance on other international institutions to deliver their commitments for them proved to be a formula that repeatedly failed.

Yet in broader terms, there are several plausible causes of the increased compliance from 2002 onward, with only some of them being the use of catalysts under the leaders' summit commitment control. Nine stand out (see also Kirton 2006). The first two are under the leaders' control at the summit, the second three are under leaders' control beyond the summit, and the final four are beyond the control of leaders and even, in some cases, the G8 system itself.

First, as suggested above, the new format with the separate and lengthy standalone chair's summary, recording only what the leaders actually talked about, more authentically allowed them to bind themselves publicly to — and signal to others — what they most wanted done; it also allowed them to express their political will more in the form of commitments, and to put commitments in this priority form. Second, the leaders began to use more compliance catalysts in each commitment.

Third, there was greater iteration of the same agenda, led by the African, terrorism, and Middle East files. Fourth, the same leaders of Africa's major democratic polities became regular summit participants, providing an external pressure group to help ensure that G8 commitments were kept. Fifth, Russia became a full equal member now allowed to host a summit of its own. Greater concert equality was thus achieved.

Sixth, greater leadership continuity, experience, and a personal, longer shadow of the future existed among G8 leaders, as political control at home allowed seven of the eight G8 leaders to come to five summits in a row. Seventh, there was greater ministerial recommitment, as the growing list of increasingly active G8 minister institutions subsequently made the same or similar commitments to those the leaders had. Eighth, the exponential expansion of the internet made it easier for civil society organisations and citizens to track commitments and compliance with them, thus encouraging democratically elected G8 leaders to ensure that promises made become promises kept. The greater usage from 2002 onward of the G8 Information Centre website (attracting more than 7 million hits in 2005) and the advent of interim compliance study monitoring in 2002 both support this judgement. Ninth, there was the reality and a sense of equalising vulnerability that came with the shock and a subsequent solidarity bred by 11 September 2001 and a steady succession of deadly terrorist shocks in Russia, Europe, and Britain.

While these candidate causes largely flow from the concert equality model, that model has previously failed to explain compliance, the only one of the five G8 governance performance functions assessed (Kirton 2004). The functions of deliberation, direction setting, decision making, and the development of global governance take place before and at the summit and are driven by forces taking place before and during it. In contrast, the functions of domestic political management, interim compliance, and, above all, final compliance take place after the summit, respectively in the following days and weeks, six months later, and then a full year later. The forces that drive final compliance are thus likely to be those that unfold in the year after the summit, rather than in the year before the summit takes place. The ability of the leader's greater compliance-catalytic behaviour at the summit to raise interim compliance six months later, far more than final compliance one year later, supports this assessment. This suggests that leaders could well address the ways in which they might remain active in the six- to twelve-month period following their summit, perhaps by conducting a formal and even multi-stakeholder implementation reviews with follow-up mechanisms at the halfway mark between summits, when the outgoing host hands off to the incoming host.

Catalysing Compliance on Health

The compliance record on an initial set of the eight highest-scoring health commitments from the period from 2000 to 2004 shows that all of these compliance catalysts save for remit mandates have been used by leaders for health during this time. The most frequently used were timetables (7), international organisations (5), and priority placement (4).

In the most general terms, the high compliance scores on the eight health commitments, averaging +81 percent (with no single score below +44 percent) and combined with the frequent use of almost all compliance catalysts, suggests that the latter have a causal effect. The four commitments that each contained four compliance catalysts had an average compliance score of +94 percent. The four commitments that each contained fewer catalysts had an average compliance score of only +69. The four commitments with the highest compliance scores most frequently used the compliance catalysts of timetable (4), target (3), specified agent (3), and international organisation (3). The four commitments with the lowest compliance scores (ranging from +44 percent to +86 percent) most frequently used the compliance catalysts of timetable (3), priority placement (3), and international organisation (3). A comparison of the two lists suggests that a target and a specified agent might be the most potent compliance catalysts in the field of health.

A broader look at a list of 22 health commitments for which final compliance information is available from 1998 to 2005 suggests that the leaders have relied most heavily on timetables (50 percent of the time), priority placement (45 percent), and international institutions (41 percent) (see Appendix 11-3). Prior to 2002 there was a heavy reliance on other international institutions rather than priority placement, whereas from 2002 onward other international institutions faded and priority placement was used a great deal. The G8 also moved away from setting targets and toward using G8-centred bodies. Compliance scores were similar for both periods. This suggests that the G8's strong shift to relying on itself for final health compliance has been as effective as its earlier reliance on others, largely in the UN system. Among the individual compliance catalysts, however, only timetables, on which there has been a reliance since 2000, appears to be associated with higher compliance. However, there are still insufficient data on compliance with health commitments to say with confidence what works in this particular policy field.

Conclusion: Prospects for Compliance with the Gleneagles Commitments

Compliance with G8 commitments has been steadily rising since 1996, as has the use of leaders-controlled compliance catalysts employed to create this effect. This higher compliance has tended to come when the G8 leaders at their summit have endowed a commitment with a priority placement in the summit communiqué's opening chapeau or the chair's summary and injected a large total number of different compliance catalysts into a commitment. The importance of priority placement also appears to have become important in inducing compliance with the G8's commitments on health, although instructions to other international organisations in earlier years and precise timetables on an ongoing basis appear to have a positive effect. For the first time there is solid evidence that the leaders themselves at their summit can do things to increase the prospects that their promises made will be promises kept. But beyond priority placement and the use of a large number of compliance catalysts, it remains unclear just what they should do at the summit to increase compliance, particularly in the field of health. And it remains even less clear how many of the causes of compliance remain under their own control at or beyond their summit, and how changing configurations of broader systemic forces might lead them to commit with different combinations of catalysts to produce the desired high compliance effect (Kirton 2006).

Amid this uncertainty, however, there were good grounds to suggest that the historic Gleneagles commitments would be complied with faithfully, at least in the fields of Africa and health. Gleneagles gave priority placement to its African-related commitments across a broad range. Of the 14 commitments in the Gleneagles chair's statement binding all G8 members, a full ten dealt with Africa.[11] These covered the issue areas of trade (three commitments), aid (two commitments), and debt (one commitment). They also embraced, with one commitment apiece, the issue areas of peacekeeping, democracy, health and education, and investment and infrastructure. In addition, these ten commitments, covering seven issue areas, were offered in the chair's summary in an order that iteratively reflected the philosophy and strategy of NEPAD, the 2002 G8 Africa Action Plan, and the 2005 report of the Commission for Africa. They also came with high degrees of leader continuity, Russian experience as a member, African and outside participation, civil society engagement, and a heightened sense of vulnerability from the shock of the terrorist attack of 7 July 2005, which occurred during the Gleneagles Summit.

Three months after the Gleneagles Summit ended, the average compliance score for the ten African-related priority commitments was 0 percent (Kirton 2005b). The health-related area of debt cancellation had been completely complied with (+100 percent). The health-related area of doubling aid stood at +25 percent. And the core health commitment reached the positive range at +17 percent.

A review of all 18 Gleneagles core health commitments further suggested that high compliance would come (see Appendix 11-4). All but two had at least one compliance catalyst. The commitment on the Global Fund had six, malaria had four, and polio had three. The core of the G8's 21st-century health agenda is thus rich with compliance catalysts. Moreover, the proven performer of priority placement occurs in 72 percent of the Gleneagles health commitments. As Russia took over the hosting responsibility for the 2006 St. Petersburg Summit, with health as one of its three thematic priorities, there seemed to be a firm foundation for keeping the health commitments of Gleneagles.

Yet this promise was not fulfilled for the two health commitments — on the Global Fund and polio — on which good evidence exists (G8 Research Group 2006b; see also Department for International Development 2006). The answer may lie in the fact that the conscious action of leaders as agents in crafting compliance catalysts needs to be supported by greater institutionalisation of the G8 system and a supportive international system. Certainly the leaders at the 2006 St. Petersburg Summit, in crafting their many health commitments, knew that innovation was necessary, for they introduced two additional measures: repeated promises encoded in the communiqué to monitor the implementation of their commitments and self-reporting through an appendix detailing what each country had done to comply with health commitments in the past. Yet, by themselves, these promises and reports were hardly convincing. More work thus needs to be done, by G8 governors and outside analysts, to understand how G8 promises made can more confidently be turned into promises kept.

Notes

1 The authors gratefully acknowledge the financial support of the Social Sciences and Humanities Research Council of Canada, the research assistance of Laura Sunderland, and the compliance assessments of Lindsay Doyle, Taleen Jakujyan, Jenevieve Mannell, Abby Slinger, Jacqueline Stillman, and members of the G8 Research Group. They are also grateful to Danielle Takacs and Nikolai Roudev for their work on the regression analysis.

2 On the G8 agenda, health is divided into two primary categories: core health, which relates to issues on the agenda that affect the maintenance of a healthy human condition and includes infectious diseases (e.g., HIV/AIDS, malaria, tuberculosis, etc.), medical research, healthcare systems, health promotion, pharmaceuticals, treatments, and resource mobilisation, and health-related issues that have a related impact on human health, including debt relief to help promote the development of a healthcare infrastructure, information

and communications technology to improve healthcare facilities, or environmental issues that affect human health (see Chapter 9).

3 See texts of final communiqués at the G8 Information Centre at <www.g8.utoronto.ca/summit>.

4 Commitments are defined as 'discrete, specific, publicly expressed, collectively agreed statements of intent: i.e., promises or undertakings by Summit members that they will take future action to move toward, meet or adjust an identified target' (Kokotsis 1999).

5 The standalone documents include Water: A G8 Action Plan (2003), Health: A G8 Action Plan (2003), Action Against Famine Especially in Africa: A G8 Action Plan (2003), Science and Technology for Sustainable Development: A G8 Action Plan (2003), G8 Commitment to Help Stop Polio Forever (2004), Ending the Cycle of Famine in the Horn of Africa (2004), and Fight Against Infectious Disease (2006).

6 Compliance is defined as national government action geared toward the domestic implementation of the necessary formal legislative and administrative regulations designed to execute summit commitments. It is therefore measured according to governmental actions intended to modify existing instruments within the executive and legislative branch to accommodate the commitments reached (Kokotsis 1999).

7 The mandate of the Global Fund is to 'attract, manage and disburse additional resources through a new public-private partnership that will make a sustainable and significant contribution to the reduction of infections, illness and death, thereby mitigating the impact caused by HIV/AIDS, tuberculosis and malaria in countries in need, and contributing to poverty reduction as part of the Millennium Development Goals' (Global Fund 2006).

8 The U.S. contribution to the Global Fund could not exceed one third of the total (see Global Fund 2004).

9 Outside of the summit itself, there are other compliance-inducing mechanisms that leaders potentially control. One is agenda continuity and commitment iteration, whereby leaders repeatedly return to the same if difficult subjects and commitments until they get the job done (Bayne 1999). Another is ministerial recommitment, whereby leaders' commitments are reinforced by the same or similar commitments made subsequently by the G8 ministerial bodies most relevant to the subject at hand.

10 Here r is the correlation coefficient between two variables; p is used to reject the null hypothesis of the t-test (that the true value of r is in fact 0); F is the value of the F-statistic, which is compared to the theoretical standard F distribution to test for the joint significance of all coefficients in a multivariate regression model; and P is the p value for the F statistic, used to reject the null hypothesis of joint insignificance of all regressors in the model.

11 This recommitment is a very strong form of priority placement.

References

Bayne, Nicholas (1999). 'Continuity and Leadership in an Age of Globalisation'. In M.R. Hodges, J.J. Kirton, and J.P. Daniels, eds., *The G8's Role in the New Millennium,* pp. 21–44 (Aldershot: Ashgate).

Bayne, Nicholas (2003). 'Impressions of the Evian Summit'. G8 Research Group. <www.g8.utoronto.ca/evaluations/2003evian/assess_bayne030603.html> (September 2006).

DATA (2006). 'The DATA Report 2006: Keep the G8 Promise to Africa'. London. <www.thedatareport.org/pdf/dataReportFull.pdf> (September 2006).

Department for International Development (United Kingdom) (2006). 'Turning Talk into Action: G8 Gleneagles One Year On'. London. <www.dfid.gov.uk/pubs/files/g8-2006.pdf> (September 2006).

G7 (1979). 'Declaration'. 29 June, Tokyo. <www.g8.utoronto.ca/summit/1979tokyo/communique.html> (September 2006).

G7 (1996). 'Economic Communiqué: Making a Success of Globalization for the Benefit of All'. 28 June, Lyon. <www.g8.utoronto.ca/summit/1996lyon/communique.html> (September 2006).

G8 (2001). 'Communiqué'. 22 July, Genoa. <www.g8.utoronto.ca/summit/2001genoa/finalcommunique.html> (September 2006).

G8 (2003). 'Health: A G8 Action Plan'. 2 June, Evian. <www.g8.utoronto.ca/summit/2003evian/health_en.html> (September 2006).

G8 (2004). 'Chair's Summary'. 10 June, Sea Island. <www.g8.utoronto.ca/summit/2004seaisland/summary.html> (September 2006).

G8 (2005a). 'Africa'. 8 July, Gleneagles. <www.g8.utoronto.ca/summit/2005gleneagles/africa.html> (September 2006).

G8 (2005b). 'Chair's Summary'. 8 July, Gleneagles. <www.g8.utoronto.ca/summit/2005gleneagles/summary.html> (September 2006).

G8 (2005c). 'Climate Change, Clean Energy, and Sustainable Development'. 8 July, Gleneagles. <www.g8.utoronto.ca/summit/2005gleneagles/climatechange.html> (September 2006).

G8 (2005d). 'Statement on the Final Day of the Summit'. 8 July, Gleneagles. <www.g8.utoronto.ca/summit/2005gleneagles/statement.html> (September 2006).

G8 Research Group (2004). '2003 Evian Final Compliance Report'. <www.g8.utoronto.ca/evaluations/2003evian_comp_final> (September 2006).

G8 Research Group (2005). '2004 Sea Island Final Compliance Report'. Toronto. <www.g8.utoronto.ca/evaluations/2004seaisland_final> (September 2006).

G8 Research Group (2006a). 'All G7/8 Commitments, 1975–2006'. <www.g8.utoronto.ca/evaluations/G8_commitments.pdf> (September 2006).

G8 Research Group (2006b). '2005 Gleneagles Final Compliance Report'. <www.g8.utoronto.ca/evaluations/2005compliance_final> (September 2006).

Global Fund to Fight AIDS, Tuberculosis, and Malaria (2004). 'Confirmation of U.S. Pledge for 2004 Boosts Global Fund Resources for Fourth Proposal Round to $900 Million'. Press release, 26 February. <www.theglobalfund.org/en/media_center/press/pr_040226.asp> (September 2006).

Global Fund to Fight AIDS, Tuberculosis, and Malaria (2006). 'Guide to the Global Fund's Policies on Procurement and Supply Management'. Geneva. <www.theglobalfund.org/en/about/procurement/policies> (September 2006).

Hodges, Michael (1999). 'The G8 and the New Political Economy'. In M.R. Hodges, J.J. Kirton, and J.P. Daniels, eds., *The G8's Role in the New Millennium,* pp. 69–74 (Aldershot: Ashgate).

Kirton, John J. (2004). 'Explaining G8 Effectiveness: A Concert of Vulnerable Equals in a Globalizing World'. Paper prepared for the International Studies Association conference, 17–20 March, Montreal. <www.g8.utoronto.ca/scholar/kirton2004/kirton_isa_040304.pdf> (September 2006).

Kirton, John J. (2005a). 'America at the G8: From Vulnerability to Victory at the Sea Island Summit'. In M. Fratianni, J.J. Kirton, A.M. Rugman, *et al.*, eds., *New Perspectives on Global Governance: Why America Needs the G8,* pp. 31–50 (Aldershot: Ashgate).

Kirton, John J. (2005b). 'A Promising Push: Complying with the Gleneagles G8 Africa Commitments and Parliamentarians' Role'. Paper prepared for a conference on Partnership Beyond 2005: The Role of Parliamentarians in Implementing NEPAD Commitments, Parliamentary Seminar on Africa, 19–22 October, London. <www.g8.utoronto.ca/scholar/kirton2005/kirton_london2005.pdf> (September 2006).

Kirton, John J. (2006). 'Explaining Compliance with G8 Finance Commitments: Agency, Institutionalizaton, and Structure'. *Open Economies Review,* vol. 17, no. 4.

Kirton, John J. and Ella Kokotsis (2005). 'Keeping Faith with Africa: Assessing Compliance with the G8's Commitments at Kananaskis and Evian'. In J.B. Atwood, R.S. Brown, and P. Lyman, eds., *Freedom, Prosperity, and Security: G8 Partnership with Africa, Sea Island 2004 and Beyond,* pp. 11–33 (Washington DC: Council on Foreign Relations).

Kokotsis, Eleanore (1999). *Keeping International Commitments: Compliance, Credibility, and the G7, 1988–1995* (New York: Garland).

Kokotsis, Ella and Joseph P. Daniels (1999). 'G8 Summits and Compliance'. In M.R. Hodges, J.J. Kirton, and J.P. Daniels, eds., *The G8's Role in the New Millennium,* pp. 75–91 (Aldershot: Ashgate).

Labonté, Ronald, Ted Schrecker, David Sanders, *et al.* (2004). *Fatal Indifference: The G8, Africa, and Global Health* (Cape Town: University of Cape Town Press).

Lewis, Stephen (2005). *Race against Time: Searching for Hope in AIDS-Ravaged Africa* (Toronto: House of Anansi).

Li, Quan (2001). 'Commitment Compliance in G7 Summit Macroeconomic Policy Coordination'. *Political Research Quarterly,* vol. 54, no. 2, pp. 355–378.

'The AIDS Fund Gets Going'. (2002). *Washington Post,* 29 April.

von Furstenberg, George M. and Joseph P. Daniels (1991). 'Policy Undertakings by the Seven "Summit" Countries: Ascertaining the Degree of Compliance'. *Carnegie-Rochester Conference Series on Public Policy,* vol. 35, pp. 267–308.

Appendix 11-1
G8 Health Compliance by Commitment and Country

Commitment and Issue	Average (overall to date)	U.S.	Japan	Germany	UK
1998 (3 of 4)[a]	+26% (26%)	+100%	–50%	–33%	+100%
1998–46[b] Aging	+0.33	+1	–	0	–
1998–23 HIV	+0.33	+1	0	0	+1
1998–24 HIV	+0.11	+1	–1	–1	+1
1999 (2 of 3)	+32% (28%)	+50	+50	–100%	+50%
1999–38 HIV	+0.63	+1	+1	–1	+1
1999–39 Infectious diseases	0.00	0	0	0	0
2000 (6 of 11)	+87% (60%)	+83%	+100%	+100%	+100%
2000–73 Aging	+0.86	+1	+1	+1	+1
2000–36 HIV	+1.00	+1	+1	+1	+1
2000–38 Malaria	+1.00	+1	+1	+1	+1
2000–37 Tuberculosis	+1.00	+1	+1	+1	+1
2000–S108 Biotechnology	+0.75	+1	+1	+1	+1
2000–23 Infectious diseases	+0.60	0	+1	–	–
2001 (1 of 3)	+75% (61%)	00%	00%	+100%	+100%
2001–26 Global Fund	+0.75	0	0	+1	+1
2002 (3 of 19)	+38% (53%)	00%	+33%	00%	+33%
2002–117 Medicines	+0.38	0	+1	0	+1
2002–11 Polio	0.00	0	0	0	0
2002–119 Global Fund	+0.25	0	0	0	0
2003 (3 of 21)	+89% (59%)	+100%	+100%	+33%	+100%
2003–13 Polio	+1.00	+1	+1	+1	+1
2003–10 Global Fund	+0.89	+1	+1	0	+1
2003–14 SARS	+0.78	+1	+1	0	+1
2004 (2 of 12)	+50% (58%)	+100%	–50%	+100%	+100%
2004–(10)1 HIV	+0.56	+1	–1	+1	+1
2004– (11)3 Polio	+0.44	+1	0	+1	+1
2005 (2 of 18)	+0.22 (55%)	+100%	00%	+50%	+50%
2005–HIV	+0.33	+1	+1	0	0
2005–Polio	+0.11	+1	–1	+1	+1
Ratio (excluding 2005)		14/20	9/19	7/19	15/18
Average (excluding 2005)	58%	70%	47%	37%	83%
Ratio (including 2005)		16/22	9/21	8/21	16/20
Average (including 2005)	55%	73%	43%	38%	80%

continued

Appendix 11-1
G8 Health Compliance by Commitment and Country, continued

Commitment and Issue	France	Italy	Canada	Russia	EU
1998 (3 of 4)[a]	+100%	–100%	+67%	–100%	+100%
1998–46[b] Aging	–	–	0	–	–
1998–23 HIV1	+1	–1	+1	–1	+1
1998–24 HIV2	+1	–1	+1	–1	+1
1999 (2 of 3)	+50%	+50%	+50%	00%	–
1999–38 HIV	+1	+1	+1	0	–
1999–39 Infectious diseases	0	0	0	0	–
2000 (6 of 11)	+100%	+100%	+83%	–50%	+100%
2000–73 Aging	+1	+1	0	–	–
2000–36 HIV	+1	+1	+1	–	+1
2000–38 Malaria	+1	+1	+1	–	+1
2000–37 Tuberculosis	+1	+1	+1	–	+1
2000–S108 Biotechnology	+1	+1	+1	–1	–
2000–23 Infectious diseases	–	–	+1	0	+1
2001 (1 of 3)	+100%	+100%	+100%	+100%	–
2001–26 Global Fund	+1	+1	+1	+1	–
2002 (3 of 19)	00%	33%	+67%	00%	–
2002–117 Medicines	0	0	+1	0	–
2002–11 Polio	0	0	0	0	–
2002–119 Global Fund	0	+1	+1	0	–
2003 (3 of 21)	+100%	+100%	+100%	+67%	+100%
2003–13 Polio	+1	+1	+1	+1	–
2003–10 Global Fund	+1	+1	+1	+1	+1
2003–14 SARS	+1	+1	+1	0	+1
2004 (2 of 12)	00%	00%	+100%	00%	+100%
2004–(10)1 HIV	+1	+1	+1	–1	+1
2004– (11)3 Polio	–1	–1	+1	+1	+1
2005 (2 of 18)	–50%	–100%	+50%	00%	+100%
2005–HIV	0	–1	0	+1	+1
2005–Polio	–1	–1	+1	–1	+1
Ratio (excluding 2005)	12/18	9/18	16/20	0/15	10/10
Average (excluding 2005)	67%	50%	80%	00%	100%
Ratio (including 2005)	11/20	7/20	17/22	0/17	12/12
Average (including 2005)	55%	35%	77%	0%	100%

Notes: Compiled by researchers at the G8 Research Group.

[a] Figures in parenthesis indicate the number of commitments monitored out of the total health commitments for that year.

[b] Identifier refers to the compilation of all G7/8 commitments produced by the G8 Research Group (2006a).

Appendix 11-2
Compliance Catalysts

Priority Placement. Priority placement refers to the presence of the commitment in the communiqué chapeau (introduction or preamble), summary (1990), or chair's statement (since 2002) to give to that particular commitment temporal primacy and prominence, emphasis through repetition, and/or the direct authority of leaders to a commitment contained documents devised elsewhere.

Target. A target is an identified, specific, and measurable welfare goal. (It provides the precisions and obligation featured by legalised liberal institutionalism.)

Timetables. A timetable is a specific target date and includes:

- an exact date, year, or season (autumn, summer, spring, winter) that is specified as the deadline for the commitment; terms such as 'over the year ahead', 'in the coming year', 'this year', or 'before the next summit' are assumed to be approximately twelve months.
- a specified meeting in forums that are not related to the G8 (e.g., at the United Nations General Assembly or a conference of parties) or in a specified G8 ministerial-level meeting.
- schedules agreed to in other forums that are reaffirmed in the commitment and are stated explicitly or implicitly (e.g., 'the timetables agreed at the end of the Uruguay Round', or 'by January 1, as decided at the United Nations General Assembly').

Specified Agency. Specified agency refers to the identification of national, intergovernmental, or other agents (individuals or organisations) responsible for putting the commitment into effect, thus suggesting a larger base of action than just the G8 on its own. Specified agency includes:

- any body, country, person, etc., specifically designated to take charge of a commitment as a representative of the G8.
- the involvement of the G8 countries along with 'all other countries', 'the international community as a whole', 'our partners', 'civil society', specified countries, etc.'; a pledge by the G8 to work with others to do something; a 'call on all countries' or pledge to work to enhance international efforts to achieve a target.

If the agent is a G8-centred ministerial or official-level institution or an international institution, it is coded in those categories rather than as an agent.

Remit Mandates. A remit mandate is a requirement to report back to the summit. (It helps provide the built-in iteration, repeated games, and long shadow of the future featured by several theories of international cooperation.) A commitment to re-examine an issue at a ministerial meeting, rather than the leaders summit, is coded as the use of a timetable, not a remit mandate.

Money Mobilised. Money mobilised refers to new money promised at the summit to put G8 commitments into effect.

continued

It includes:

- money committed by the G8;
- money committed by another agency, group, institution, etc.;
- reaffirmations of previously committed money.

A commitment to provide 'the necessary resources' or 'sufficient resources' for a target is not considered money mobilised.

Other Institutions. Other institutions refers to instructions to an international institution other than the G8 or a G8-centred ministerial and official-level body. Such institutions include:

- any international organisation other than the G8 that is specifically designated to take charge of the commitment;
- any institution or its ministerial meetings indicated (e.g., United Nations, Organisation for Economic Co-operation and Development, etc.) or the codes, rules, standards, conventions, system, work, etc., of a particular institution (e.g., the United Nations conventions against drugs) that are mentioned to emphasise the commitment without specifically asking the international institution to implement it.
- references to how the G8 plans to change, provide resources, or means to help fulfil a mandate to a specific international institution, without asking that institution to take control of the commitment.
- general mentions of 'all relevant international organisations', the international financial institutions', 'other international forums', etc.

G8 Institutions. G8 institutions refers to the creation of new G8-centred ministerial and official-level bodies for implementation, or direction to existing G8 institutions to take action on implementing the new commitment. This can include:

- an institution created by the G8 to take charge of the commitment (as suggested by legalisation's delegation and by the democratic institutionalist model of G8 governance);
- an existing G8 body that is mandated to take charge of the commitment;
- a request by the G8 or a reminder to the G8 members to take into consideration or build on the work or recommendations of an existing G8-centred ministerial or official-level institution;
- a commitment by the G8 to improve, strengthen, replenish, or otherwise increase the effectiveness of a previously existing G8-centred ministerial or official-level institution.

Appendix 11-3
Compliance-Generating Precursors for Health Commitments, 1998–2005 (Cases = 22)

Commitment and Issue	Priority Placement	Target	Timetable	Remit Mandate	Money
1998–23[a] HIV	–	–	–	–	–
1998–24 HIV	–	–	–	–	–
1998–46 Aging	–	–	–	–	–
1999–32 Infectious diseases	–	–	–	–	–
1999–38 HIV	–	–	–	–	–
2000–23 Infectious diseases	–	–	–	–	–
2000–36 HIV	–	Yes	Yes	–	–
2000–37 Tuberculosis	–	Yes	Yes	–	–
2000–38 Malaria	–	Yes	Yes	–	–
2000–73 Aging	–	–	–	–	–
2000–S108 Biotechnology	Yes	–	Yes	–	–
2001–26 Global Fund	–	–	Yes	–	Yes
2002–11 Polio	Yes	Yes	Yes	–	–
2002–117 Medicine	Yes	–	–	–	–
2002–119 Global Fund	Yes	–	–	–	–
2003–10 Global Fund	Yes	–	Yes	–	–
2003–13 Polio	Yes	Yes	Yes	–	–
2003–14 SARS	Yes	–	–	–	–
2004(10)–1 HIV	Yes	–	–	–	–
2004(11)–3 Polio	Yes	–	Yes	–	–
2005–42 Global Fund	Yes	Yes	Yes	–	Yes
2005–44 Polio	–	–	Yes	–	Yes
Total	10/22	6/22	11/22	0/20	3/22
Percentage	45%	27%	50%	00%	14%

continued

Appendix 11-3
Compliance-Generating Precursors for Health Commitments, 1998–2005, continued

Commitment and issue	Agent	G8-Centred Body	International Institution	Total	Score
1998–23[a] HIV	–	–	Yes	1	+0.33
1998–24 HIV	–	Yes	–	1	+0.11
1998–46 Aging	–	–	–	0	+0.33
1999–32 Infectious diseases	–	–	–	0	0.00
1999–38 HIV	–	–	–	0	+0.63
2000–23 Infectious diseases	–	–	–	0	+0.60
2000–36 HIV	Yes	–	Yes	4	+1.00
2000–37 Tuberculosis	Yes	–	Yes	4	+1.00
2000–38 Malaria	Yes	–	Yes	4	+1.00
2000–73 Aging	–	–	–	0	+0.86
2000–S108 Biotechnology	–	–	Yes	3	+0.86
2001–26 Global Fund	–	Yes	Yes	4	+0.75
2002–11 Polio	–	–	–	3	0.00
2002–117 Medicine	Yes	–	–	2	+0.38
2002–119 Global Fund	–	–	–	1	+0.25
2003–10 Global Fund	Yes	Yes	Yes	5	+0.88
2003–13 Polio	–	–	–	3	+1.00
2003–14 SARS	–	–	–	1	+0.78
2004(10)–1 HIV	–	Yes	–	2	+0.56
2004(11)–3 Polio	Yes	–	–	3	+0.44
2005–42 Global Fund	–	Yes	Yes	6	+0.33
2005–44 Polio	–	–	Yes	3	+0.11
Total	6/22	5/22	9/22	50/22	+55%
Percentage	27%	23%	41%	2.3/commitment	

Note: [a] Identifier refers to the compilation of all G7/8 commitments produced by the G8 Research Group (2006a).

Appendix 11-4
Compliance Catalysts in Health Commitments, 2005

Commitment and Issue (Total)	Compliance Score	Priority Placement	Target	Timetable
2005–5[a] Africa disease (1)		Yes		–
2005–9 Immunisation		Yes	–	–
2005–32 African health (1)		Yes	–	–
2005–33 Health workers (2)		Yes	–	–
2005–34 Healthy future (2)		Yes	–	–
2005–35 Teachers' AIDS (2)		Yes	–	–
2005–38 Health systems (2)		Yes	–	–
2005–39 Health capacity (1)		Yes	–	–
2005–40 HIV (2)		–	–	Yes
2005–41 AIDS orphans (2)		Yes	–	–
2005–42 Global Fund (6)	+0.33	Yes	Yes	Yes
2005–43 Biotechnology (0)		–	–	–
2005–44 Polio (3)	+0.11	–	–	Yes
2005–45 Malaria (4)		Yes	Yes	Yes
2005–46 Tuberculosis (3)		Yes	–	Yes
2005–47 Water (2)		–	–	–
2005–48 Famine (0)		–	–	–
2005–54 Health/food (1)		–	–	–
TOTAL	+22%	12/18	5/18	5/18
Percentage		67%	27%	27%

Commitment and Issue (Total)	Remit Mandate	Money	Agent	G8-Centred Body	International Institutions
2005–5[a] Africa disease (1)	–	–	–	–	–
2005–9 Immunisation	–	–	Yes	–	–
2005–32 African health (1)	–	–	–	–	–
2005–33 Health workers (2)	–	–	Yes	–	–
2005–34 Healthy future (2)	–	–	Yes	–	–
2005–35 Teachers' AIDS (2)	–	–	Yes	–	–
2005–38 Health systems (2)	–	–	Yes	–	–
2005–39 Health capacity (1)	–	–	–	–	–
2005–40 HIV (2)	–	–	–	–	Yes
2005–41 AIDS orphans (2)	–	–	Yes	–	–
2005–42 Global Fund (6)	–	Yes	–	Yes	Yes
2005–43 Biotechnology (0)	–	–	–	–	–
2005–44 Polio (3)	–	Yes	–	–	Yes
2005–45 Malaria (4)	–	–	Yes	–	–
2005–46 Tuberculosis (3)	–	–	–	Yes	–
2005–47 Water (2)	–	–	–	Yes	Yes
2005–48 Famine (0)	–	–	–	–	–
2005–54 Health/food (1)	–	–	Yes	–	–
TOTAL	–	2/18	8/18	3/18	4/18
Percentage	00%	11%	44%	17%	22%

Note: Even if an international institution is mentioned in two or more contexts within the same commitment, it is counted as one.

[a] Identifier refers to the compilation of all G7/8 commitments produced by the G8 Research Group (2006a).

Chapter 12

Breaking Faith with Africa: The G8 and Population Health after Gleneagles

Ted Schrecker, Ronald Labonté, and David Sanders

The G8 summit at Gleneagles was preceded by unprecedented popular culture rhetoric (the Live 8 concerts and the Make Poverty History wristband campaign) and also by the release of two major research syntheses on the topic. The United Nations Millennium Project was established in 2002 as an advisory body to the UN secretary general, under the directorship of economist Jeffrey Sachs, to explore policy options for achieving the Millennium Development Goals (MDGs) (Sachs and McArthur 2005; UN Millennium Project 2005). The Commission for Africa was established and chaired by Britain's prime minister Tony Blair in support of an African development focus for the summit (see Commission for Africa 2005).[1] Nevertheless, the author of the August/September 2005 cover story in *African Business* wondered: 'So, after the sound and fury of Gleneagles, what are we left with? Have there been any decisive policy changes that will ultimately lead most of Africa out of poverty?' (Versi 2005). The conclusion: 'One must say, reluctantly given the well-meaning intentions, that there were not.'

If one accepts this view of the Gleneagles outcome, as reflected in the content of summit commitments themselves and in subsequent policy developments, including the 2006 G8 St. Petersburg Summit, then it can be viewed as continuing a recent pattern of commitments and policies affecting health in the region: some commitments are fulfilled, others are compromised by uncoordinated initiatives or inadequate resources, and still others incorporate policy prescriptions that are actually destructive of health and human well-being (Labonté and Schrecker 2004; Labonté *et al.* 2004; Labonté and Schrecker 2005, 2006). Despite several genuinely positive outcomes from Gleneagles, the departure from a past pattern of 'fatal indifference' (Labonté *et al.* 2004) must be viewed as incremental rather than fundamental. Furthermore, there is concern about the sustainability of that departure in the uncertain world of G8 summitry. This concern is deepened by the limited attention paid to African issues at St. Petersburg beyond a rather self-congratulatory 'update on Africa', by the lack of progress on such key long-standing issues as secure financing for the Global Fund to Fight AIDS, Tuberculosis, and Malaria, and by the apparent collapse of the development round of World Trade Organization (WTO) negotiations just weeks after St. Petersburg.

This approach taken in this chapter is distinctive in several respects. First, it is concerned with policies that affect health, but not only with health care. A substantial body of research, to which Canadians have been important contributors, demonstrates that various aspects of social and economic systems are at least as relevant to the health status of a particular population as is its access to health care (Evans and Stoddart 1990, 2003; Evans, Barer, and Marmor 1994; Heymann *et al.* 2005). These are referred to generically as social determinants of health, and are the focus of a multinational commission established in 2005 by the World Health Organization (see WHO 2006b). Second, the chapter is concerned not only with whether the G8 fulfilled or failed to fulfil its summit commitments with respect to Africa, but also — indeed, primarily — with the adequacy of those commitments when measured against the scale of the region's needs and their appropriateness in view of what is known about the social determinants of health. These determinants are shaped by the broader social and economic policy context, which has been referred to as 'those central engines in society that generate and distribute power, wealth, and risks' (Diderichsen, Evans, and Whitehead 2001).[2] The approach taken here therefore incorporates a critique of the effects on the social determinants of health of the dominant development policy model that has been adopted with respect to Africa.

The G8 made a commitment at the 2001 Genoa Summit to 'make globalisation work for all [its] citizens and especially the world's poor' (G8 2001). Immediately following this statement was the claim that 'drawing the poorest countries into the global economy is the surest way to address their fundamental aspirations'. This formulation sidesteps the crucial question of on what terms (and on whose terms) such countries are to be integrated. The operative model has been described as the Washington consensus, after John Williamson's (1990) codification of the development policy wisdom of the time; it has alternatively been referred to as neo-liberal globalisation, in its representation of a retreat from post-war norms of at least partial social provision to the 'non-redistributive laissez faire liberalism of the seventeenth and eighteenth centuries, which held that the main function of government was to make the world safe and predictable for the participants in a market economy' (Jaggar 2002, 425). Regardless of terminology, little serious disagreement exists on either the broad outlines of the model, emphasising the liberalisation of trade (especially imports) and financial flows, deregulation, privatisation of state-owned economic entities, the scaling back of government subsidies, and a retreat from other forms of social provision on the grounds that even if affordable they encourage economic inefficiency, or the consistency with which key institutions in the industrialised world promoted it throughout most of Africa.[3]

The governments of G7 countries were not alone in promoting this model, of course, and the lead role was often assumed by multilateral institutions: the World Bank, the International Monetary Fund, and, more recently, the WTO.[4] However, the G8 nations 'account for 48% of the global economy and 49% of global trade, hold four of the United Nations' five permanent Security Council seats, and boast majority shareholder control over the International Monetary Fund (IMF) and the World Bank'

(G8 Research Group 2005). They also account for roughly 75 percent of the annual value of development assistance expenditure, and their deep pockets are among the resources that provide them with formidable advantages in trade negotiations and dispute resolution proceedings, both within and outside the framework provided by the WTO (Jawara and Kwa 2003). Hence, there is a third respect in which the approach taken here is distinctive, and explains the title of this chapter. 'Breaking faith' implies the existence of an obligation (in this case, on the part of the G7/8 countries) that has not been lived up to, whether the obligation is derived from a previous promise or from some other source. One can identify at least four such sources, in addition to specific commitments that were made at annual summits.

Population Health and the G8: Why Care?

First, obligations may be said to arise from the sheer disparity between the resources available to the world's affluent minority and the modest cost of medical and public health interventions that would save literally millions of human lives per year. On this line of argument, 'radical inequality' is ethically reprehensible both because simple arithmetic suggests that it is so easily avoidable (Pogge 2005b) and because of the incommensurability of needs that remain unmet for millions and wants that are easily satisfied by the winners in the global economy: 'One person's desire for an additional jar of caviar is not equal in urgency to another person's need for an additional bowl of black beans' (Shue 1996, 10). The argument is broadly analogous to the rule of rescue (McKie and Richardson 1982), with the distinction that the lives in question are 'statistical lives' that do not belong to identifiable individuals. Although popular acceptance neither validates nor vitiates an ethical argument, it should be noted that the extent to which an obligation to provide access to health care or key social determinants of health on grounds of disparities and affordability would be accepted by G8 electorates even with respect to their fellow nationals is unclear and varies among the countries in question. Solidarity, for example, is widely invoked in discussions of access to health services in some European jurisdictions, but is absent from the vocabulary used in Canadian discussions of the same issue (Flood, Stabile, and Tuohy 2002; Giacomini *et al.* 2004). This point is revisited at the end of the chapter.

Second, the international community, to the extent that the membership of the United Nations General Assembly (UNGA) fits that description, has committed support for achievement of the MDGs by specified target dates, usually 2015 (see Appendix). Three of the goals involve reducing child and maternal mortality and reversing the spread of HIV/AIDS, malaria, and other communicable diseases; these are explicitly related to health. Four others directly address crucial social determinants of (ill) health, such as extreme poverty, undernourishment, living in slums, the subordination of women, and lack of access to education, safe water, and basic sanitation. An assessment prepared for a WHO forum held in 2004 is typical in its conclusion that 'even if economic growth accelerates … and even if progress toward the gender and water goals is substantially accelerated, the developing world is likely to wake up on the morning of January 1, 2016, some way from the health targets; in Sub-Saharan Africa, it may be a long way' (Wagstaff and Claeson 2004, 42). More recent syntheses of available evidence have offered similar prognoses, at least in the absence of greatly intensified policy efforts on the part of the industrialised world (UN 2005; WHO 2005b). Given the dominant role of the G8 in the global economic and geopolitical order, it seems reasonable to ascribe to them a substantial share of the responsibility for this impending policy failure.

Third, in a world in which an increasingly dense network of trade and investment flows and 'government networks' links rich and poor across national borders, it may be reasonable to search for loci of past and current causal responsibility (who makes what happen?) in that set of networks (see Slaughter 2005). Thomas Pogge has developed an extensive corpus of work elaborating this line of argument with specific reference to the global persistence of poverty. His position can be summarised as follows:

> We are not bystanders who find ourselves confronted with foreign deprivations whose origins are wholly unconnected to ourselves. In fact, there are at least three morally significant connections between us and the global poor. First, their social starting positions and ours have emerged from a single historical process that was pervaded by massive grievous wrongs … Second, they and we depend on a single natural resource base, from the benefits of which they are largely, and without compensation, excluded … Third, they and we coexist within a single global economic order that has a strong tendency to perpetuate and even to aggravate global economic inequality (Pogge 2001, 14–15; see also Pogge 2002; Pogge 2005a, 2005b).

Two elements of that order are singled out for special attention by Pogge: the 'resource privilege', which describes the international community's willingness to allow rulers to dispose of natural resources within their borders with scant concern for the well-being of their subjects (as in the appropriation of billions of dollars in resource revenues by Mobutu Sese Seko and Sani Abacha, among others), and the 'borrowing privilege', which maintains the collectibility of debts incurred by rulers on behalf of the countries they govern, without scrutiny of the extent to which subjects have consented to those financial obligations. This latter privilege has quite specific implications for development policy, as indicated in the subsequent discussion of the issue of odious debt. 'Given these connections,' concludes Pogge (2001, 15), 'our failure to make a serious effort toward poverty reduction may constitute not merely a lack of beneficence, but our active impoverishing, starving, and killing millions of innocent people by economic means'.

Fourth, obligations related to development and population health may also arise from international human rights law. Key texts include the 1948 Universal Declaration of Human Rights, which states that 'everyone has the right to a standard of living adequate for the health and well-being of himself and of his family' (UN 1948, art. 25); the 1966 International Covenant on Economic, Social, and Cultural

Rights, never ratified by the United States, which specifies the 'right of everyone to the enjoyment of the highest attainable standard of physical and mental health' (Office of the High Commissioner for Human Rights 1966, art. 12); and General Comment 14 of the UN Economic and Social Council (2000, para. 33), which sets out states' specific legal obligations 'to *respect, protect* and *fulfil'* the right to health.[5] Even apart from the 1966 covenant, Pogge argues that specific duties follow from article 28 of the Universal Declaration of Human Rights: 'Everyone is entitled to a social and international order in which the rights and freedoms set forth in this Declaration can be fully realized.' At present, no effective supranational mechanisms analogous to the institutions of trade policy and law exist to ensure respect for these requirements, which represents a glaring asymmetry in the world of international relations. Nevertheless, this source of obligations cannot be dismissed as irrelevant, and is indeed the focus of increased attention within the UN system, notably the appointment of a special rapporteur on the right to health (Hunt 2003, 2004, 2005; Office of the High Commissioner for Human Rights 2006).

African Development, Poverty, and Health: Some Necessary Background

Even apart from the scrutiny of compliance with commitments made at G8 summits, then, several sets of reasons exist for ascribing responsibility to the G8, individually and collectively, for changes in the social determinants of health in Africa. The most basic and omnipresent term of the equation is poverty, however defined. According to the World Bank's figures, in sub-Saharan Africa 313 million people, or almost half the population, live below a standardised poverty line of US$1 or less per day (Chen and Ravallion 2004). Caution is in order about the use of these figures. It has been argued that the way in which market income figures are adjusted for purchasing power parity bears little relation to real-world prices of basic necessities (Reddy and Pogge 2005). David Satterthwaite (2003) notes that this disconnect may be especially acute in the case of major urban areas, even in the poorest countries: rapid urbanisation in the developing world may therefore mean that the extent to which the World Bank's estimates understate the global extent of inability to meet basic needs is actually increasing over time. And poverty, when treated as a dichotomous variable (poor/non-poor), has the disadvantage of implying that different kinds of redistributive obligations apply to people depending on whether they fall just to one side or the other of a largely arbitrary divide. The World Bank figures are nevertheless useful in the African context for highlighting the fact that sub-Saharan Africa is the only region of the world in which, according to this admittedly flawed measurement, the number of people living in extreme poverty has increased — indeed, almost doubled between 1981 and 2001. This reflects a disastrous failure of development policy, with far-reaching implications for population health.

Interactions between poverty and ill health are pernicious everywhere. They are pervasive throughout the developing world, particularly in Africa. Inadequate health care sets 'medical poverty traps' at the household level, because of medical costs (user fees, but also costs of transport to often distant medical facilities) and loss of income resulting from inability to work (Whitehead, Dahlgren, and Evans 2001). At the national level, the fundamental finding of the Commission on Macroeconomics and Health (2001), established by the WHO as its first exploration of the linkages between economic development and health, was that improved health can make a substantial contribution to economic growth. Low-cost, demonstrably effective interventions that could save millions of lives per year throughout the developing world are available (Commission on Macroeconomics and Health 2001; Jha *et al.* 2002; Bryce *et al.* 2005). However, a minimal level of health-system functioning is required to deliver even relatively simple interventions such as childhood immunisation; a higher level of both physical and human infrastructure, although still rudimentary by standards of the industrialised world, is required for such services as effective HIV prevention and antiretroviral treatment (ART) (Travis *et al.* 2004; Sanders, Chopra, and Todd 2005). In the words of the Commission for Africa (2005, 188, 190), 'massive under-investment, along with unsystematic responses to single diseases and unpredictable financing, have left health care delivery at the point of collapse. Poor people are the worst affected' as 'health care delivery systems are in danger of disintegrating beyond repair.'

As one illustration of the consequences, immunisation coverage with the six basic vaccines of childhood (against tuberculosis, polio, diphtheria, pertussis, tetanus, measles) has stagnated at a dismal 50 percent to 60 percent in the region (WHO 2005a). The seemingly intractable 'brain drain' of health professionals from sub-Saharan Africa is now recognised as perhaps the single most immediate contributor to health system crisis (Chen *et al.* 2004; Friedman 2004; Joint Learning Initiative 2004; WHO 2006a); according to one estimate it costs countries in the region US$0.5 billion per year in health training investment (Commission for Africa 2005, 192). One recent study indicated that 'sub-Saharan countries must nearly triple their current numbers of workers by adding the equivalent of 1 million workers through retention, recruitment, and training if they are to come close to approaching the MDGs for health' (Chen *et al.* 2004). A recent study estimated that the 600 or more South African–trained physicians who have been licensed to practice in Canada since 1993 represented a loss in South Africa's public training costs approaching CA$1 billion; or a savings of some CA$3 billion to CA$5 billion in foregone Canadian training costs (Labonté, Packer, and Klassen 2006).

The effects of the brain drain are compounded by losses of health professionals to HIV/AIDS and by the internal brain drain of health professionals into the private healthcare sector and into vertical, donor-supported initiatives that address specific diseases or deliver specific interventions, such as the U.S.-funded President's Emergency Program for AIDS Relief. These programmes, which have historically been favoured by G8 donor countries, routinely offer better salaries and working conditions than are available in healthcare institutions funded from national revenue budgets.

Health Care and Health Systems

The G8 did not rise to this set of challenges at Gleneagles, most conspicuously in their failure to provide adequate financing for the Global Fund to Fight AIDS, Tuberculosis, and Malaria. AIDS and malaria alone are responsible for approximately 3.5 million deaths per year in Africa. The Global Fund, announced by the G8 in 2001 with rhetoric about 'a quantum leap in the fight against infectious diseases', estimates that it will need US$7.1 billion in 2006 and 2007 to fund new projects and continuations of existing work, but had pledges in hand for those years of just US$1.45 billion at the time of the Gleneagles Summit (G8 2001; Global Fund 2005a; Global Fund 2006a). The effect was, and is, to create tight constraints on the value of grants that can be approved even after scientific merit has been demonstrated in the fund's competitive technical review process, since the fund 'can only approve grants if the full amount required for the first two years is covered by pledges from donors in the calendar year of the approval' (Global Fund 2005a, 34). The September 2005 replenishment meeting raised the total value of funds pledged for 2006–07 to US$3.73 billion, or just over half the anticipated funding requirement (Global Fund 2005b). This can hardly be seen as the basis for a quantum leap. More fundamentally, the G8 can be faulted for failing to move forward on the need to secure longer term financial support for the Global Fund, which now estimates that funding requirements could be as high as US$7–8 billion per year, as an alternative to the current practice of periodic replenishment meetings at which the fund, in effect, passes around a hat (Global Fund 2005a, 32; Commission for Africa 2005, 196). At the St. Petersburg Summit, the G8 would commit only to 'work with other donors and stakeholders in the effort to secure funds needed for the 2006–2007 replenishment period and call upon all concerned to participate actively in the development of a four-year strategy, aimed at building a solid foundation for the activities of the Fund in the years ahead' (G8 2006).

Programs such as the Global Fund and the Global Alliance for Vaccines and Immunization (GAVI), although valuable, tend to emphasise funds for specific technical interventions such as new drugs and vaccines. The Global Fund (2006b), for example, targets 49 percent of its expenditure on drugs and commodities, such as ART and new anti-malarials, but only 20 percent on human resources and training; GAVI began by spending 90 percent of its disbursements on vaccines and injectables but only 10 percent on health-system strengthening (Hardon 2001); this ratio has since changed to approximately two thirds and one third (GAVI Alliance 2006). More generally, support for 'vertical' programmes, often provided without long-term donor commitments, is unaccompanied by support for strengthening health systems. The Commission for Africa (2005, 196–195) placed special emphasis on this need, arguing for an immediate increase of US$10 billion in donor support for African health systems including 'long-term and predictable compensatory funding' needed to eliminate all user fees for basic health care but excluding the costs of responding to the HIV/AIDS crisis and delivered 'predominantly through national budgets' rather than project-specific funding. In making this recommendation, the commission was arguably responding to long-standing criticisms of how user fees and 'cost recovery' programmes undermine access to health care for the poor and of how donor practices and policies compromise the effectiveness of development assistance for health by fragmenting national efforts to develop integrated health systems and increasing opportunity costs for already overstretched ministries of health (see Lister 2005). Continued lack of a detailed response on the part of the G8, which at past summits has announced highly specific action plans on other topics, is a troubling indication both of the relatively low priority attached to health care as a human right and a lack of understanding of the critical role of health in economic development.

Official Development Assistance

One of the two highest-profile outcomes of Gleneagles was a commitment to increasing official development assistance (ODA) to Africa by US$25 billion by 2010, driven primarily by pre-summit announcements by France, Britain, and the European Union to raise their aid spending to the long-standing UN target of 0.7 percent of each industrialised country's gross national income (GNI), originally floated in 1970 and cautiously reaffirmed at the United Nations Conference on Financing for Development in Monterrey in 2002. Conversely Canada, the United States, and Japan were conspicuous by refusing to state timetables for reaching the 0.7 percent target. The Gleneagles development assistance commitment can be read as a direct response to the reports of the UN Millennium Project and, in particular, the Commission for Africa, each of which recommended an approximate doubling of the current value of ODA. Some civil society organisations, notably Jubilee Research (2005), were strongly critical of this commitment on the basis that much of it involved not genuinely new money, but rather recycled announcements made in advance of the summit. This is perhaps a less serious limitation than several others.

First, no specific financing mechanisms were described, leaving the prospect that the commitments will fall by the wayside as other, domestic priorities take over the attention of governments. The International Financing Facility (IFF), which was promoted by Britain and recommended both by the Commission for Africa (2005, 333–335) and the UN Millennium Project (2005, 256), was not endorsed at Gleneagles. The IFF would provide new funds for ODA by issuing bonds backed by national governments' pledges of funds up until 2015, although the term of the bonds would be much longer. The proposal has numerous problems, notably the possibility of a major drop in post-2015 development assistance flows and the fact that raising funds through new borrowing rather than taxation would transfer US$220 billion to presumably wealthy bondholders over a 30-year period (Moss 2005); however, it has the advantage of offering clear assurance that aid commitments will actually be fulfilled. Thus the G8 can be faulted for neither adopting the proposal nor offering a clear alternative that would provide a comparable degree of predictability in terms of the availability of ODA funds. Second, some of the new spending may come in the form of additional debt relief (as noted below), or may simply offset substantial revenue losses from import liberalisation by developing countries, for instance as a result of the economic partnership agreements now being negotiated between the EU and African countries.[6] Third, no specific priorities are indicated for aid — as would be suggested by the preceding discussion of the need to strengthen health systems and by the UN Millennium Project's strong critique of current aid priorities as not being aligned with the MDGs. It estimated that just 35 percent of aid to low-income countries, and 20 percent of aid to middle-income countries, provides direct support for achieving the MDGs (UN Millennium Project 2005, 199). The lack of specific priorities for aid may respond to calls for expanded opportunities for recipient countries to select their own priorities, but this has not been a major concern of most aid suppliers historically, and the lack of explicit commitment to supporting the MDGs (or any other set of core objectives related to basic needs) stands in striking contrast to the long history and current persistence of detailed economic policy conditionalities attached to structural adjustment lending and debt relief.

Conversely, the civil society critiques neglect an important positive dimension of the Gleneagles aid commitment: it can be read as rejecting, as did the UN Millennium Project and the Commission for Africa, a scepticism about the value of ODA that is fashionable in some circles.[7] While properly directing attention to the internal politics and political economy of African countries, the sceptical position fails to attach enough importance to external factors such as the willingness of industrialised world financial institutions to facilitate capital flight, the industrialised world's hunger for natural resources (*cf.* Pogge's discussion of the resource privilege), and the debilitating effects of structural adjustment conditionalities.[8] In an important shift of the assignment of responsibility, the UN Millennium Project and the Commission for Africa each emphasised donor policies and practices as constraints on aid effectiveness. The UN Millennium Project (2005, 202) argued that 'the notion of taking the [Millennium Development] Goals seriously remains highly unorthodox among development practitioners' because of a lack of financial support from the industrialised world; it identified numerous ways in which aid suppliers should realign their activities with support for the MDGs. Furthermore, in a direct challenge to received wisdom that weak governance or absorptive-capacity constraints seriously limit the potential benefits from short-term increases in ODA, its discussion of Africa argued that the quality of governance in African countries is comparable to that in other regions with similarly low per capita incomes. Incomes are a necessary consideration for comparison purposes because 'good governance requires resources for wages, training, information systems, and so forth' (146) — resources that may simply not be available.

Debt Relief

Perhaps the most serious constraint on aid's effectiveness is that 'dozens of heavily indebted poor and middle-income countries are forced by creditor governments to spend large parts of their limited tax receipts on debt service, undermining their ability to finance investments in human capital and infrastructure. In a pointless and debilitating churning of resources, the creditors provide development assistance with one hand and then withdraw it in debt servicing with the other' (UN Millennium Project 2005, 35). Between 1970 and 2002, African countries borrowed US$540 billion from foreign sources, paid back US$550 billion (in principal and interest), but still owe US$295 billion, according to the United Nations Conference on Trade and Development ([UNCTAD] 2004, 19).

Over the past ten years, the G8 has led the industrialised world in committing a total of US$58 billion to the partial cancellation of the debts of up to 40 countries, 32 of them in Africa, under the Enhanced Heavily Indebted Poor Countries (HIPC) Initiative. Some G7 members have gone farther in terms of offering the cancellation of debts owed to their governments alone. Although this initiative has made possible increased public spending on health and education in a number of recipient countries (Gupta *et al.* 2002), it has also been widely criticised on several grounds. First, debt relief is often also used simply to pay off other creditors. For example, between 2002 and 2005 almost two thirds of the revenue freed by debt relief for Zambia went to reduce debts owed to other creditors, leaving only a third for investing in poverty-reducing programmes including health and education (IMF and World Bank 2005, 35).

Second, according to one pre-Gleneagles estimate, half the debts of the HIPCs would remain unpaid and uncancelled even if all countries received the full amount of debt relief for which they were eligible (Martin 2004). Despite receiving debt relief, two African countries (Malawi and Mozambique) have actually seen increases in their debt service costs, while Uganda and Senegal have seen reductions of less than 25 percent (UN Department of Economic and Social Affairs 2005, 148).

Third, the conditions attached to debt relief for HIPCs, notably the requirement that a Poverty Reduction Strategy Paper (PRSP) be approved by the World Bank and the IMF, have been criticised as replicating an earlier pattern of conditionalities attached to structural adjustment loans (Cheru 2001; Gottschalk 2004). These often increased economic inequality, reduced access to health care, led to deterioration in the social determinants of health, and almost certainly accelerated the spread of HIV infection (Cornia, Stewart, and Jolly 1987; Bijlmakers, Bassett, and Sanders 1999; Cheru 1999; Schoepf *et al.* 2000; Kim *et al.* 2000; Sanders and Sambo 1991; De Vogli and Birbeck 2005). The report of the UN Millennium Project added a further dimension to the critique of PRSPs by noting that 'very few PRSPs are ambitious enough to achieve the [Millennium Development] Goals, *largely because* they have been prepared in a context of insufficient donor assistance' (UN Millennium Project 2005, 49 [emphasis added]).

Fourth, the process of granting debt relief under the Enhanced HIPC Initiative still gives priority to minimising creditors' losses rather than meeting basic needs in debtor countries: at the insistence of the G7 a sustainable debt load has been defined with reference to forecasts of future export earnings (Martin 2004). The UN Millennium Project incorporated many earlier critiques in recommending that '"debt sustainability" should be redefined as "the level of debt consistent with achieving the Millennium Development Goals," arriving in 2015 without a new debt overhang. For many heavily indebted poor countries, this will require 100 percent debt cancellation. For many heavily indebted middle-income countries, this will require more debt relief than has been on offer' (UN Millennium Project 2005, 207–208).

At Gleneagles, the G8 agreed to a proposal that had been previously accepted by the G7 finance ministers to cancel an additional US$40 billion to US$56 billion of debts owed by HIPCs to the World Bank, the IMF, and the concessional arm of the African Development Bank (AfDB). This commitment, which has now been formalised as the Multilateral Debt Relief Initiative (MDRI), was a welcome and overdue next step, as was a separate partial debt cancellation deal for Nigeria estimated to be worth US$31 billion (World Bank 2006; Elliott and Wintour 2005). However, questions remain about reliability, since as of early 2005 US$12.3 billion of commitments under the existing Enhanced HIPC Initiative remained unfunded (UN Department of Economic and Social Affairs 2005, 146). The Gleneagles response also may be inadequate. Notably, it fails to address the debts owed by low-income non-HIPCs other than Nigeria, including those owed to private creditors (Commission for Africa 2005, 328). Development assistance to countries that receive additional debt relief under the MDRI will be reduced by some portion of the amount (IMF 2005), thus repeating the pattern in which ODA declined substantially in the late 1990s after the start of the original HIPC Initiative (Killick 2004, 6–7). As a further indication of the persistence of this pattern, Britain's Department for International Development (DfID) conceded in April 2006 that its inflation-adjusted spending on development assistance had actually declined between 2004 and 2005 if one subtracted the value of Britain's contribution to debt relief for Nigeria and Iraq (Gow 2006).

Perhaps of most immediate concern are the conditions that are likely to be attached to debt cancellation. For example, the Nigerian debt deal requires acceptance of 'intensive surveillance of its economy by the International Monetary Fund' (Elliott and Wintour 2005). Given Nigeria's record of corruption and misallocation of resource revenues, such surveillance is not intrinsically undesirable, but the IMF's past record is grounds for scepticism about whether it will focus on how effectively the Nigerian government directs resources toward basic needs. Since Gleneagles the World Bank expressed concern that the G8 debt cancellation announcement 'offered no mechanism for suspending debt relief if a debtor country deviated from economic and social reforms' prescribed by it and the IMF — presumably reforms at least partly like those characteristic of the earlier era of structural adjustment (Wroughton 2005). So far 19 countries have reached the 'completion point' under the Enhanced HIPC Initiative, meaning they have already been through multiple stages of approvals by the IMF and World Bank; only these countries are eligible for the additional debt relief offered in 2005. Adding new conditions indicates that these institutions and the G8 members that together command effective voting majorities in both are not prepared to relinquish control over the economic and social policies of recipient countries, opting instead for a more extended period of what can only be called forced integration into the global economy.

Finally, the Gleneagles and St. Petersburg summits continued a long-standing refusal to address the question of odious debts (Kremer and Jayachandran 2002; King, Khalfan, and Thomas 2003). The Commission for Africa (2005, 114) correctly pointed out that during the Cold War era, 'dictators who were enriching themselves through their countries' oil, diamonds and other resources … siphoned billions of dollars out of their country [*sic*] using the financial systems of developed countries' — an illustration of the pernicious interaction of the resource and borrowing privileges identified by Pogge — and cited an estimate 'that stolen African assets equivalent to more than half of the continent's external debt are held in foreign bank accounts' (150).[9] However, neither the commission nor the G8 seriously proposed that public debts incurred (for example) by Zaire (now the Democratic Republic of the Congo) under Mobutu Sese Seko, Kenya under Daniel arap Moi, Nigeria under Sani Abacha, or South Africa under the National Party between 1948 and 1994 should be regarded as uncollectible.[10] The G8 has never addressed this issue, although it is surely not beyond members' individual and collective forensic ingenuity to compile an inventory of odious debts and criminalise attempts to collect them by natural or legal persons within their jurisdictions, including both public and private creditors.

Trade Policy

A development policy failure with comparably destructive effects on equitable access to the social determinants of health involves trade. Recent trade policy has required that developing countries accept minimal gains as the price of major concessions, which may foreclose policy flexibilities that the now-industrialised countries used in earlier stages of their own economic development (Chang 2002, 2005). Many developing countries have destroyed their domestic economic sectors, such as textiles and clothing in Zambia (Jeter 2002) and poultry in Ghana (Atarah 2005), by lowering trade barriers and accepting the resulting social dislocations as the price of global integration. Import liberalisation was a key element of structural adjustment programmes; one study found that PRSPs may include 'trade-related conditions that are more stringent, in terms of requiring more, or faster, or deeper liberalisation, than WTO provisions to which the respective country has agreed', thus underscoring the continuity of macroeconomic policy prescriptions (Brock and McGee 2004, 20).

Development policy protagonists who disagree about much else agree on the desirability of drastically improving access to industrialised world markets for developing country exports, and in particular on the need to reduce market-distorting agricultural subsidies, often citing estimates issued by the Organisation for Economic Co-operation and Development ([OECD] 2004) that support for agricultural producers amounts to more than US$300 billion annually. Five years after the commencement of WTO negotiations that were described by the G8 leaders and others in terms of a development agenda, negotiations apparently collapsed in July 2006 — ironically, just weeks after the St. Petersburg Summit — largely because of industrialised country intransigence on agricultural subsidies ('In the Twilight of

Doha' 2006; International Centre for Trade and Sustainable Development [ICTSD] 2006).

Admittedly, the relations between agricultural subsidies as defined by the OECD and prospects for development are more complicated than acknowledged by many participants in the debates.[11] No one-to-one correspondence exists between the value of subsidies, as defined by the OECD, and income lost by agricultural producers outside the OECD. Model-based estimates of the 'welfare gains' from worldwide elimination of agricultural subsidies fail to distinguish winners and losers within developing countries and regions, and in some cases the losses would be substantial, thus undermining the claimed pro-poor, pro-development effect of subsidy cuts. Although improved market access in the developing world may increase the incomes of agricultural producers who are already part of the cash economy, it is likely to have little benefit for larger numbers of producers who are primarily oriented toward subsistence, with occasional local market sales — the problem of 'two agricultures', one of which requires selective domestic subsidy as well as other policy supports if it is to remain viable (Howell 2005; see also Cousins 2006). Finally, some of the most serious, negative trade-related impacts on producers of specific crops are attributable only in part to developed country subsidies. Indiscriminate liberalisation of agricultural imports, which may be part of a larger governmental strategy of embracing the global marketplace even at high cost to particular economic sectors, is also implicated; so too is the increased control of agricultural commodity chains by multinational corporations (MNCs) based in the industrialised world, which tend to maximise profits on a global scale with little concern for the viability of local economies (Weatherspoon and Reardon 2003; McMichael 2005).

This is not to let the G8 off the hook with respect to specific destructive subsidies, but to suggest that the entire issue requires 'a more fine-grained approach, which would differentiate among crops and countries', with more sensitivity to incidence of costs and benefits within developing countries than has been evident in the course of recent multilateral trade negotiations and G8 summits (Stiglitz and Charlton 2005, 45). The events of the summer of 2006 suggest that prospects for implementing such an approach in a development-friendly way have taken a turn for the worse. These events also suggest problems ahead for acting on the tension between provisions in trade agreements and developing countries' need for 'policy space' within which to implement social and economic policies that meet the needs of their own citizens — or, at least, their governments' interpretation of those needs (Chang 2002, 2005; South Centre 2005).[12] One mechanism for providing that flexibility, but not the only one, is the special and differential treatment (SDT or S&DT) provision in trade agreements, which has existed since the founding of the General Agreement on Tariffs and Trade (GATT).[13] WTO members, including the G7, agreed in 2001 to review 'all special and differential provisions … with a view to *strengthening* them and making them more precise, effective and operational' (WTO 2001, para. 44 [emphasis added]). However, a 2004 assessment noted flatly that 'efforts since then to achieve these objectives have come to naught' because of deep differences between developed and developing countries (Hoekman 2004).

From a development policy perspective, 'it is important to see S&DT as a mechanism to deal with systemic imbalances in the trading system. It is not charity, but rather dealing with the reality of an unequal playing field resulting from rules designed by negotiations by unequal partners' (ICTSD 2003, 17). One observer notes that the fundamental question is whether such provisions should be considered temporary measures to facilitate the integration of developing economies into global exchange relationships characterised by dramatic disparities in resources and bargaining power, or whether 'the bottom-line question for the WTO should be what it can do to facilitate development, not what it is willing to allow to ease adjustment' (Garcia 2004, 300). The Commission for Africa (2005, 280–281) similarly mooted the idea of applying to selected WTO commitments a 'development test' that 'would focus on the likely net effects of not implementing WTO rules in favour of more development-orientated trade policy and on negative spillovers, and would allow greater discussion of development concerns, rather than merely the implementation of the rule of law.

The events of July 2006 suggest that such measures are highly unlikely if they would create substantial costs for any politically significant domestic constituency in the industrialised world, unless there are also very substantial benefits for comparably influential actors. Further concerns arise from the proliferation of bilateral and regional trade negotiations and agreements, in which disparities between industrialised and developing countries in bargaining power and resources may be even more glaring (World Bank 2004, 27–56). 'WTO-plus' provisions emerging from these settings may vitiate whatever gains in terms of market access and domestic policy flexibility African countries, and others in the developing world, are able to secure within the WTO framework (Shadlen 2005). Unless the WTO negotiating process can be quickly and decisively revitalised, it is likely that the industrialised countries will simply 'go bilateral' or regional, arguably with negative impacts on all developing countries save those few with special bargaining advantages.

Such tensions within trade policy are not surprising. The criticisms of G8 offered here, and in fact the entire concept of the trade negotiations that began in 2001 as a 'development round', imply the desirability of 'a fundamental departure from the system of mercantilism towards a collectively agreed global social welfare function. However, there has been almost no discussion, let alone agreement, on what that function should be' (Stiglitz and Charlton 2004, 496). Still less has trade policy acknowledged the need to incorporate the issues of fairness and distribution that are an integral part of linking trade with development, or with attaining shared objectives such as the MDGs (Stiglitz and Charlton 2005).

Conclusion: What to Expect from the G8?

As noted earlier, it is important to situate these observations in the context of what is known about the social determinants of health — more specifically, with reference to fact 'that many of the most devastating problems that plague the daily lives of billions of people are problems that emerge from a single, fundamental source: the consequences of poverty and inequality' (Paluzzi and Farmer 2005, 12; see also Farmer 2003). The preceding discussion of the health implications of recent G8 policies and summit commitments is far from exhaustive. For example, no discussion of hunger and food insecurity is provided, although this is one of the most clearly poverty-related determinants of health and more than 800 million people — including 240 million in Africa — are chronically undernourished and a substantially larger number suffer from serious micronutrient deficiencies (UN Standing Committee on Nutrition 2000, 23–32; Food and Agriculture Organization 2005). Neither does this chapter address such crucial issues as lack of regulation of the trade in small arms manufactured in the G8 countries or brokered by individuals or firms within their jurisdiction — a persistent failure of the international community and one with special significance for much of Africa. However, the analysis provided here suffices to raise some fundamental questions about the role of the G8 in a globalising world, and also to demonstrate the value of an explicitly normative approach to the G8 and population health.

To what extent is it reasonable to expect leadership from the G8 on development and global health? The G8 originated as the G6 in response to the economic crises of the 1970s as an effort to restore the profitability of private investment by coordinating macroeconomic policy (Webb 2000) — what Stephen Gill (1999, 131) calls 'part of an attempt to institutionalize a new form of transnational capitalist hegemony, and to reinforce the power of certain social forces within an emergent transnational civil society'. Political institutions like the G8 of course evolve in response to both internal and external influences, and heightened recent concern with African development issues is a matter of record. However, expecting leadership from the G8 on issues related to the determinants of health outside the industrialised world may be asking too much, for two related reasons.

First, the fact that summit agendas are determined by the host country is not necessarily conducive to building momentum for complex issues that inherently require high levels of policy coordination, except in the case where a high degree of agreement already exists among G8 governments. This is almost certainly not the case with respect to reshaping development policy in ways that are conducive to widely shared improvements in population health — especially not given the current trend of unilateralism and aggressive defence of national economic interests on the part of the United States. On the other hand, early press reports on the agenda for the 2007 Heiligendamm Summit in Germany indicate that poverty and African issues will both be on the agenda (G8 Research Group 2006). Thus the potential may exist for regaining whatever momentum remains from the grand words at Gleneagles — and, crucially, an opportunity may exist for the Commission on Social Determinants of Health to foreground the linkages among poverty, development, and population health.

Second, domestic politics enter the equation. The G8 are formal democracies, in the sense that they operate on the basis of peaceful transfers of power among leaders based on periodic, reasonably open competitions for political office. Political leaders can try to shape the policy preferences of their electorates, as Prime Minister

Tony Blair did in advance of Gleneagles. At the same time, they must continue to appeal to some combination of interests that together comprise a decisive electoral plurality. They must also keep in mind the limits that an integrated global economy imposes even on the rich countries (Fourcade-Gourinchas and Babb 2002; Tanzi 2002). They must also consider the fact that political leaders are by no means the only ones able to engage in value shaping: one such example is Jeffrey Sachs and the mass media exposure of the campaign against poverty (Sachs 2005), but another is Fox News, other elements of Rupert Murdoch's media empire, and the global concentration of media ownership (McChesney and Schiller 2003). When G8 governments fail to engage adequately with the imperatives identified earlier in this chapter, they cannot be assumed to be acting either in isolation from or in opposition to domestic constituencies. A key question therefore becomes, as transnational economic integration (globalisation) widens the divide between economic winners and losers, both within and across national borders, under what conditions is it possible to exercise political leadership and mobilise domestic coalitions in support of a global development and health agenda that explicitly assigns priority to such values as achieving the MDGs?

Notes

1 Commissioners included finance ministers from Canada and the United Kingdom, the former director of the International Monetary Fund (Michel Camdessus), several African leaders, and entertainment entrepreneur Bob Geldof. Although the establishment of the commission was initially met with cynicism by development activists and African civil society organisations, its final report was strongly critical of the industrialised countries' past policies on aid, trade, and debt relief. Many of its recommendations, released a few months before the Gleneagles Summit, resembled the more sweeping reform calls of the Make Poverty History civil society campaign.

2 The analytical framework set out by Finn Diderichsen and his colleagues (2001) has, with modifications, been adopted by the WHO Commission on Social Determinants of Health (see Solar and Irwin 2005).

3 See, for example, Michael Barratt Brown (1995), David Simon *et al.* (1995), Brooke Schoepf *et al.* (2000). Disagreement persists on the relative contribution to development failures in Africa of external factors, including the Washington consensus, and internal factors such as neo-patrimonial systems of rule even in formally democratic states. Notably, Nicolas van de Walle (2001) argues that primary causal responsibility should be ascribed to the latter — a view that closely parallels, if it does not actually inspire, some of the harsher critics of the Commission for Africa's proposals for major increases in development assistance (Killick 2005; de Renzio 2005). Historically, many of the G8 governments have been complicit in supporting these systems of rule (notably during the Cold War); the interdependencies created between many of the G8 countries and African nations by, first, colonisation and, second, global market integration, should caution against dichotomous argumentation on this point. Without minimising the extent of African responsibility for the continent's current health and economic problems, this chapter focusses on the role played by G8 countries in creating or mitigating those problems.

4 Reference to the G7 in this context reflects the fact that Russia was not involved in the promotion of market-based economic development models throughout the 1980s and 1990s.

5 For an explication, see Audrey Chapman (2002) and the WHO (2002).

6 See Christopher Stevens and Jane Kennan (2005, 4), who note that 'three-quarters of the ACP', i.e., the African, Caribbean, and Pacific countries with which these agreements are being negotiated, 'could lose 40% or more of their tariff revenue from the EU, and for over one-third it could be 60% or more'. Their paper indicates that the impact of this loss will depend on the speed and sequencing of trade liberalisation, and does not provide a regional breakdown of impacts.

7 For key statements of the sceptical position see the Overseas Development Institute (2005), Tony Killick (2005), and Nicolas van de Walle (2001); for counterarguments see, for example, Mick Foster (2004); Diana Conyers and Rob Mellors (2005), and Howard White (2005). The sceptical position also involves a distinct normative claim about the appropriate uses of aid. Thus, while the UN Millennium Project emphasises the importance of using aid more effectively in support of the MDGs, Killick (19) actually argues that less attention should be paid to the MDGs and poverty reduction, and more to 'promoting the development of directly productive sectors'.

8 On this last point, one recent study applied standard econometric modelling to the counterfactual: What would economic growth have been in sub-Saharan Africa over the past 20 years had its countries not been forced to liberalise their economies by the international financial institutions (IFIs) and conditions attached to aid (Kraev 2005)? Based on results from a sample of 22 African countries, the study implies costs of roughly US$272 billion — about the same amount the continent received in aid during this time. According to Christian Aid (2005, 2), the organisation that commissioned the study, 'effectively, this aid did no more than compensate African countries for the losses they sustained by meeting the conditions that were attached to the aid they received'.

9 Even this estimate understates the economically debilitating effect of capital flight, much of which may admittedly have occurred through legal channels. James Boyce and Léonce Ndikumana (2001) estimate that value of flight capital from 25 African countries between 1970 and 1996, plus imputed interest earnings, was considerably higher than the entire value of the combined external debt of those 25 countries in 1996.

10 The Swiss government's decision in September 2005 to return US$485 million of Nigerian funds deposited in Swiss bank accounts is 'a significant step toward the return of funds which have been looted from Africa', even though this represents only a small portion of the estimated value of resource revenues looted by Abacha and his circle (World Bank 2005).

11 This discussion draws in particular on Timothy Wise (2004), Philip McMichael (2005), and John Howell (2005).

12 This qualifier is added because numerous examples exist of situations in which developing country governments have adopted policies that actually increased domestic inequalities and potentially undermined access to social determinants of health. Whatever the industrialised world's appropriate role in such matters, it is difficult to envision a role for trade policy beyond ensuring that flexibilities needed for development are not compromised.

13 For description and analysis, see ICTSD (2004), Peter Kleen and Sheila Page (2005), and, for more recent developments, the ICTSD (2005).

References

Atarah, Linus (2005). 'Playing Chicken: Ghana vs. the IMF'. 14 June, CorpWatch. <www.corpwatch.org/article.php?id=12394> (September 2006).

Barratt Brown, Michael (1995). *Africa's Choices: After Thirty Years of the World Bank* (Boulder: Westview).

Bijlmakers, Leon A., Mary T. Bassett, and David Sanders (1999). *Socioeconomic Stress, Health, and Child Nutritional Status in Zimbabwe at a Time of Economic Structural Adjustment: A Three-Year Longitudinal Study* (Uppsala: Nordiska Afrikainstitutet).

Boyce, James K. and Léonce Ndikumana (2001). 'Is Africa a Net Creditor? New Estimates of Capital Flight from Severely Indebted Sub-Saharan African Countries, 1970–96'. *Journal of Development Studies,* vol. 38, no. 2, pp. 27–56.

Brock, Karen and Rosemary McGee (2004). 'Mapping Trade Policy: Understanding the Challenges of Civil Society Participation'. Institute for Development Studies, Brighton. <www.ids.ac.uk/ids/bookshop/wp/wp225.pdf> (September 2006).

Bryce, Jennifer, Robert E. Black, Neff Walker, *et al.* (2005). 'Can the World Afford to Save the Lives of 6 Million Children Each Year?' *Lancet,* vol. 365, no. 9478, pp. 2154–2156.

Chang, Ha-Joon (2002). *Kicking Away the Ladder: Development Strategy in Historical Perspective* (London: Anthem Press).

Chang, Ha-Joon (2005). 'Policy Space in Historical Perspective, with Special Reference to Trade and Industrial Policies'. Paper presented at Queen Elizabeth House 50th Anniversary Conference on the Development Threats and Promises, 4–5 July, Oxford. <www.qeh.ox.ac.uk/pdf/qehconf/chang.pdf> (September 2006).

Chapman, Audrey R. (2002). 'Core Obligations Related to the Right to Health'. In A.R. Chapman and S. Russell, eds., *Core Obligations: Building a Framework for Economic, Social, and Cultural Rights,* pp. 185–215 (Antwerp: Intersentia).

Chen, Lincoln, Timothy Evans, Sudhir Anand, *et al.* (2004). 'Human Resources for Health: Overcoming the Crisis'. *Lancet,* vol. 364, no. 9449, pp. 1984–1990.

Chen, Shaohua and Martin Ravallion (2004). 'How Have the World's Poorest Fared since the Early 1980s?' *World Bank Research Observer,* vol. 19, no. 2, pp. 141–169.

Cheru, Fantu (1999). 'Effects of Structural Adjustment Policies on the Full Enjoyment of Human Rights'. E/CN.4/1999/50, 24 February, United Nations Economic and Social Council, New York. <www.unhchr.ch/Huridocda/Huridoca.nsf/TestFrame/f991c6c62457a2858025675100348aef?Opendocument> (September 2006).

Cheru, Fantu (2001). 'The Highly Indebted Poor Countries (HIPC) Initiative: A Human Rights Assessment of the Poverty Reduction Strategy Papers (PRSP)'. E/CN.4/2001/56, 19 January, United Nations Economic and Social Council, New York. <www.unhchr.ch/Huridocda/Huridoca.nsf/(Symbol)/E.CN.4.2001.56.En?Opendocument> (September 2006).

Christian Aid (2005). 'The Economics of Failure: The Real Cost of "Free" Trade for Poor Countries'. Briefing paper, London <www.christianaid.org.uk/indepth/506liberalisation/Economics%20of%20failure.pdf> (September 2006).

Commission for Africa (2005). 'Our Common Interest'. Report of the Commission for Africa, London. <www.commissionforafrica.org/english/report/thereport/english/11-03-05_cr_report.pdf> (September 2006).

Commission on Macroeconomics and Health (2001). 'Macroeconomics and Health: Investing in Health for Economic Development'. World Health Organization, Geneva. <www.cid.harvard.edu/cidcmh/CMHReport.pdf> (September 2006).

Conyers, Diana and Rob Mellors (2005). 'Aid Ineffectiveness in Sub-Saharan Africa: The Problem of Donor Capacity'. *IDS Bulletin,* vol. 36, no. 3, pp. 83–89.

Cornia, Giovanni Andrea, Frances Stewart, and Richard Jolly (1987). *Adjustment with a Human Face.* Vol. 1, *Protecting the Vulnerable and Promoting Growth* (Oxford: Clarendon Press).

Cousins, Ben (2006). 'Agrarian Reform and the "Two Economies": Transforming South Africa's Countryside'. In L. Ntsebeza and R. Hall, eds., *The Land Question in South Africa: The Challenge of Transformation and Redistribution* (Cape Town: HSRC Press).

de Renzio, Paolo (2005). 'Increased Aid vs. Absorptive Capacity: Challenges and Opportunities Towards 2015'. *IDS Bulletin,* vol. 36, no. 3, pp. 20–27.

De Vogli, Roberto and Gretchen L. Birbeck (2005). 'Potential Impact of Adjustment Policies on Vulnerability of Women and Children to HIV/AIDS in Sub-Saharan Africa'. *Journal of Health Population and Nutrition,* vol. 23 no. 2, pp. 105–120.

Diderichsen, Finn, Timothy Evans, and Margaret Whitehead (2001). 'The Social Basis of Disparities in Health'. In T. Evans, M. Whitehead, F. Diderichsen, *et al.*, eds., *Challenging Inequities in Health: From Ethics to Action,* pp. 12–23 (New York: Oxford University Press).

Elliott, Larry and Patrick Wintour (2005). 'Biggest African Debt Rescue Saves Nigeria £17.3bn'. *Guardian,* 1 July. <www.guardian.co.uk/hearafrica05/story/0,,1518961,00.html> (September 2006).

Evans, Robert G. and Gregory L. Stoddart (1990). 'Producing Health, Consuming Health Care'. *Social Science & Medicine,* vol. 31 no. 12, pp. 1347–1363.

Evans, Robert G. and Gregory L. Stoddart (2003). 'Consuming Research, Producing Policy?' *American Journal of Public Health,* vol. 93, no. 3, pp. 371–379.

Evans, Robert G., Morris L. Barer, and Theodore R. Marmor, eds. (1994). *Why Are Some People Healthy and Others Not? The Determinants of Health of Populations* (New York: Aldine DeGruyter).

Farmer, Paul (2003). *Pathologies of Power: Health, Human Rights and the New War on the Poor* (Berkeley: University of California Press).

Flood, Colleen M., Mark Stabile, and Caroline Tuohy (2002). 'The Borders of Solidarity: How Countries Determine the Public/Private Mix in Spending and the Impact on Health Care'. *Health Matrix,* vol. 12, no. 2, pp. 297–356.

Food and Agriculture Organization (2005). 'The State of Food Insecurity in the World 2005: Eradicating World Hunger — Key to Achieving the Millennium Development Goals'. Rome. <www.fao.org/docrep/008/a0200e/a0200e00.htm> (September 2006).

Foster, Mick (2004). 'MDG-Orientated Sector and Poverty Reduction Strategies: Lessons from Experience in Health'. Paper prepared for the High-Level Forum on the Health MDGs, December, Abuja. <www.hlfhealthmdgs.org/Documents/MDGorientedPRSPs-Final.pdf> (September 2006).

Fourcade-Gourinchas, Marion and Sarah L. Babb (2002). 'The Rebirth of the Liberal Creed: Paths to Neoliberalism in Four Countries'. *American Journal of Sociology,* vol. 108, no. 3, pp. 533–379.

Friedman, Eric A. (2004). 'An Action Plan to Prevent Brain Drain: Building Equitable Health Systems in Africa'. Physicians for Human Rights, Boston. <www.phrusa.org/campaigns/aids/pdf/braindrain.pdf> (September 2006).

G8 (2001). 'Communiqué'. 22 July, Genoa. <www.g8.utoronto.ca/summit/2001genoa/finalcommunique.html> (September 2006).

G8 (2006). 'Fight Against Infectious Disease'. 16 July, St. Petersburg. <www.g8.utoronto.ca/summit/2006stpetersburg/infdis.html> (September 2006).

G8 Research Group (2005). 'The G8 and Africa Final Report: An Overview of the G8's Ongoing Relationship with African Development from the 2001 Genoa Summit to the 2005 Gleneagles Summit'. <www.g8.utoronto.ca/evaluations/csed/g8africa_050624.html> (September 2006).

G8 Research Group (2006). 'The Prospective Agenda for the 2007 G8 Heiligendamm Summit'. <www.g8.utoronto.ca/evaluations/2007heiligendamm/2007agenda061215.html> (September 2006).

Garcia, Frank J. (2004). 'Beyond Special and Differential Treatment'. *Boston College International and Comparative Law Review,* vol. 27 no. 2, pp. 291–317.

GAVI Alliance (2006). 'Questions and Answers about GAVI and the GAVI Fund'. Geneva. <www.gavialliance.org/General_Information/About_alliance/FAQ/qanda.php> (September 2006).

Giacomini, Mita, Jeremiah Hurley, Irving Gold, *et al.* (2004). 'The Policy Analysis of "Values Talk": Lessons from Canadian Health Reform'. *Health Policy,* vol. 67, no. 1, pp. 15–24.

Gill, Stephen (1999). 'Structural Changes in Multilateralism: The G7 Nexus and the Global Crisis'. In M. Schecter, ed., *Innovation in Multilateralism* (New York: St. Martin's Press).

Global Fund to Fight AIDS, Tuberculosis, and Malaria (2005a). 'Addressing HIV/AIDS, Malaria, and Tuberculosis: The Resource Needs of the Global Fund 2005–2007'. Geneva. <www.theglobalfund.org/en/files/about/replenishment/Resource%20Needs%20-%20February%202005.pdf> (September 2006).

Global Fund to Fight AIDS, Tuberculosis, and Malaria (2005b). 'Global Fund Receives Pledges of US$3.7 Billion for 2006–2007'. Press release, 6 September, Geneva. <www.theglobalfund.org/en/media_center/press/pr_050906.asp> (September 2006).

Global Fund to Fight AIDS, Tuberculosis, and Malaria (2006a). 'Pledges and Contributions to the Global Fund'. Geneva. <www.theglobalfund.org/en/files/pledges&contributions.xls> (July 2005).

Global Fund to Fight AIDS, Tuberculosis, and Malaria (2006b). 'Distribution of Funding after Five Rounds'. Geneva. <www.theglobalfund.org/en/funds%5Fraised/distribution> (September 2006).

Gottschalk, Ricardo (2004). 'The Macroeconomic Policy Content of PRSPs: How Much Pro-Growth, How Much Pro-Poor?' Paper prepared for the North-South Institute. <www.ids.ac.uk/ids/global/pdfs/RGPRSPpaper.pdf> (September 2006).

Gow, David (2006). 'British Government Accused of Inflating Aid Figures'. *Guardian,* 4 April. <politics.guardian.co.uk/development/story/0,,1746398,00.html> (September 2006).

Gupta, Sanjeev, Benedict Clements, Maria Teresa Guin-Siu, *et al.* (2002). 'Debt Relief and Public Health Spending in Heavily Indebted Poor Countries'. *Bulletin of the World Health Organization,* vol. 80 no. 2, pp. 151–157.

Hardon, Anita (2001). 'Immunisation for All? A Critical Look at the First GAVI Partners Meeting'. *HAI-Lights,* vol. 6, no. 1. <www.haiweb.org/pubs/hailights/mar2001/mar01_lead.html> (September 2006).

Heymann, Jody, Clyde Hertzman, Morris L. Barer, *et al.* (2005). *Healthier Societies: From Analysis to Action* (New York: Oxford University Press).

Hoekman, Bernard (2004). 'Policy Space, Coherence, and Economic Development: Options for the WTO'. Mimeo, Yale University, New Haven. <www.ycsg.yale.edu/core/forms/Project_terms_Reference.doc> (September 2006).

Howell, John (2005). 'Farm Subsidies: A Problem for Africa Too'. Opinions, September, Overseas Development Institute, London. <www.odi.org.uk/publications/opinions/47_farm_subsidies_sept05.pdf> (September 2006).

Hunt, Paul (2003). 'Economic, Social, and Cultural Rights: The Right of Everyone to the Enjoyment of the Highest Attainable Standard of Physical and Mental Health'. 13 February, E/CN.4/2003/58, United Nations Economic and Social Council, New York. <www.unhchr.ch/Huridocda/Huridoca.nsf/0/9854302995c2c86fc1256cec005a18d7> (September 2006).

Hunt, Paul (2004). 'Economic, Social, and Cultural Rights: The Right of Everyone to the Enjoyment of the Highest Attainable Standard of Physical and Mental Health—Addendum'. 8 March, E/CN.4/2004/49/Add.1, United Nations Economic and Social Council, New York. <www.unhchr.ch/Huridocda/Huridoca.nsf/(Symbol)/E.CN.4.2004.49.Add.1.En?Opendocument> (September 2006).

Hunt, Paul (2005). 'The Right of Everyone to the Enjoyment of the Highest Attainable Standard of Physical and Mental Health'. Report to the United Nations General Assembly. 12 September, A/60/348, United Nations Economic and Social Council, New York. <daccess-ods.un.org/access.nsf/Get?Open&DS=A/60/348&Lang=E> (September 2006).

'In the Twilight of Doha' (2006). *Economist*, 29 July, pp. 63–64.

International Centre for Trade and Sustainable Development (2003). 'Making Special and Differential Treatment More Effective and Responsive to Development Needs'. Chavannes-de-Bogis, Switzerland, 6–7 May. Draft meeting report, Geneva. <www.ictsd.org/dlogue/2003-05-06/Dialogue-draft-meeting-report.pdf> (September 2006).

International Centre for Trade and Sustainable Development (2004). 'Special and Different Treatment'. Doha Round Briefing Series: Developments since the Cancun Ministerial Conference, vol. 3, no. 13. <www.ictsd.org/pubs/dohabriefings/Vol3/V3_13.pdf> (September 2006).

International Centre for Trade and Sustainable Development (2005). 'Special and Differential Treatment in the Multilateral Trading System'. ICTSD-FES Independent Analytical Track Meeting, 1–2 July, Lausanne. <www.ictsd.org/dlogue/2005-07-01/2005-07-01-docu.htm> (September 2006).

International Centre for Trade and Sustainable Development (2006). 'Doha Round Suspended Indefinitely After G6 Talks Collapse'. *Bridges Weekly,* vol. 10, no. 27. <www.ictsd.org/weekly/06-07-26/story1.htm> (September 2006).

International Monetary Fund (2005). 'Development Committee Communiqué'. 25 September, Washington DC. <www.imf.org/external/np/cm/2005/092505.htm> (September 2006).

International Monetary Fund and World Bank (2005). 'Zambia: Enhanced Initiative for Heavily Indebted Poor Countries — Completion Point Document'. IMF Country Report No. 05/137, Washington DC. <www.imf.org/external/pubs/ft/scr/2005/cr05137.pdf> (September 2006).

Jaggar, Alison (2002). 'Vulnerable Women and Neo-Liberal Globalization: Debt Burdens Undermine Women's Health in the Global South'. *Theoretical Medicine,* vol. 23, no. 6, pp. 425–440.

Jawara, Fatoumata and Eileen Kwa (2003). *Behind the Scenes at the WTO: The Real World of International Trade Negotiations* (London: Zed Books).

Jeter, Jon (2002). 'The Dumping Ground: As Zambia Courts Western Markets, Used Goods Arrive at a Heavy Price'. *Washington Post,* 22 April.

Jha, Prabhat, Anne Mills, Kara Hanson, *et al.* (2002). 'Improving the Health of the Global Poor'. *Science, Technology, and Human Values,* vol. 295, no. 5562, pp. 2036–2039.

Joint Learning Initiative (2004). 'Human Resources for Health: Overcoming the Crisis'. Global Equity Initiative, Harvard University, Cambridge MA. <www.globalhealthtrust.org/report/Human_Resources_for_Health.pdf> (September 2006).

Jubilee Research (2005). 'The G8 2005: What Are the Lessons?' 11 July. <www.jubileeresearch.org/latest/g8110705.htm> (September 2006).

Killick, Tony (2004). 'Politics, Evidence, and the New Aid Agenda'. *Development Policy Review,* vol. 22, no. 1, pp. 5–29.

Killick, Tony (2005). 'Don't Throw Money at Africa'. *IDS Bulletin,* vol. 36, no. 3, pp. 14–19.

Kim, Jim Yong, Aaron Shakow, Jaime Bayona, *et al.* (2000). 'Sickness Amidst Recovery: Public Debt and Private Suffering in Peru'. In J.Y. Kim, J.V. Millen, J. Gershman, *et al.*, eds., *Dying for Growth: Global Inequality and the Health of the Poor,* pp. 127–154 (Monroe ME: Common Courage Press).

King, Jeff, Ashfaq Khalfan, and Bryan Thomas (2003). 'Advancing the Odious Debt Doctrine'. CISDL Working Paper, Centre for International Sustainable Development Law, Montreal <www.odiousdebts.org/odiousdebts/publications/Advancing_the_Odious_Debt_Doctrine.pdf> (September 2006).

Kleen, Peter and Sheila Page (2005). 'Special and Differential Treatment of Developing Countries in the World Trade Organization'. Ministry for Foreign Affairs, Sweden, Stockholm. <www.egdi.gov.se/pdf/study/40725_Gl%20Dev%20Stud%202.pdf> (September 2006).

Kraev, Egor (2005). 'Estimating GDP Effects of Trade Liberalisation on Developing Countries'. Centre for Development, Policy and Research, School of Oriental and African Studies, London <www.christianaid.org.uk/indepth/506liberalisation/FinalPaper4.pdf> (September 2006).

Kremer, Michael and Seema Jayachandran (2002). 'Odious Debt'. April. International Monetary Fund, Washington DC. <www.imf.org/external/np/res/seminars/2002/poverty/mksj.pdf> (September 2006).

Labonté, Ronald and Ted Schrecker (2004). 'Committed to Health for All? How the G7/8 Rate'. *Social Science and Medicine,* vol. 59, no. 8, pp. 1661–1676.

Labonté, Ronald and Ted Schrecker (2005). *The G8, Africa, and Global Health: A Platform for Global Health Equity for the 2005 Summit* (London: Nuffield Trust).

Labonté, Ronald and Ted Schrecker (2006). 'The G8 and Global Health: What Now? What Next?' *Canadian Journal of Public Health,* vol. 97, no. 1, pp. 35–38.

Labonté, Ronald, Corinne Packer, and Nathan Klassen (2006). 'The "Brain Drain" of Health Professionals from Sub-Saharan Africa to Canada: Findings and Options'. South African Migration Project, Queen's University, Kingston.

Labonté, Ronald, Ted Schrecker, David Sanders, *et al.* (2004). *Fatal Indifference: The G8, Africa, and Global Health* (Cape Town: University of Cape Town Press).

Lister, John (2005). *Driving the Wrong Way? A Critical Guide to the Global "Health Reform" Industry* (London: Middlesex University Press).

Martin, Matthew (2004). 'Assessing the HIPC Initiative: The Key HIPC Debates'. In J.J. Teunissen and A. Akkerman, eds., *HIPC Debt Relief: Myths and Realities* (The Hague: FONDAD).

McChesney, Robert W. and Dan Schiller (2003). 'The Political Economy of International Communications: Foundations for the Emerging Global Debate about Media Ownership and Regulation'. Technology, Business, and Society Programme Paper No. 11, United Nations Research Institute for Social Development.

McKie, John and Jeff Richardson (1982). 'The Rule of Rescue'. *Social Science and Medicine,* vol. 56, no. 1212, pp. 2407–2419.

McMichael, Philip (2005). 'Global Development and the Corporate Food Regime'. In F.H. Buttel and P. McMichael, eds., *New Directions in the Sociology of Global Development* (Amsterdam: Elsevier).

Moss, Todd (2005). 'Ten Myths of the International Finance Facility'. Working Paper No. 60, Center for Global Development. <ssrn.com/abstract=800706> (September 2006).

Office of the High Commissioner for Human Rights (1966). 'International Covenant on Economic, Social, and Cultural Rights'. <www.unhchr.ch/html/menu3/b/a_cescr.htm> (September 2006).

Office of the High Commissioner for Human Rights (2006). 'Special Rapporteur of the Commission on Human Rights on the Right of Everyone to the Enjoyment of the Highest Attainable Standard of Physical and Mental Health'. <www.ohchr.org/english/issues/health/right> (September 2006).

Organisation for Economic Co-operation and Development (2004). *Agricultural Policies in OECD Countries at a Glance* (Paris: Organisation for Economic Co-operation and Development).

Overseas Development Institute (2005). 'Scaling Up versus Absorptive Capacity: Challenges and Opportunities for Reaching the MDGs in Africa'. Briefing paper, London. <www.odi.org.uk/publications/briefing/bp_may05_absorptive_capacity.pdf> (September 2006).

Paluzzi, Joan E. and Paul Farmer (2005). 'The Wrong Question'. *Development,* vol. 48, no. 1, pp. 12–18.

Pogge, Thomas (2001). 'Priorities of Global Justice'. *Metaphilosophy,* vol. 32, no. 1/2, pp. 6–24.

Pogge, Thomas (2002). *World Poverty and Human Rights* (Cambridge: Polity Press).

Pogge, Thomas (2005a). 'World Poverty and Human Rights'. *Ethics and International Affairs,* vol. 19, no. 1.

Pogge, Thomas (2005b). 'Human Rights and Global Health'. *Metaphilosophy,* vol. 36, no. 1-2, pp. 182–209.

Reddy, Sanjay G. and Thomas W. Pogge (2005). 'How Not to Count the Poor'. Columbia University, New York. <papers.ssrn.com/sol3/papers.cfm?abstract_id=893159> (September 2006).

Sachs, Jeffrey (2005). 'The End of Poverty'. *Time,* 14 March, pp. 44–54.

Sachs, Jeffrey and J. W. McArthur (2005). 'The Millennium Project: A Plan for Meeting the Millennium Development Goals'. *Lancet,* vol. 365, pp. 347–353.

Sanders, David and Abdulrahman Sambo (1991). 'AIDS in Africa: The Implications of Economic Recession and Structural Adjustment'. *Health Policy and Planning,* vol. 6, no. 2, pp. 157–165.

Sanders, David, Mickey Chopra, and Charles Todd (2005). 'Confronting Africa's Health Crisis: More of the Same Will Not Be Enough'. *British Medical Journal,* vol. 331, no. 7519, pp. 755–758.

Satterthwaite, David (2003). 'The Millennium Development Goals and Urban Poverty Reduction: Great Expectations and Nonsense Statistics'. *Environment and Urbanization,* vol. 15 no. 2, pp. 181–190.

Schoepf, Brooke G., Claude Schoepf, Joyce V. Millen*, et al.* (2000). 'Theoretical Therapies, Remote Remedies: SAPs and the Political Ecology of Poverty and Health in Africa'. In J.Y. Kim, J.V. Millen, J. Gershman*, et al.*, eds., *Dying for Growth: Global Inequality and the Health of the Poor,* pp. 91–126 (Monroe ME: Common Courage Press).

Shadlen, Kenneth C. (2005). 'Exchanging Development for Market Access? Deep Integration and Industrial Policy under Multilateral and Regional-Bilateral Trade Agreements'. *Review of International Political Economy,* vol. 12, no. 5, pp. 750–775.

Shue, Henry (1996). 'Environmental Change and the Varieties of Justice'. In F.O. Hampson and J. Reppy, eds., *Earthly Goods: Environmental Change and Social Justice,* pp. 9–29 (Ithaca: Cornell University Press).

Simon, David, Wim van Spengen, Chris Dixon, *et al.*, eds. (1995). *Structurally Adjusted Africa: Poverty, Debt, and Basic Needs* (London: Pluto Press).

Slaughter, Anne-Marie (2005). 'Government Networks, World Order, and the L20'. In J. English, R. Thakur, and A.F. Cooper, eds., *Reforming from the Top: A Leaders' 20 Summit,* pp. 281–295 (Tokyo: United Nations University Press).

Solar, Orielle and Alec Irwin (2005). 'Towards a Conceptual Framework for Analysis and Action on the Social Determinants of Health'. Discussion paper for the Commission on Social Determinants of Health, World Health Organization, Geneva. <www.who.int/entity/social_determinants/resources/framework.pdf> (September 2006).

South Centre (2005). 'Policy Space for the Development of the South'. Trade Policy Brief No. 1, November, Geneva. <www.southcentre.org/info/policybrief/01PolicySpace.pdf> (September 2006).

Stevens, Christopher and Jane Kennan (2005). 'EU-ACP Economic Partnership Agreements: The Effects of Reciprocity'. Institute of Development Studies, Sussex. <www.dfid.gov.uk/aboutdfid/organisation/epas-effects-reciprocity.pdf> (September 2006).

Stiglitz, Joseph and Andrew H. Charlton (2004). 'Common Values for the Development Round'. *World Trade Review,* vol. 3, no. 3, pp. 495–506.

Stiglitz, Joseph and Andrew Charlton (2005). 'A Development Round of Trade Negotiations?' In F. Bourguignon, B. Pleskovic, and A. Sapir, eds., *Are We on Track to Achieve the Millennium Development Goals? Annual World Bank Conference on Development Economics: Europe 2005,* pp. 31–60 (New York: Oxford University Press).

Tanzi, Vito (2002). 'Globalization and the Future of Social Protection'. *Scottish Journal of Political Economy,* vol. 49, no. 1, pp. 116–127.

Travis, Phyllida, Sara Bennett, Andy Haines, *et al.* (2004). 'Overcoming Health-Systems Constraints to Achieve the Millennium Development Goals'. *Lancet,* vol. 364, no. 9437, pp. 900–906.

United Nations (1948). 'Universal Declaration of Human Rights'. <www.un.org/Overview/rights.html> (September 2006).

United Nations (2005). 'The Millennium Development Goals Report 2005'. New York. <millenniumindicators.un.org/unsd/mi/pdf/MDG%20Book.pdf> (September 2006).

United Nations Conference on Trade and Development (2004). 'Economic Development in Africa: Debt Sustainability, Oasis, or Mirage?' <www.unctad.org/Templates/Download.asp?docid=5457&lang=1&intItemID=3246> (September 2006).

United Nations Department of Economic and Social Affairs (2005). 'World Economic and Social Survey 2005: Financing for Development'. United Nations, New York.

United Nations Economic and Social Council (2000). 'The Right to the Highest Attainable Standard of Health'. E/C.12/2000/4, 11 August. <www.unhchr.ch/tbs/doc.nsf/(symbol)/E.C.12.2000.4.En?OpenDocument> (September 2006).

United Nations Millennium Project (2005). 'Investing in Development: A Practical Plan to Achieve the Millennium Development Goals'. United Nations Development Programme, New York. <www.unmillenniumproject.org/reports/fullreport.htm> (September 2006).

United Nations Standing Committee on Nutrition (2000). 'Fourth Report on the World Nutrition Situation: Nutrition Throughout the Life Cycle'. <www.unsystem.org/scn/Publications/rwns/4RWNS.html> (September 2006).

van de Walle, Nicolas (2001). *African Economies and the Politics of Permanent Crisis, 1979–1999* (Cambridge: Cambridge University Press).

Versi, Anver (2005). 'The G8 Pledges: What Happens Next?' *African Business*, August/September, pp. 14–20.

Wagstaff, Adam and Mariam Claeson (2004). 'The Millennium Development Goals for Health: Rising to the Challenges'. World Bank, Washington, DC

Weatherspoon, Dave D. and Thomas Reardon (2003). 'The Rise of Supermarkets in Africa: Implications for Agrifood Systems and the Rural Poor'. *Development Policy Review,* vol. 21, no. 3, pp. 333–355. <papers.ssrn.com/sol3/papers.cfm?abstract_id=410968> (September 2006).

Webb, Michael (2000). 'The Group of Seven and Political Management of the Global Economy'. In R. Stubbs and G. Underhill, eds., *Political Economy and the Changing Global Order,* pp. 141–151 (Don Mills: Oxford University Press Canada).

White, Howard (2005). 'The Case for Doubling Aid'. *IDS Bulletin,* vol. 36, no. 3, pp. 8–12.

Whitehead, Margaret, Gïran Dahlgren, and Timothy Evans (2001). 'Equity and Health Sector Reforms: Can Low-Income Countries Escape the Medical Poverty Trap?' *Lancet,* vol. 358, pp. 833–836.

Williamson, John (1990). 'What Washington Means by Policy Reform'. In J. Williamson, ed., *Latin American Adjustment: How Much Has Happened?,* pp. 5–38 (Washington DC: Institute for International Economics).

Wise, Timothy A. (2004). 'The Paradox of Agricultural Subsidies: Measurement Issues, Agricultural Dumping, and Policy Reform'. Tufts University, Medford MA. <ase.tufts.edu/gdae/Pubs/wp/04-02AgSubsidies.pdf> (September 2006).

World Bank (2004). *Global Economic Prospects 2005: Trade, Regionalism, and Development* (Washington DC: World Bank).

World Bank (2005). 'With World Bank Assistance, Stolen Funds Deposited in Swiss Banks Are Returned to Nigeria'. News, 27 September, Washington DC.

World Bank (2006). 'The Multilateral Debt Relief Initiative'. 29 June, Washington DC. <www.worldbank.org/html/extdr/thematic.htm » Debt Issues> (September 2006).

World Health Organization (2002). '25 Questions and Answers on Health and Human Rights'. World Health Organization, Geneva.

World Health Organization (2005a). 'Global and Regional Immunization Profile: African Region'. <www.who.int/immunization_monitoring/data/data_AFR/en> (September 2006).

World Health Organization (2005b). 'Health in the Millennium Development Goals'. Geneva. <www.who.int/entity/mdg/publications/MDG_Report_revised.pdf> (September 2006).

World Health Organization (2006a). 'World Health Report 2006: Working Together for Health'. World Health Organization, Geneva. <www.who.int/whr/2006/en> (September 2006).

World Health Organization (2006b). 'Commission on Social Determinants of Health'. <www.who.int/social_determinants/en> (September 2006).

World Trade Organization (2001). 'Ministerial Declaration'. 14 November, Doha. <www.wto.org/english/thewto_e/minist_e/min01_e/mindecl_e.htm> (September 2006).

Wroughton, Lesley (2005). 'World Bank Report Calls for Changes to G8 Debt Plan'. *Reuters,* 3 August.

Chapter 13

Global Health and Universal Human Rights: The Case for G8 Accountability

Colleen O'Manique

'Unlike certain other social animals, we have no collective social instinct or biological solidarity that is automatically aroused by the destruction of our fellow kind,' Mike Davis (2005, 3) writes in his book about the global threat of avian influenza. Global communications have brought the fate of our fellow kind into full view, with contradictory effects. On the one hand, it has normalised human tragedy in distant places, whether emerging from natural disasters, war, famine, or pandemic disease. But, on the other hand, it has brought home the message that we are interdependent, that security at home is affected by events far away. Recent pandemics have made it clear that public health crises cross borders and we are all vulnerable; it is clear that global health challenges require global responses. In this context, the G8 — the world's richest and most powerful countries — in partnership with the International Monetary Fund (IMF), the World Bank, and the World Trade Organization (WTO) — has emerged as a major player in shaping global health policy, prompting a growing scholarly debate concerning the G8's role and influence in the global health arena. As John Kirton and Jenevieve Mannell write in Chapter 9, the 'debate ranges widely from the critics who think the G8 has done too little, done too much of the wrong thing, or failed to deliver the good promises it has made through to supporters who claim the G8 has already filled some gaps, has the potential to do much more, and is already delivering a new generation of health governance for a globalising world'. Other concerns range from questions of accountability, transparency, and democratic process in G8 decision making to more complex questions about the relationship between the deepening privatisation of power accompanying the neo-liberal market model of development supported and sustained by the G8 and the international financial institutions (IFIs) and the exercise of human rights, including the right to health.

In many of the 'distant places' where poverty and poor health go hand in hand, the expansion of market relations has trumped the right of access to the basic constituents of human health — food, water, work, land, shelter, bodily integrity, medical care, and education. The context within which sick bodies find themselves profoundly shapes disease distribution and premature mortality, a context that in the past three decades has become ever more subject to geopolitics, market forces, and the privatisation of power (Brysk 2005). In today's increasingly borderless world, it becomes ever more difficult to untangle the complex relationships among the community, national, and international structures within which people's daily lives are embedded and that shape the exercise of human rights and, by extension, health and well-being. A growing consensus is emerging that global health and social reproduction cannot be de-linked from policies governing finance, trade, debt, intellectual property, labour, and national security.[1] Despite the heightened globalisation of disease, we do not all share the same vulnerability.

What ought to be the responsibility of the G8 with regard to global health? In other words, what are the obligations of those who play a central role in global governance to protect the exercise of the human right to health? This chapter argues that the success of institutions of governance ought to be measured by whether policies and laws enhance the conditions for the exercise of human rights and the provision of basic human needs for all people. Health is foundational to the exercise of a range of basic rights and it is a measure of human development in its broadest conceptualisation. Hence the links between health and global governance provide a window into analysing the relationship among global governance, the global political economy, and human rights, and, ultimately, whether the globalisation regime in place is indeed ethical. The state of the health of people on the planet is thus a window into broader questions of global justice and human rights.

Without denying that the nation-state holds responsibility for ensuring the exercise of the human rights of its citizens, this chapter argues for broader accountability beyond the nation-state and, in particular, for G8 accountability for economic policies, regulatory frameworks, laws, and military interventions that spill over national borders and indirectly and directly affect human security in its broadest sense — on the individual body, bodily integrity, and the destruction of infrastructures and ecosystems upon which human life depends. As other authors in this collection have illustrated, certain health benefits and innovations in the global governance of health have accompanied economic globalisation. But the issue here extends beyond whether the G8 is delivering on its stated commitments to global health to a consideration of whether the G8's specific policies outside of the 'health box' of the analytical model — whether they govern the behaviour of public or private actors — are linked to violations of the exercise of the right to health. Rather than providing policy prescriptions, the objective of this chapter is to broaden the contours of the debate.

Human Rights: Universal and Inalienable?

The starting point for this chapter is the position that health is a basic and universal human right. If the concept of human rights is to include the concepts of universality and inalienability, then it will be acceptable only if the claims it justifies are claims for what is genuinely needed for human development. They must be the requirements of *all humans* for human development, regardless of age, race, sex, class, nation, or ability. Hence the essence of a human right is a fundamental requirement for human development. As humans, everyone has biological needs, as well as purely human needs that transcend the biological. What is required for human development can, at least in principle, be observed and empirically determined. Fundamental requirements for human development include the following: nutritious food, shelter, security, a non-threatening environment, health care, and education. The legitimacy of rights linked to transcendent human needs can also be verified empirically; the human need for control over one's destiny, for community, and for self-determination, can also be confirmed through the social sciences and psychology. The recognition of fundamental human rights within communities implies obligation or duty on the part of members of that community; rights and obligations cannot be separated, because for rights to be exercised, responses to that right by members of the community are required.[2]

The term 'universal human rights' and an emergent global consensus about human rights (as codified for example in recent human history in resolutions adopted by members of the United Nations Universal Declaration of Human Rights) is at least partly rooted in globalisation and an emerging 'cosmopolitan' consciousness. According to Alison Brysk (2005), a discourse of cosmopolitan values is now evolving and expresses the equal dignity and worth of all human beings, the reconnection of international law and morality, and an emerging understanding that many problems transcend nation-state boundaries and require global solutions.

But there is great variability among different societies as to what constitutes human rights. Understandings of rights and responses to rights claims are highly variable and historically contingent. Susan Eckstein and Timothy Wickham-Crowley (2003, xii) suggest that 'people within and among different societies may conceive of their rights differently and they may reconstruct their views of such rights over time, and not in predictable sequences or with characteristic end states. Even certain rights around which a global consensus has emerged can be interpreted variably, depending on the context.' Furthermore, even in contexts where fundamental development needs are understood and accepted as basic human rights, the application of each need to specific individuals and communities can be less than straightforward.[3]

Rights have been conceptualised in many different ways, but principally through theist and rationalist accounts. The recognition of human rights is generally understood as having evolved in three stages. The core rights that constitute human rights, Gary Teeple (2005) observes, evolved in transition from feudalism to capitalism and represent the principles of the emerging world order in the 17th and 18th centuries. The early conceptions of the 'rights of man' in the 17th century were understood as rights of particular individuals against each other and against the states under which they lived. The French Declaration of the Rights of Man and Citizen (1789) and the American Bill of Rights (1791) were the first codifications of these rights. But, as Teeple points out, the exercise of these rights was far from universal and absolute: it did not extend to women, certain racial and religious groups, particular strata and classes, or colonised people. These 'first-generation rights' were consistent with the political philosophy of liberal individualism and the related economic and social doctrine of laissez-faire (2005, 3). Conceived of as negative rights to protect individuals from the excesses of the state and from other individuals, they are the classic liberal rights of individual liberty: freedom of expression, religion, and the right to own property and not to be deprived of it arbitrarily. This western liberal conception of human rights is featured in almost every constitution of today's states and dominates the majority of the international declarations and covenants adopted since World War II.

A particular set of assumptions about the nature of 'man' underlies first-generation rights. From Hobbes to Kant, Rawls, and Nozick — the most significant representatives of the western perspective — valid moral laws are the products of pure reason, and cannot be tarnished by experience; their foundations are not in human experience (O'Manique 2003). Essential human characteristics are reason/autonomy and isolation, with the tendency to define autonomy as freedom from constraints — as independence, self-control, and freedom from external influence. Teeple (2005) points out that there is no vision of community in these declarations beyond the mutual interdependence of buyers and sellers, that members of society are related to each other as isolated individuals with competitive interests, with this interdependence mediated by commercial exchange: 'With the atomized individual as the basic social unit, human relations were transformed into relations mediated by money, and humans were defined as embodiments of private exclusive rights' (3). Martha Nussbaum (2000) and others have demonstrated that most of humanity does not fit this description of the isolated, autonomous individual; if one considers babies and children, the elderly, the sick, those with disabilities, and many women during certain stages of reproduction, one can see that there are times in life when one is more or less dependent upon others within the community.

The counterpoint to first-generation civil and political rights, second-generation rights, emerged later, the impetus coming largely from the global economic South as a response to the abuses of colonialism as well as capitalist development and its underlying conception of individual liberty that legitimated the exploitation of workers and colonised peoples. The International Covenant on Economic, Social, and Cultural Rights, which entered into force in 1976, gives further expression to the second-generation rights found in the UN Universal Declaration in articles 22–27 (UN 1948; Office of the High Commissioner for Human Rights [OHCHR] 1966). (It is worth noting that the United States has not ratified this agreement.) Largely considered positive rights, these are largely understood as 'rights to' rather than 'freedoms from'. Rights to social security, work, rest and leisure, education, and health are included. The right to health, as well as other second-generation rights, reflects the heightened understanding of government responsibility for the welfare of its citizens. A familiar incantation about second-generation rights is that these positive rights or rights-to are burdensome and expensive to the extent that they imply a duty or an obligation of society to provide secure access to public goods such as social services, health care, education, and so on. With regard specifically to the right to health, the right has rarely been interpreted as the right to the conditions that would optimise human health, but as a right to access to health care or health protection when one is sick. And even the latter is rarely interpreted as an enforceable individual entitlement, but as a policy directive that sets goals (Chapman 2002, 193). In much of the South, investments in public health and other social entitlements have taken a backseat to neo-liberal economic restructuring and national budgetary priorities established largely by IFIs, with the notion that social spending will follow once debts are paid and the full growth potential of economies is realised through trade.

Moreover, the distinction between positive and negative rights is not so clear-cut. The exercise of second-generation rights involves both positive and negative dimensions and depends on freedom from the negative impacts of the behaviour of state and non-state actors (for example, corporations, individuals) that undermine the conditions under which human rights can be exercised. To illustrate, the exercise of the right to food is codified in article 25 of the Universal Declaration of Human Rights (UN 1948), article 11 of the International Covenant on Economic, Social, and Cultural Rights (OHCHR 1966), and articles 24 and 27 of the Convention on the Rights of the Child (OHCHR 1989); it implies freedom from the conditions — political, cultural, and economic — that render that right impossible to exercise. Such conditions might include below-subsistence wages, enforced policies of agricultural deregulation, competition by industrial agribusiness that undermines local food production, discriminatory land tenure policies, and human destruction of local ecosystems. It is often possible to locate the undermining of the exercise of the right to food in the policies or practices of private and public actors. But it is also the case that the exercise of the right to healthy food might involve a 'positive claim' on other members of the community to provide food. If we were all isolated, autonomous individuals, then it would be difficult to make that claim; people could fend for themselves. Implicit in second-generation rights is the notion that humans are not isolated and autonomous but are interdependent and live in communities, and that claims based on obligation and need are met within families and the broader community.

Today, it is increasingly recognised that that community is global. Article 28 of the Universal Declaration of Human Rights states that 'everyone is entitled to a social and international order in which the rights and freedoms set forth in this Declaration can be fully realized' and article 30 states that 'nothing in this Declaration may be interpreted as implying for any State, group or person any right to engage in any activity or to perform any act aimed at the destruction of any of the rights and freedoms set forth herein' (UN 1948). But the main responsibility for the protection of human rights has been nested within the nation-state, the protection of human rights historically a function of national citizenship. Despite the rather dramatic shift in the role and function of the state *vis-à-vis* global actors and the elevation of private power, it is still the sovereign state that is the main institution that administers and enforces rights, even those conceived as universally held (Shafir 2004, 11). Article 2 of the Declaration on the Right and Responsibility of Individuals, Groups, and Organs of Society to Promote and Protect Universally Recognized Human Rights and Fundamental Freedoms (adopted by the UN General Assembly resolution 53/144 of 9 December 1998) reads: 'Each State has a prime responsibility and duty to protect, promote and implement all human rights and fundamental freedoms, inter alia, by adopting such steps as may be necessary to create all conditions necessary in the social, economic, political and other fields, as well as the legal guarantees required to ensure that all persons under its jurisdiction, individually and in association with others, are able to enjoy all those rights and freedoms in practice' (UN 1999). But trade law can restrict the capacity of states to do just that; health and environmental standards and labour laws are non-tariff barriers to free trade and open to legal challenge when it is deemed that they limit the 'rights' of capital.

A Right to Health?

The human right to health is set out in a broad range of human rights instruments. According to the World Health Organization (WHO), every country in the world is now party to at least one human rights treaty that addresses health-related rights, including the right to health, as well as a number of rights related to conditions necessary for health. The human right to health has been recognised in a range of conventions and declarations (including the Universal Declaration of Human Rights, the 1978 Declaration of Alma-Ata, the International Covenant on Economic, Social, and Cultural Rights, and the Convention on the Rights of the Child, among others). With specific regard to health, article 25 of the Declaration of Human Rights states that: '1) Everyone has the right to a standard of living adequate for the health and well-being of himself and of his family, including food, clothing, housing and medical care and necessary social services, and the right to security in the event of unemployment, sickness, disability, widowhood, old age or other lack of livelihood in circumstances beyond his control; 2) Motherhood and childhood are entitled to special care and assistance. All children, whether born in or out of wedlock, shall enjoy the same social protection' (UN 1999). The International Covenant on Economic, Social, and Cultural Rights recognises 'right of everyone to the enjoyment of the highest attainable standard of physical and mental health' (OHCHR 1966, art. 12). The right to the highest attainable standard of health is reflected, for example, in General Comment No. 14 of the Committee on Economic, Social, and Cultural Rights adopted in May 2000 (UN Economic and Social Council 2000). Chapman (2002, 195) explains that the document interprets the right to health as extending beyond the availability of timely and appropriate health care to incorporate sanitation, an adequate supply of safe food, healthy occupational and environmental conditions, and access to health-related education and information; furthermore, it emphasises the importance of the participation of the population in all health-related decision making at the community, national, and international levels, and it articulates the need for a gender perspective an the elimination of discrimination against women.

Sofia Gruskin and Daniel Tarantola (2000, 1) argue that the structural connections between health and human rights more broadly are beginning to emerge:

> The development of a 'health and human rights' language in the last few years has allowed for the connections between health and human rights to be explicitly named, and therefore for conceptual, analytical, policy and programmatic work to begin to bridge these disparate disciplines and to move forward. In the last few years human rights have increasingly been at the center of analysis and action in regard to health and development issues. The level of institutional and stated political commitment to health and human rights has, in fact, never been higher. This is true within the work of the United Nations system but, even more importantly, can also be seen in the work of governments and non-governmental organizations (NGOs) at both the national and international level.

If one accepts the broad WHO definition of health as 'a state of complete physical, mental and social well-being and not merely the absence of disease or infirmity', it is easy to conclude that the exercise of the right to health is one of the least secure and protected (WHO 1994). The fundamental requirements for health mirror many of the requirements for human development that are codified in the Universal Declaration of Human Rights: food, water, shelter, security, a non-threatening physical environment, education, and self-determination. The right to health can be interpreted as a right to secure access to the basic constituents of health (clean water, healthy food, an unpolluted and secure environment), a right to health knowledge, a right to bodily autonomy and integrity, a right to health care and medicines, a right to informed consent, a right to rest and leisure, and a right to participate in shaping how health services are to be delivered.

It is difficult to move from the more inclusive discourse of a human right to health to an understanding of the concrete conditions required for enhanced exercise of that right. The dominant lens through which most view health remains biomedical, and the vast bulk of the knowledge comes from the 'West' and is still firmly within the domain of the clinical, which pays little attention to the social and economic determinants of health. Health policy in the industrialised world remains principally focussed on after-the-event curative care, paying little attention to what makes people sick in the first place. Public health specialists have tended to share the underlying assumptions of biomedicine to the extent that public health campaigns are largely about individual behaviour modification. Today, biomedicine is largely a commodity in the free market to be purchased by those who can pay, or available to those with public or private insurance policies. And pharmaceuticals are commodities like any other, their development principally determined by market demand and profitability. Drugs are not considered public goods, essential to human health and thus distributed based on need, but are a multi-billion dollar industry; research on drugs focusses overwhelmingly on drugs that will secure high profits. But it is not just drugs and medical care that are subject to the market mechanism: access to all life necessities is increasingly commodified and subject to the 'rules' of supply and demand, including water, food, and other essentials.

Even within the emergent framework of the social determinants of health, the dominant understanding is that poor countries are simply too strapped for cash to extend those determinants to their populations; hence the onus is on the wealthy countries to finance the gap and provide social safety nets for the most wretchedly poor.[4] Notable exceptions include the contribution by Ted Schrecker, Ronald Labonté, and David Sanders in Chapter 12, which explicitly interrogates the specific terms on which countries in sub-Saharan Africa are being integrated into the global neo-liberal order, and links trade and debt with the undermining of health. Paul Farmer and Nicole Gastineau Campos (2004) point to a selective silence within the field of medical ethics about the ethical dilemmas of the poor and make a compelling case for re-socialising medical ethics away from the dominant individualist readings of health and medical problems, as part of a broader project that includes a critique of the dominant modes of thinking in a variety of fields, and for connecting health and medical research with the interests of the destitute sick. In the field of medical ethics, they state, 'the question of who shall live is not even on the radar screen'. Re-socialising medical ethics would involve, in their view, a turn toward disciplines such as anthropology, history, and political economy to illuminate complex transnational ethical problems shared by subaltern populations, the systematic participation of the destitute sick in shaping medical ethics, and the linking of research with interventions that are demanded by the poor or otherwise marginalised. Such an approach would need to begin with the principle that health is indeed a human right, universal and inalienable.

Globalisation and Human Rights

A paradox of human rights in the current era of neo-liberal globalisation is that while, on the one hand, a new 'cosmopolitan consciousness' that people are all fully human and entitled to the exercise of human rights is emerging, on the other, the capacity of states in the South to protect and enhance the exercise of human rights within their borders is increasingly limited by challenges to state sovereignty and by the increasing fragmentation of political authority among state and non-state actors at all levels. A growing share of the global and national economies is now governed through the IMF, the WTO, bilateral and multilateral trade agreements, and private business, while responsibility for the protection and enhancement of the 'social' or second-generation rights remains at the level of the nation-state. Corporations have become increasingly powerful *vis-à-vis* states and, particularly in weak or fragile states, can evade the authority of governments with impunity, or in some cases act in partnership with corrupt elites; the past activities of Shell in Nigeria and the Canadian energy company Talisman in Sudan are perhaps the most well-known examples on the African continent. As Janine Brodie (2003, 60) states, 'neoliberal globalization simultaneously maximizes the need for social intervention in the name of human security, while at the same time minimizes the political spaces and strategic instruments necessary to achieve this public good'. She also says that

> international debt repayment schemes, SAPS [structural adjustment programmes], PRSPs [Poverty Reduction Strategy Papers] turn binding control over designated national policy

> fields to external constitution-like agreements that facilitate the mobility of capital, and often trump the decisions of national democratic bodies. These are binding for an indefinite future, and define a new set of negative freedoms from democratic interventions for global capital operating in national spaces (Brodie 2003, 57).

Isabella Bakker and Stephen Gill (2003, 20) characterise the recent transformations of the global governance order as a movement away from social citizenship, secured and supported by nation-states to market citizenship, where citizens become responsible for helping themselves in a more privatised social order. They view the emerging global governance order emerging from the G7/8 and IFIs as one that guarantees the security of capital at the expense of human security. While providing maximum security for the owners of capital, the 'new constitutionalism', the evolution of new juridical frameworks — laws, rules, standards, trade agreements enforced through the WTO, states, and conditionality frameworks — have removed the state of responsibility for the maintenance of basic conditions for the exercise of human rights. Stable conditions for social reproduction are being undermined by the global accumulation of capital within the framework of global governance emerging from the G7 and the international financial institutions (IFIs) (27).

David Held (2003, 123) presents a slightly less pessimistic picture of the transformations in the nature of the state under economic globalisation. Transformations in global governance and the global political economy have been accompanied by a shift to the language of democracy and human rights; in his view, legitimate authority has become linked in moral and legal terms with the maintenance of human rights and democratic standards. This is an evolution of new frameworks of global governance and international law, reflected in new binding rules set out in conventions on biodiversity, climate change, and genocide. These new frameworks represent a movement toward international rules that entrench basic humanitarian values, a regime that consists of overlapping national, regional, and global conventions and institutions. Changes in human rights law are placing individuals, governments, and nongovernmental organisations (NGOs) under new systems of legal regulation that, in principle, transcend nation-state boundaries. The development of an 'emergent liberal universal constitutional order' is a significant indicator of the distance that has been travelled from the classic, state-centric conception of sovereignty to what amounts to a new formulation for the delimitation of political power on a global basis (Held 2003). However, the discourse of human rights and democracy remains largely abstracted from the heightened power of capital in governing the global economy. A competing self-evident truth backed up by a variety of powerful (some would say hegemonic) institutions such as the World Bank and the IMF is that markets improve the poor's access to rights and aspirations, and that poor nations can trade their way to prosperity.[5] What this means for how mechanisms evolve for the protection of human rights remains to be seen. States have given up certain domains of governance to market principles and non-democratic institutions, which in essence means that the so-called rights of capital often supersede the human rights of people. One need not look far for evidence of this. The overarching rules of neo-liberal globalisation are rarely subject to scrutiny from a human rights perspective.

The G8

The G8 informally manages these transformations. Some regard the G8 as the legitimate and effective rulers of the global economy; others ask whether the preferences and interests of the most powerful states take precedence. What is clear is that the G8 is not a single hegemonic power, and within the G8 are competing visions and articulations of national and regional interests. It is still the case that individual nation-states first and foremost enact policies to maintain their own competitive position within the global order; significant tensions inevitably arise between the imperatives of global governance and perceived national interest. As a group of the most powerful nation-states, the G8 has a vested interest in a global governance regime that maintains the primacy of those nation-states; to what extent can there be mutual interest shared by the G8 and the poorest countries? Some view the Millennium Development Goals (MDGs) as providing 'a set of specific benchmarks that can be used as mobilizing devices for scaling up policies, resources, and efforts by all actors to change the patterns of globalization' (Cheru and Bradford 2005, 14). Others remain more guarded about their outlook for the future, given that it is within the broad parameters of free trade, capital mobility, currency speculation, odious debt, and the continued polarisation of wealth that the MDGs are to be reached. The global health agenda still reflects the unequal Westphalian divisions of political sovereignty and global structural inequalities in power and wealth. To this extent, the G8's record with regard to global health must be analysed in the broader context of the collateral damage caused by its members' attachment to the specific policies governing the global political economy and their enforcement by the IFIs, as well as by the effects and impacts outside their borders of their national and global security policies. What is the responsibility of states to persons outside their jurisdiction? And what is their responsibility with regard to governing private actors whose jurisdiction and activities transcend the boundaries of the nation-state?

A few key issues illustrate the point that policies emerging from the G8 can have profound and direct cross-border impacts on human health and the exercise of health rights. What are some of the specific features of the current global order that can be linked to the violation of people's exercise of their human right to health?

Oil Security and the Right to Health

The G8 model of economic development remains critically dependent on the natural resources of the global economic South. The recent war in Iraq has prompted an expansion of U.S.-led oil exploration in eleven African states as it seeks alternative supplies from non–Middle Eastern sources; sub-Saharan Africa could supply one quarter of U.S. oil by 2015, up from 16 percent today (Somerville 2002). A legitimate issue is whether western oil security is a threat to the exercise of the human right to health. This is a complex question, and one that cannot be answered here. But it points to the need to expand the analysis of core obligations to protect the right to health to laws, policies, and corporate and state behaviour that undermine the basic conditions for social reproduction upon which human health depends. Evidence suggests that often the activities of western-based oil companies in sub-Saharan Africa, supported by their governments, have undermined the exercise of human rights of the local inhabitants. Cyril Obi (2001) describes the situation in the Niger Delta, the region of Nigeria that has been transformed into a local site for global accumulation through a partnership between oil multinationals and the Nigerian state. The entire region was militarised to provide the order necessary to produce oil, 'while complaints have been ignored, protests violently crushed, villages sacked, and thousands killed, exiled, or displaced by armed forces' (179). The inhabitants of the region have received no benefits from the oil extracted from their lands and waters, yet have suffered the effects of eco-systemic crisis:

> Most of the oil communities lack electricity, piped water, and basic infrastructure. There is virtually no development, with people torn between a life of subsistence and the stark reality of unemployment. Worse still, these pauperized villagers bear the full costs of pollution and degradation arising from oil production. In some instances, multinational oil companies directly govern in the sense of exercising power and allocating resources in the oil producing communities, patronizing local chiefs and opinion leaders, and influencing the decisions of local authorities (Obi 2001, 179).

Local democratic and opposition groups through international human rights organisations brought the crisis of the Ogoni people in the Niger Delta to the global stage, challenging global oil capital and the complicity of the Nigerian state, yet the fact remains that apart from the most grotesque human rights abuses that might result in a drop in share prices or a loss of market share, mining and oil MNCs continue to violate the exercise of basic human rights, and often with impunity. The increased emphasis on global corporate responsibility and voluntary codes of conduct has perhaps, in some cases, led to marginal improvements in the lives of local people. But the fundamental issue is one of the injustice of a system in which human life is secondary to market freedom and western oil security.

Other examples abound. Today, Equatorial Guinea — one of the world's most repressive regimes, where 90 percent of the population lives in misery — is being courted by the Bush administration and the oil industry as a new investment hot spot for ExxonMobil, Chevron, and other American oil companies that have invested a collective US$5 billion. Equatorial Guinea is a country where upward of half of the population has no access to clean water, basic sanitation, and health care. According to UNAIDS, the influx of migrant labour for the booming oil industry coupled with poverty and inequality are favourable factors for the spread of HIV, which stood at 7.2 percent in 1999, and where the response is in its 'initial stages' due to 'poor mechanisms for the allocation of funds and insufficient human resources'

(UNAIDS 2005). Several oil-producing countries in Africa receive U.S. arms under the Pentagon's Excess Defense Articles Program, among them Angola, Nigeria, Cameroon, Chad, Gabon, and Congo-Brazzaville. Military security is key to encourage investment by foreign firms (Klare 2004, 177). One could argue that the onus is on local African states to monitor the activities of oil companies operating within their borders and to ensure that they are complying with international human rights standards. But when evidence suggests that states are failing to do so, for a variety of reasons (including weak regulatory infrastructures, corrupt government officials, and pressure to encourage foreign investment at all costs), should the onus rest only with the host state? MNCs work in partnership with host governments and, in the case of the oil industry, closely with their home governments; hence the analysis of their conduct must be situated in the global rules-based framework within which they operate. As Joyce Millen and Timothy Holtz (2000) argue, MNCs cannot be considered as something other than what they have collectively been enabled to be, as actors operating in a global system of market competition that impels countries to offer them the lowest possible labour and environmental standards and allows them to operate in ways that maximise profit while undermining basic rights. Should not the rules of global trade and investment be extended to govern the relationship among corporations, citizens, and the state? From a human rights perspective, it seems self-evident that the rules of global trade and foreign investment should extend to the protection of needs for human survival.

The Corporate Food Regime and the Right to Health

Another complex issue directly relevant to human health is food security. To what extent does the current global corporate food regime undermine the exercise of the right to health? In the 2002 report 'WTO Agreements and Public Health', a meaningful discussion of the relationship between trade and household food security was conspicuously omitted 'because of its complexity' (WHO and WTO 2002, 125). It acknowledged that malnutrition and undernutrition are responsible for about one third of the disease burden in sub-Saharan Africa, and that 'the great majority of the burden of disease associated with under-nutrition arises from chronic nutrition as a result of household food insecurity' (125). (One could add that even within food-secure households, all members of the household might not be receiving enough nutrition for sound human health; typically female children and women eat less.) Yet the report chooses to focus only on national food security, predictably stating that agricultural trade liberalisation helps to improve export growth 'thus providing more foreign exchange with which to import essential imports' (125).

Philip McMichael (2003) argues that the 1995 WTO Agreement on Agriculture, which advocated universal reductions in trade protection, farm subsidies, and government intervention, shares this logic and has institutionalised the meaning of food security. States no longer have the right to food self-sufficiency as a national strategy, but the 'minimum market access rule' guarantees the 'right to export,' consolidating a position of primacy to multinational agribusiness. Jagjit Plahe (2005) argues that the Agreement on Agriculture fails to recognise key factors that affect food-insecure countries and has established conditions that perpetuate food insecurity. Currently 15 of the 20 countries that are chronically food insecure (where more than 35 percent of the population is food insecure) are members of the WTO. The *raison d'être* of the Agreement on Agriculture is to liberalise trade in agriculture following the neoclassical assumption that the market will address problems of food security. To this end, according to Plahe, the agreement fails to consider the reality of declining terms of trade for primary products; countries that are chronically food insecure primarily export raw materials that increasingly face declining terms of trade on the world market. She writes:

> In terms of food security, the WTO's AoA [Agreement on Agriculture] does not acknowledge nation states' food security obligations or needs. A state can no longer automatically take measures to protect the right to food, but it must negotiate for this right at the WTO. How, when and if states can regulate trade to uphold the right to food will be determined by international trade rules, and not by international human rights standards (Plahe 2005, 11).

The undermining of the conditions within which local communities have been able to satisfy their basic subsistence needs has a long and complex history dating back to colonial times. But recent analyses by Farshad Araghi (1995), Deborah Bryceson (1999), and Ankie Hoogvelt (2001) point to 'depeasantization' (in Araghi's words) as a manifestation of the negative consequences of structural adjustment and economic liberalisation that have intensified food insecurity and have undermined subsistence economies. The consolidation of small into large holdings and the competition of industrial-style agribusiness — along with HIV/AIDS losses in productivity and drought-related famine (this in itself a consequence of western-induced global warming) and patriarchal 'law' and development practices governing women's access to land and resources — have continued the movement toward the elimination of rural small holders. Mike Davis (2004, 16), in *Planet of Slums,* details this movement of 'surplus' rural labour to urban slums, where no infrastructure or employment opportunities await the new migrants, who join the 'informal sector' in such occupations as rag picking, prostitution, street sweeping, and street vending. 'Quite apart from the incidence of HIV/AIDS plague,' he writes, 'the UN considers that two out of five African slum dwellers live in a poverty that is literally life threatening' (16). They also live in an ideal environment for the spread of disease. The burgeoning slums provide perfect conditions for the incubation of disease: population densities that defy imagination, coupled with an absence of the basic constituents of human life — clean water, sanitation, shelter, and public health systems. In the WHO's 'worst-case scenario' for avian influenza, according to Davis, upward of 98 percent of the victims will be the poor city dwellers of urban slums of the developing world (150).

Military Security and the 'War on Health'

The health toll emerging from the militarisation of the planet and the seemingly endless 'war on terrorism' reveals the contradiction between national security and human health and security. Rosalind Petchesky (2003, 251) points out that dramatic gaps in the U.S. public health system have been exposed by the 2001 'bioterrorist' scares of anthrax, which some had hoped might lead to the restoration of decent funding after 15 years of privatisation and cutbacks; instead, a new US$11 billion bioterrorism industry has emerged alongside reductions in Medicaid and other cutbacks to healthcare mechanisms for the poor and people with disabilities in a context where more than 40 million Americans remain without health insurance. She asks whether a globalised state of permanent war and ubiquitous police surveillance can ever be compatible with equity and justice in access to health:

> Is the 'war against terrorism' ultimately a war against health and all forms of social justice — an 'enemy of the poor' and especially women? Will we allow human rights and women's empowerment to get buried under the ashes of 11 September? I believe a worse danger than terrorism now is that all the resources that might be channelled toward reducing misery; eliminating maternal mortality; treating, preventing and curing AIDS; and promoting equality will be diverted into the waging and deflecting of violence … I have to wonder whether this endless war and all its ancillary security production will sap the energies and budgets for health, education, and racial and gender justice for years to come — meanwhile inflaming the global hostility and terror it was supposed to curtail (Petchesky 2003, 252).

Meanwhile, the potential global threat of avian influenza goes largely unnoticed in the South; the threat perhaps too ominous in a global context of gaping holes in the most basic public health coverage and disease surveillance. In sub-Saharan Africa, communities already coping with HIV/AIDS epidemics can hardly worry about a hypothetical virus. The most recent report of the WHO on avian influenza preparedness in the region paints a bleak picture (WHO 2005). Surveillance for avian disease is non-existent, nutrition of poultry is poor, and high mortality is common, increasing the likelihood that outbreaks will be missed. Few governments are in a position to offer support for disease control — let alone compensate farmers for destroyed birds, which discourages early and open reporting. Deaths of large numbers of poultry would deprive already impoverished populations of an important source of dietary protein. The occurrence of human cases would create huge challenges for health systems and services that are already fragile and overburdened. Surveillance systems are weak and unlikely to pick up cases of a disease with symptoms similar to illness from many other common causes. Health capacity and human and financial resources are already overwhelmed by the demands of AIDS, tuberculosis, and malaria. Laboratory confirmation of human infections of highly pathogenic avian influenza is technically challenging, expensive, and demanding on human resources, and infection control in most hospitals is difficult to introduce and sustain.

Sporadic cases of infection and the frequent reluctance of residents to comply with recommended reporting and isolation measures during outbreaks of severe disease could push fragile health systems close to the brink of collapse. Surveillance systems, with rare exceptions, are not sufficiently sensitive to pick up clusters of human cases — a critical early warning signal that the virus is improving its transmissibility.

Global Health, Human Security, and Social Reproduction

Oil, food, and military security are just three of the many dimensions of security that have a bearing on the human right to health. They illustrate how the health of the poor is shaped by the current vacuum in the governance of the global life economy. They also provide a window into the value system underpinning the present global order, which protects the entitlements of capital at the expense of the exercise of human rights and the protection of the ecosystem upon which present and future life depends. Today, global markets are in place not to meet human needs, but to generate growth and profit, abstractly understood as good in and of themselves. This is not an argument against globalisation or trade liberalisation *per se*, but a critique of the rules-based system that governs markets and the activities of states and private actors and that allows for the violation of basic human rights. The impacts of globalisation are often abstracted and aggregated in ways that obscure an understanding of their very real effects on human and other populations. Micro analyses of the health impacts of specific policies and activities illustrate these effects; more of this work is being carried out, and much remains to be done. This research points to the fact that the exercise of the right to health depends both on a functioning public health system and on an ecosystem and economy in which the exercise of basic human rights is secured and nurtured.

Health crises are often crises of social reproduction within households and local communities. Indeed, it is the case that 'nature itself imposes limitations on health' and 'depends not only on state responsibilities … but also upon the actions of other individuals in the society and the behaviour of the individual himself or herself' (Chapman 2002, 188). That being said, sound health is secured largely within the private sphere of the household and the surrounding community, the maintenance of the health of members of a household being typically the responsibility of women. In much of the global economic South, this provisioning entails the labours of subsistence food production, historically assigned household chores, birthing and suckling labours, tending to young and old bodies, and socialising children — what Ariel Salleh (2000) describes as the 'labour transactions between humanity and nature'. On top of these labours, women also participate in the wage economy, in sub-Saharan Africa almost exclusively as informal sector workers or micro-entrepreneurs. The satisfying of daily needs, the social provisioning necessary for human health, remains largely invisible; 'in conventional political economy, where the production of objects for exchange is prioritized, the reproduction of daily needs and the reproduction of future generations is taken as an essential backdrop to production' (31).

The taken-for-grantedness of women's caring labours is a deeper reflection of the devalorisation of the tasks of social reproduction (carried out by both males and females) that under capitalism are largely performed within the privatised household. The relationship between health and gender equality in the South, then, is about much more than educating women and empowering women in the marketplace and ending discrimination, as some UN and bilateral gender units would have one believe. It is about recognising and valorising the centrality of social reproduction in reproducing and nurturing our species against all odds. The undermining of the conditions needed for social reproduction and the exercise of basic human rights has largely gone unnoticed in recent decades of global restructuring. The undermining of public health infrastructures where they have in the past existed, or the failure to provide basic services in new human settlements, has meant an increasein the intensity of the largely invisible labours of social reproduction, particularly of women and girls. The undermining of the resources, social entitlements, and ecosystems upon which this labour depends is the collateral damage of an economic model that is largely disconnected from people's real, daily needs. The ontology of neo-liberal globalisation is specific — all persons are autonomous, isolated individuals with equal power in the marketplace. For those who, by accident of birth, live outside of market relations or whose subsistence labours have been undermined by markets, or who are incorporated into markets as sub-subsistence wage earners, securing the basic conditions for human health and flourishing is extremely difficult. The destruction of the ecological and biological structures that sustain life is also linked to free markets and intensified commodification, environmental destruction — now just one of the costs of doing business. The privileged elite who shape global health policy live in the G8 countries, where the basic constituents of health are now largely taken for granted.

This chapter has sought to broaden the contours of the debate about G8 responsibility for global health to include as central to the analysis of G8 health performance a consideration of its governance of the global political economy more generally. Is it life enhancing and sustaining, or is it destructive of human health? If it is agreed that all, by virtue of being born, are fully human, and that by virtue of their humanity all have human rights to survive and to develop, then global governance should evolve to protect and enhance the exercise of those human rights. If the health promises made at the various G8 summits are undermined by the more general failure to regulate the activities of private and public actors that undermine the conditions for human health and social reproduction, then those promises are likely to have little impact on the health and well-being of the global poor. Although all humans do not share the same vulnerability, today they depend on a single global ecosystem and are interdependent members of the same global community.

Notes

1 Social reproduction is defined by feminist scholars as including biological reproduction as well as the reproduction of humans on a daily basis: the nurturing, caring, feeding,

educating, and carrying out other labours that reproduce humans (and their labour power) on a daily and generational basis. The labours of social reproduction under capitalism are largely confined to the private household, but can also be provided by the public sphere. On the subject of this consensus, see, for example, Jim Yong Kim and colleagues (2000).

2 John O'Manique (1990, 476) argues that most accounts of human rights, whether theistic or rationalist, are not sufficient to support the principles of universality and inalienability; the positivist claims that rights are the creation of powerful agents, usually states, are simply entitlements granted by an authority. The concept of 'human dignity', the basis for human rights in United Nations covenants, is subjective and variable. The questions O'Manique answers are the following: What are the basic elements of a concept of universal and inalienable rights? And what would cause human beings to accept this concept and behave accordingly? Some argue that empirically validated needs restrict rights to the minimal physiological level. Yet O'Manique suggests that what is needed for the specifically human dimensions of development can also be inferred from empirically confirmed premises:

> In the case of distinctly human needs, validation must come from the social and psychological sciences. The existence of such needs for human development — the need for some association with other human beings, for self-expression, for some control over one's destiny, and even the need for love and beauty — can all be observed and even empirically determined within the social sciences and psychology. The confirmation of the need for association and for love will, of course, not have the precision or specificity of the confirmation of physiological needs.

3 Different groups have different claims for the protection and exercise of basic rights on the basis of their subject position. For example, women require different protections and entitlements than men in order to exercise their human rights given that certain aspects of reproductive and sexual health are specific to women. Rosalind Petchesky (2003, 8) identifies four principles of a feminist ethical perspective on reproductive and sexual rights: '(1) bodily integrity, or the right to dignity and respect for one's physical body and to be free from abuses and assaults, including unwanted pregnancy and unwanted sex; (2) personhood, which is closely associated with bodily integrity and implies the right to self determination and respect in one's decisions about reproduction and sexuality; (3) equality in access to health services and all social resources, not only of women with men (gender equality) but of women with one another across lines of class, race, ethnicity, age, marital status, sexual orientation, physical ability, and other common social dividers; and (4) diversity, or the right to be respected in one's group affinities and cultural differences, in so far as these are freely chosen and women are empowered to speak on their own behalf, not subordinated to group claims in the name of tradition'.

4 On the social determinants of health, see the WHO (2006).

5 See, for example, 'A Discussion on Ethical Globalization' (Yale Center for the Study of Globalization 2003) as well as Martin Wolf (2004).

References

Araghi, Farshad (1995). 'Global Depeasantization: 1945–1990'. *Sociological Quarterly,* vol. 36, no. 2, pp. 337–368.

Bakker, Isabella and Stephen Gill (2003). 'Ontology, Methods, and Hypothesis'. In I. Bakker and S. Gill, eds., *Power, Production, and Social Reproduction: Human In/Security in the Global Political Economy,* pp. 17–42 (Basingstoke: Palgrave Macmillan).

Brodie, Janine (2003). 'Globalization, In/Security, and the Paradoxes of the Social'. In I. Bakker and S. Gill, eds., *Power, Production, and Social Reproduction: Human In/ Security in the Global Political Economy,* pp. 47–65 (Basingstoke: Palgrave Macmillan).

Bryceson, Deborah (1999). 'African Rural Labour, Income Diversification, and Livelihood Approaches: A Long-Term Development Perspective'. *Review of African Political Economy,* vol. 26, no. 80, pp. 171–189.

Brysk, Alison (2005). *Human Rights and Private Wrongs: Constructing Civil Society* (New York: Routledge).

Chapman, Audrey R. (2002). 'Core Obligations Related to the Right to Health'. In A.R. Chapman and S. Russell, eds., *Core Obligations: Building a Framework for Economic, Social, and Cultural Rights,* pp. 185–215 (Antwerp: Intersentia).

Cheru, Fantu and Colin I. Bradford Jr. (2005). 'The Planet at Risk: Mobilizing Resources for Global Human Security'. Working Paper for the Track on the Global Economic Agenda, Helsinki Process on Globalisation and Democracy, Helsinki.

Davis, Mike (2004). 'Planet of Slums'. *New Left Review,* vol. 26 (March-April), pp. 5–34. <newleftreview.org/A2496> (September 2006).

Davis, Mike (2005). *Monster at Our Door: The Global Threat of Avian Flu* (New York: New Press).

Eckstein, Susan and Timothy Wickham-Crowley, eds. (2003). *Struggles for Social Rights in Latin America* (New York: Routledge).

Farmer, Paul and Nicole Gastineau Campos (2004). 'Rethinking Medical Ethics: A View from Below'. *Developing World Bioethics,* vol. 4, no. 1, pp. 17–41.

Gruskin, Sofia and Daniel Tarantola (2000). 'Health and Human Rights'. Working Paper No. 10, François-Xavier Bagnoud Center, Boston. <www.hsph.harvard.edu/fxbcenter/FXBC_WP10—Gruskin_and_Tarantola.pdf> (September 2006).

Held, David (2003). 'The Changing Structure of International Law: Sovereignty Transformed?' In D. Held and A. McGrew, eds., *The Global Transformations Reader,* pp. 162–166 (Cambridge: Polity Press).

Hoogvelt, Ankie (2001). *Globalization and the Postcolonial World: The New Political Economy of Development* (Baltimore: Johns Hopkins University Press).

Kim, Jim Yong, Joyce V. Millen, John Gershman, *et al.*, eds. (2000). *Dying for Growth: Global Inequality and the Health of the Poor* (Monroe ME: Common Courage Press).

Klare, Michael (2004). 'Blood for Oil: The Bush-Cheney Energy Strategy'. In L. Panitch and C. Leys, eds., *Socialist Register 2004: The New Imperial Challenge,* pp. 166–185 (Monmouth: Merlin Press).

McMichael, Philip (2003). 'Food Security and Social Reproduction: Issues and Contradictions'. In I. Bakker and S. Gill, eds., *Power, Production, and Social Reproduction: Human In/Security in the Global Political Economy,* pp. 169–188 (Basingstoke: Palgrave Macmillan).

Millen, Joyce V. and Timothy H. Holtz (2000). 'Dying for Growth, Part 1: Transnational Corporations and the Health of the Poor'. In J.Y. Kim, J.V. Millen, J. Gershman, *et al.*, eds., *Dying for Growth: Global Inequality and the Health of the Poor,* pp. 177–223 (Monroe ME: Common Courage Press).

Nussbaum, Martha (2000). *Women and Human Development: A Capabilities Approach* (New York: Cambridge University Press).

Obi, Cyril I. (2001). 'Global, State, and Local Intersections: Power, Authority, and Conflict in the Niger Delta Oil Communities'. In T. Callaghy, R. Kassimir, and R. Latham, eds., *Interventions and Transnationalism in Africa: Global–Local Networks of Power,* pp. 173–196 (Cambridge: Cambridge University Press).

Office of the High Commissioner for Human Rights (1966). 'International Covenant on Economic, Social, and Cultural Rights'. <www.unhchr.ch/html/menu3/b/a_cescr.htm> (September 2006).

Office of the High Commissioner for Human Rights (1989). 'Convention on the Rights of the Child'. <www.unhchr.ch/html/menu3/b/k2crc.htm> (September 2006).

O'Manique, John (1990). 'Universal and Inalienable Rights: A Search for Foundations'. *Human Rights Quarterly,* vol. 12, no. 4, pp. 465–485.

O'Manique, John (2003). *The Origins of Justice* (Philadelphia: University of Pennsylvania Press).

Petchesky, Rosalind (2003). *Global Prescriptions: Gendering Health and Human Rights* (London: Zed Books).

Plahe, Jagjit Kaur (2005). 'Globalizing Trade in Agriculture: The Implications of the WTO Agricultural Agreement on the Right to Food in Developing Countries'. Paper prepared for the conference on Human Rights in a Globalizing Era?, 4–6 August, Windsor ON.

Salleh, Ariel (2000). 'The Meta-Industrial Class and Why We Need It'. *Democracy and Nature,* vol. 6, no. 1, pp. 27–36.

Shafir, Gershon (2004). 'Citizenship and Human Rights in an Era of Globalization'. In A. Brysk and G. Shafir, eds., *People out of Place: Globalization, Human Rights, and the Citizenship Gap,* pp. 11–25 (New Haven: Routledge).

Somerville, Keith (2002). 'U.S. Looks to Africa for "Secure Oil"'. BBC News Online. <news.bbc.co.uk/2/hi/africa/2255297.stm> (September 2006).

Teeple, Gary (2005). 'Honoured in the Breach: Human Rights as Principles of a Past Age'. Paper prepared for a conference on Human Rights in a Globalizing Era?, 4–6 August, Windsor ON.

UNAIDS (2005). 'Equatorial Guinea'. <www.unaids.org/en/geographical+area/by+country?equatorial+guinea.asp> (June 2005).

United Nations (1948). 'Universal Declaration of Human Rights'. <www.un.org/Overview/rights.html> (September 2006).

United Nations (1999). 'Declaration on the Right and Responsibility of Individuals, Groups, and Organs of Society to Promote and Protect Universally Recognized Human Rights and Freedoms'. A/RES/53/144, 8 March. <www.unhchr.ch/huridocda/huridoca.nsf/(Symbol)/A.RES.53.144.En?OpenDocument> (September 2006).

United Nations Economic and Social Council (2000). 'The Right to the Highest Attainable Standard of Health'. E/C.12/2000/4, 11 August. <www.unhchr.ch/tbs/doc.nsf/(symbol)/E.C.12.2000.4.En?OpenDocument> (September 2006).

Wolf, Martin (2004). *Why Globalization Works* (New Haven: Yale University Press).

World Health Organization (1994). 'Constitution of the World Health Organization'. Geneva. <www.who.int/about/en » WHO Constitution> (September 2006).

World Health Organization (2005). 'Avian Influenza and the Pandemic Threat in Africa: Risk Assessment for Africa'. 28 October, Geneva. <www.who.int/csr/disease/avian_influenza/riskassessmentAfrica/en> (September 2006).

World Health Organization (2006). 'Commission on Social Determinants of Health'. <www.who.int/social_determinants/en> (September 2006).

World Health Organization and World Trade Organization (2002). 'WTO Agreements and Public Health: A Joint Study by WHO and the WTO Secretariat'. Geneva. <www.wto.org/English/res_e/booksp_e/who_wto_e.pdf> (September 2006).

Yale Center for the Study of Globalization (2003). 'A Discussion on Ethical Globalization'. 15 January. <www.yaleglobal.yale.edu/article.print?id=751 > (September 2006).

PART V
Conclusion

Chapter 14

Toward Innovation in Global Health Governance

Andrew F. Cooper, John J. Kirton, and Ted Schrecker

This book has addressed three central questions: What are the major health challenges and crises the global community confronts in the 21st century? How well have the world's dominant international institutions and their defining ideas responded to these challenges and crises and why? And what innovations does the global community need to create a healthier world and where should it start to bring such a future to life?

The analyses in the preceding chapters have together provided clear answers to all three questions. The real world of global health, disease, and illness is rapidly changing in ways that compound the challenges and crises with which the world must cope. The institutions and ideas relied on by the world's global governance system to respond to these challenges are still catching up to these often grim and deadly realities. While many innovations are available and starting to be introduced, there is still much work to do in redesigning global health governance and its underlying values for the 21st-century world.

Challenge

The challenges to global health are great and growing. Despite advances in some areas, the optimism fuelled by the faith in modern medicine that dominated the 20th century and delivered the eradication of smallpox has, as Mark Zacher highlights, now largely gone. The hope that new vaccines and microbicides will win the global war against HIV/AIDS is important in spurring intensified research efforts at present. But the realisation of the promise of products that will be delivered to save the lives of those who need them is still many years away. And even where antiretroviral treatment (ART) is available, making the drugs affordable and accessible through properly equipped healthcare systems to all those who need them is a campaign that remains far from won, and one demands major increases in the available resources.

Meanwhile, the body count is rising inexorably on so many fronts. Diseases such as polio, on the verge of extinction only a few years ago, are making a comeback in a growing number of countries and continents, even though they have known cures and elaborate health organisations and networks eager to deliver the vaccines. Long-known chronic diseases such as malaria and tuberculosis (TB) remain major causes of death in much of the developing world, even though the global community has accumulated more than a century of experience in combating them. The HIV/AIDS pandemic is proliferating. Exotic emerging and re-emerging infectious diseases, led by severe acute respiratory syndrome (SARS), Ebola, and the Marburg virus, are erupting frequently. Diseases are spreading in unknown and untreatable ways from animals to humans, threatening an avian influenza pandemic that is moving from its Asian incubator into birds and humans in Europe and endangering other far less well-defended areas of the world, with far fewer resources available to address the medical, economic, and social crises that would result from such a pandemic. To these diseases of the poor are added increases in the incidence of cancer, obesity, asthma, and cardiovascular disease that often defy the stereotypical view of such conditions as diseases of affluence (see, for example, Monteiro *et al.* 2004; Ezzati *et al.* 2005). Furthermore, the possibility continues to exist that terrorists will deliberately use biological agents to deadly effect in some of the healthiest and best-guarded countries on earth.

At the centre of the current global health crisis is the HIV/AIDS pandemic. Now almost a quarter of a century old, and under control in most G8 countries, it continues to have a compounding devastating effect on human life around the world. As James Orbinksi highlights, HIV/AIDS is creating a September 11 every day in Africa. It is penetrating the so-called emerging economies of Asia, where countries such as China and India now seem to be the great growth locomotives for the future. It is also ripping through Russia, which, as John Kirton and Jenevieve Mannell show, now leads the G8 countries as having the most new HIV/AIDS infections among the G8 countries. If HIV/AIDS does to Russia, India, China, and Brazil — the emerging powers of tomorrow — over the next two decades what it has done to South Africa and the rest of that continent over the past two decades, the world will be a much poorer, more deadly, and less politically stable place.

Compounding the severity of the assault from so many individual diseases on so many fronts are the complex interconnections among them, and between their physical processes and the human communities within which they work. The health of animals and humans is now tightly linked in an age of SARS and avian influenza. Nick Drager and Laura Sunderland, Ted Schrecker, Ron Labonté, and David Sanders, and Colleen O'Manique all highlight a growing recognition of the importance of the social determinants of health — a recognition underscored by the World Health Organization's (WHO) establishment of the Commission on Social Determinants of Health (WHO 2006). There is also an emerging awareness of the ecological determinants of health, as Lee-Nah Hsu shows in the case of asthma. And there is a sudden and now well-entrenched realisation of the security implications, as David Fidler argues in the case of anthrax. When these linkages are taken together, under the current principles, policies, and practices, Colin Bradford and Chantal Blouin both show that there is little chance of achieving any of the health-related Millennium Development Goals (MDGs).

Also intensifying are the deadly feedback loops, described by Margaret Whitehead, Gïran Dahlgren, and Timothy Evans (2001) as 'medical poverty traps'. Poor health makes it more difficult for societies to be well fed, to be treated by government with high-quality healthcare facilities, to become well educated in ways that reduce risky sexual behaviour and reduce the economic pressures for such behaviour, to protect their natural environments, and to remain free of terrorists and civil strife. The upward virtuous spirals that took place in Europe, North America, and Japan over the past two centuries are now working in reverse as deadly, downward, grave-digging vortexes in many countries of the developing world.

The more comprehensive and complex global health challenge acquires even larger dimensions in an age of globalisation. The discouraging possibility is that the world may now have gone through a first generation of globalisation, which was on the whole beneficial in terms of population health. The globalisation of finance made many governments and peoples more wealthy and thus able and willing to invest in good health. The globalisation of the internet and information technology, as Zacher notes, gave rise to much better disease surveillance networks beyond the control of suspicious sovereign governments, and brought new opportunities for telemedicine. And freer trade, as Blouin notes, held forth the promise that medicines, medical equipment, and other health-promoting goods and services could be made more affordably available in many places of the world.

Yet with the Asian-turned-global financial crisis starting in 1997, a second generation of intense, post–Cold War globalisation began. It had a much more negative effect on global health. The financial crisis destroyed the ability of many governments and citizens in the afflicted areas to provide and secure the heath care they needed. Trade brought health risks in the forms of invasive species and illegal trade. In 2005 avian influenza invaded Britain through an infected imported parrot, which was caught and contained by the 800-year-old political technology of national quarantine laws. Trade liberalisation, the globalisation of finance, and technological advances combined to facilitate the global reorganisation of production, often in ways that undermined the livelihoods of substantial numbers of people. The globalisation of airline travel has meant that infectious diseases are only one plane ride away from anywhere. Moreover, it can arrive in one country even before its incubation period ends to make its threat known in its country of origin. And demographic globalisation in the form of (legal and illegal) migration can bring disease into all those G8 countries, save Canada, that border poorer states with desperate people to the south. As Obijiofor Aginam evocatively notes, we are now swimming in the same microbial sea.

Post–Cold War globalisation has given rise to additional threats that compound the global health challenge. One is failed and failing states where domestic conflict and economic insecurity undermine the most basic determinants of health, with no public healthcare systemhealthcare systems from the state or even the voluntary sector to provide basic treatment. The rise of religious fundamentalism may be a force for good in some cases, as American faith-based coalitions have done much to push the United States and the G8 to do more to govern global health and directly delivered health care in some of poorest places in the world. However, Islamic fundamentalism in Nigeria has also prevented state authorities from providing the treatment necessary to eradicate polio there and stop its spread. Some Christian evangelicals and those of other faith groups may undermine HIV prevention efforts based on condom use, both in programme delivery and through their influence on national policies. In other places the grip of the past still overwhelms the health-inducing openness that globalisation brings. In non-democratic China, the secrecy and slow response to SARS and avian influenza have encouraged its spread to neighbouring countries, in what some might see as a form of medical aggression, whether intended or not. And in Swaziland and South Africa, attachments to old traditions or suspicions of imperialist practices have significantly hampered the campaign to stop the spread of HIV/AIDS (Lewis 2005).

Response

These challenges have led to several changes in the dominant approach to global health governance, in the realms of both ideas and institutions. But in both realms the response has encountered resistance and remained incomplete.

In the realm of ideas, the dominant principles and norms that govern global health have long gone beyond the narrow bio-medical model of old. But here, as Colleen O'Manique argues, the new philosophy at the top, accepted as long ago as 1978, has done little to filter down to how global health is done and delivered on the ground. And laterally, all international institutions may now recognise the economic determinants of health and, increasingly, the reciprocal principle of health for development. But in the cognate field of the social determinants of health, progress has been slower, especially where gender equality and intergenerational equality — starting with today's children, especially those being raised as AIDS orphans — is concerned. Acceptance of the many complex links between the environment and health also remains narrow and localised.

The recurrent claim that health is a human right, as powerfully set forth by O'Manique, still has little appeal beyond the human rights community. It has almost none for the many major power governments that do not domestically recognise a national right to health. G8 members such as Japan and emerging global giants such as China do not have political cultures where the appeal to inalienable individual self-evident rights from a Franco-American revolutionary tradition has much normative appeal. Nor is there any agreement on, or even strong recognition of, the way to arbitrate the conflicts among rights that arise when they compound and thus conflict — for example, when Africa's healthcare professionals exercise their right to leave their home countries for better jobs in the rich North, as they are doing in volumes. And a vast array of rights claimed by everyone may leave too few individuals or institutions willing to accept the responsibilities of meeting the many rights-based demands.

In the field of security, the terrorist attacks of 11 September 2001 and after may have restored faith in the public sector, especially in the post-securitisation era described by Fidler. But many do not recognise the value of the new impulse toward the securitisation of health, while others actively resist on normative grounds (cf. O'Manique 2005). And military models of health delivery, such as dispatching attack aircraft carrier squadrons to save lives in the wake of a devastating tsunami, may be more effective, if costly, instruments of curative reaction than prevention.

Temporally, most accept the need for prevention, treatment, and promotion as parts of an integrated strategy to deliver global health. But major debates remain over the emphasis to be placed on each components and about the appropriate techniques — abstinence or condoms for AIDS prevention, bed nets or vaccines for malaria prevention. In particular, interventions to alter the socioeconomic determinants of health are dismissed by some prominent health researchers as 'romantic but impracticable notions' (Jha *et al.* 2005). Similarly, as Orbinski and Drager and Sunderland show, most have acknowledged the capacity of many actors to meet the global health challenges, from many international institutions and national governments to the private sector, voluntary sector, philanthropists, and professional communities. But there are still sometimes bitter debates over privatisation, public-private partnerships, and the concept of health as a commodity and the value of markets in supporting health.

Perhaps the slowest ideational response comes in the reluctance of the United Nations–centred intergovernmental system to surrender the core Westphalian principle of non-interference by outside actors in the internal affairs of sovereign states. At the UN's 2005 World Summit the leaders did move in the traditional security field to accept a new principle of the 'responsibility to protect' innocent civilians when their own national governments cannot or will not protect them from deliberate deadly threats (UN General Assembly 2005). But they did nothing in the field of health to forward a principle of the responsibility of the international community to protect the many more innocent civilians who are dying of unintended but easily preventable disease.

In the realm of institutions, there is a similar sequence of advance and adjustment, resistance and inadequate response. As Drager and Sunderland show, the WHO has now broadened its activities and institutional structures to deal routinely with the socioeconomic determinants of health. However, as an institution, the WHO remains constrained by its deference to the national sovereignty of its members, its confederal culture, its slow decision-making process, and its failure to convince its many members to invest the major money required to meet the new global health threats.

In the relationship between health and trade, as Orbinski and Blouin both argue, the World Trade Organization (WTO) has responded to the global health crisis by invoking those rules that suspend normal trade discipline on intellectual property to allow the transfer of affordable and accessible drugs to poor countries and poor peoples in the world. But Aginam emphasises that few G8 countries have changed their national legislation to take full advantage of these rules. And there is much more that the WTO could do, in both trade-liberalising and trade-restricting directions, to support global health. However, the apparent collapse of the Doha development round shortly after the 2006 G8 St. Petersburg Summit does not augur well for such responses, at least over the short term.

In the fields of development and finance, the World Bank has come in for much deserved criticism about how its structural adjustment programmes (SAPs) in the 1980s forced poor countries seeking loans to reduce state expenditures on education and health. To be sure, the International Monetary Fund (IMF) and the World Bank are now complying with the G8's 2005 instruction to cancel the debt of the world's poorest countries so that they might have more of their own money left at home to devote to health. Yet the World Bank on its own has not mounted the health programmes required to make up for the damage done to public health systems in the past. And the IMF remains almost completely unconcerned with health.

In the health and environment fields, the desirable necessary links are inhibited by the absence of a World Environmental Organization (WEO) to deal as an equal with the long-established WHO (Biermann and Bauer 2005). Thus the WHO is left to reach out by way of the many weak, widely dispersed institutional fragments responsible for climate change, biodiversity, desertification, and animal health. In the field of health security, the UN Security Council (UNSC) has not done much other than hold the odd discussion. And the UN as a whole, through its General Assembly (UNGA), has done little, beyond giving a rhetorical recognition at its 2005 World Summit that under no circumstances is terrorism justified.

Some governance flaws cut across all individual global intergovernmental institutions and their interconnections. One is their failure to give the many stakeholders now involved in global health governance a legitimate and substantial role in the governance of the institutions themselves, starting with the formula pioneered by the International Labour Organization (ILO) a century ago. Another is the need for better internal and external mechanisms for monitoring compliance with commitments, to ensure that decisions are delivered in the intended way at the intended time. Kirton and Mannell show that with the creation of the Global Fund to Fight AIDS, Tuberculosis, and Malaria, the G8 has pioneered the use of the multi-stakeholder model for mobilising and disbursing money for health. But Kirton and Ella Kokotsis confirm that despite a relatively good compliance record, even the G8 leaders have not yet found a way to ensure that all their health promises made are health promise kept. And O'Manique and Schrecker and his colleagues powerfully argue that even with complete compliance G8 health governance is inappropriate for or inadequate to the global health challenge that continues to grow.

Two larger issues arise from these analyses. The first is how to transform the global health governance system from its prevailing conservative tendency to respond to real world crises and institutional failures into a strategic, proactive system that can anticipate and prevent. The second is how to secure overall coherence and central direction in a world where so many actors and policy issues are now involved. Can the world continue to rely on the old institutions to reform themselves, or ask governors of last resort such as the G8 to ride in to cope with their failures? Or is there a growing need for a constitutional moment when the world's leaders assemble to redesign the system as a whole?

Increasingly, the latter alternative commands attention. The deliberately fragmented, incomplete, unbalanced functional system of the UN architecture, designed for the world of the 1940s, still stands at the centre of the world's global health governance system today. Although bearing the legacy of the League of Nations before it (most notably with the ILO), the UN system was created in a 'big bang' more than half a century ago. The layer created first was the most powerful Bretton Woods institutions — the World Bank and the IMF, born in 1944–45. The UN in the form of UNGA, the UNSC, the United Nations Educational, Scientific, and Cultural Organization (UNESCO), and the secretariat were created a year later, as weaker and deliberately separated parts with no summit-level creation above. A year later came the still weaker institutions at the heart of today's global system — the WHO, the General Agreement on Tariffs and Trade (GATT) (upgraded in 1995 to the World Trade Organization [WTO]). and the human rights bodies. They remain third-tier players, unable to deliver the extended agenda that Drager and Sunderland and Bradford properly highlight. The UN system in its very design has become increasingly inappropriate for an ever more integrated 21st-century world. The 2005 UN World Summit offered an architectural opportunity to redesign the global health governance system to meet the new imperatives encoded in the UN's MDGs. But that opportunity was missed.

In contrast to the UN, the G8 system offers comprehensiveness, interconnectedness, soft law flexibility, overall capabilities, and intense summit-level attention. Kirton and Mannell argue that it has done much in the 21st century to bring in the leading democratic African and systemically important powers as regular participants, and to involve civil society as well. But its governors remain only a small part of a rapidly globalising world. And it has still to create a ministerial-level institution to deal with global health.

Beneath these central global institutions stands an array of plurilateral bodies that embrace rich and poor countries from many different parts of the world. Among the more prominent are the old Commonwealth and newer Francophonie, and also the Asia-Pacific Economic Cooperation (APEC) forum. At its autumn 2005 leaders meeting, APEC took up the issue of avian influenza and authorised useful actions in response. But, on the whole, the plurilateral institutions have left global health governance to the UN-based multilateral system of old.

The global community is also equipped with regional bodies for health governance. Here the Pan American Health Organization (PAHO) stands out as one of the more powerful bodies, historically performing valuable service in combating geographically specific diseases such as yellow fever. But as its long experience indicates, its presence and power can be a way for consequential countries such as the U.S. to avoid a full-strength participation in the global institutions. In the most afflicted countries such as Africa, regional health organisations remain very weak. Few regional organisations have the comprehensive, balanced, integrated functional coverage and coherent guidance that the UN system lacks. And a reliance on a network of regional institutions seems inappropriate as the desirable dominant model for global governance in a rapidly globalising age.

Innovation

The growing body count from both infectious and non-communicable diseases strongly suggests that all the globe's dominant ideas and institutions have failed in varying degrees. There is thus a strong and pressing need for innovation beyond existing institutional boundaries.

Several broad, fundamental, even revolutionary innovations warrant consideration. The largest is to address the entire comprehensive, interlinked change of conceptions and institutions advanced by Schrecker and his colleagues and by O'Manique. To get a start, in the realm of ideas, it is important to make the social determinants of health — now the focus of the WHO's commission — a dominant part of the policy paradigm. The G8 should find it easy to do so, given that its core mission is the global promotion of social advance. Another ideational advance is to replace abstract claims based on health as a right, forwarded as a rhetorical redistributional demand, with a claim to health as a basic human need from which a concrete and tightly connected set of priority claims and responsibilities can derive. The latter is likely to have a far greater appeal beyond the already rich and relatively healthy North.

It is also useful to identify a win-win agenda, in which greater trade liberalisation can combine with greater security provision in ways that promote health. As a start, quite apart from other matters on the now-stalled development agenda, as a matter of priority the WTO could liberalise barriers to the freer and more affordable imports of all health goods and services — such as bed nets — known to promote health, especially that of the poor. And a shift in focus from development as conventionally defined to development with health as its core might prove a fruitful way to restart the negotiations that began at Doha in 2001 and apparently collapsed in 2006.

While the military is routinely used in response to natural disaster to deliver clean water and treat those hurt, there is an urgent need, in today's tsunami-, hurricane-, earthquake-afflicted world for a standing international rapid reaction force to intervene instantly and rapidly to save the lives of survivors when a natural disaster strikes. And military professionals can be mobilised in more systemic ways as healthcare providers and enhancers in their peacekeeping and post-conflict peacebuilding roles. Although it is not strictly relevant to the international frame of reference, the failure of U.S. government agencies to mobilise effectively in response to the damage wrought by Hurricane Katrina demonstrates the importance of such considerations.

Perhaps most important is a strategy to extend the fledgling principle of responsibility to protect from narrow security to the broader human health security field — a predisposition that was much in evidence in the outputs from St. Petersburg, despite a continued lack of specific commitments on such matters as the financing of the Global Fund. Here in the wake of the SARS assault and the approach of avian influenza, the environmentalist's precautionary principle can provide a platform on which to build.

International institutions are in equal need of innovation. The starting point is the IMF. It is still the world's most powerful institution, both for finance and for trade for most of those countries that have had their trade policies determined by SAPs. Yet it is the body least sensitive to issues of environment and health. A 'finance for health' agenda should be part of the current review of its future mission. Here, important partners could be the WHO as well as a new WEO. In the field of health security the Global Health Security Initiative (GHSI), composed of the G7 members and Mexico, has emerged since 2001. But the subject could usefully be taken up in a broader, regular forum of the systemically important countries and international institutions of the world.

A further need for innovation lies among and above the individual institutions. As more institutions and other stakeholders move into governing global health, the chances increase for greater capacity, balance, invigorating competition, experimentation, and innovation. Drager and Sunderland note that much is to be gained from improved informal coordination. But too many players can lead to an unhealthy competition for scarce resources, systematic duplication and costly administrative overhead, underfunding of everyone, turf wars, and checkmate. This is especially the case, as Bradford notes, if there is no single superior source of governance to ensure coherence overall.

Also important is the need to introduce innovative measures to give civil society a more prominent role. On a regional basis, the old tripartite model — joining together business, labour, and government — of the ILO and the Organisation for Economic Co-operation and Development (OECD) has been joined by regional arrangements in Europe and North America where a broader array of civil society representatives have a much stronger place at the core of the international institutions. Better use can be made of the university and research communities, where public authorities have long had a major role in discovering and deploying medicines as has the for-profit private sector.

Recommendations for Action

To help put these innovations into immediate action, the authors in this volume have assembled a large and impressive array of proposals, with varying degrees of practicality and ambition, for what can be done — and should be done — in the years ahead. These recommendations for action embrace both ideas and institutions and are aimed at international institutions, national governments, and civil society alike.

Ideas

In an age when the health challenges are great and growing, the resources relatively scarce, and the security frame here to stay, Fidler recommends the use of an 'epi-elasticity' approach, in which the risks from individual diseases are assessed according to their mobility and material advantage. More broadly, Drager and Sunderland suggest the development of a consensus on fundamental ethical principles such as universalism, health as a human right, justice, dignity, and development. On this foundation would be built a system to 'address factors that cross, and even ignore, the geographical boundaries of the state' and to employ a multisectoral perspective on the determinants of health.

Institutions

In regard to the international institutions at the core of the multilateral UN system, Drager and Sunderland recommend a definition of leadership and authority for global health governance, a pooling of state sovereignty in collective action, sufficient resources and dual-track budgets distributed according to agreed priorities and effective monitoring, accountability, and enforcement mechanisms. There is also a need for a better link between trade and health led by ministries of health as well as instruments and incentives that foster trust and continuity, systems to get accurate evidence and assessments of financial implications, and measures to evaluate progress and adjust course.

In regard to the G8, O'Manique and Schrecker and his colleagues recommend the adoption of a fundamentally different set of principles to guide governance in all interrelated realms. Kirton and Mannell recommend that at its next summit the G8 produce the money to fulfill its outstanding central health commitments to the Global Fund, the WHO's failed '3 by 5' initiative, and the eradication of polio, and that the G8 create a health ministers institution to work with stakeholders on a comprehensive agenda. Kirton and Kokotsis point to how G8 leaders can use many catalysts, in particular priority placement, targets, and even timetables, to increase compliance with their commitments, without relying on the mobilisation of new money and, above all, without counting on other international institutions to do the job. Bradford also believes in the power of plurilateral, institutionalised, summit-driven institutions to bring about the needed innovative change. But he calls for a broader group of 20 at the leaders level (L20), based on the members of the G20 systemically significant countries, to convene, coordinate, and manage the three forums for health, education, and the environment, at the levels of the ministers and officials who would draft the actions plans needed to realise the core MDGs.

National Governments

National governments are also the target of several recommendations. Blouin wants those in developing countries to assess the impact of health tourism before using it as a key export sector, and adjust their strategy as a result. Unless they are capable of strong regulatory and redistributive policies, they should adopt a cautious approach to foreign direct investment (FDI) or trade in health services, and rely more on public funding for health, civil society engagement to defend the right to health, and increased inflows of official development assistance (ODA) and technical assistance from international institutions to achieve the health MDGs. In response to the HIV/AIDS crisis, Aginam calls for all the G8 governments to follow Canada's lead and take practical legislated steps to allow their national generic drug companies to negotiate contracts for the production and export of patented drugs to developing countries based on need.

Civil Society

In recognition of its increasing importance, civil society can also be improved in several ways. Drager and Sunderland call on civil society groups to become more transparent and accountable and engaged at any earlier stage. Aginam asks that civil society organisations and citizens constantly remind the G8 and the WTO of their duty to those dying of AIDS. And Orbinski offers several axioms to strengthen civil society effectiveness: accept no sacred cows, understand and use the global context, create advocacy coalitions, marshal evidence to support moral and legal claims, and engage in opportunism.

References

Biermann, Frank and Steffen Bauer, eds. (2005). *A World Environmental Organization: Solution or Threat for Effective International Environmental Governance* (Aldershot: Ashgate).

Ezzati, Majid, Stephen Vander Hoorn, Carlene M.M. Lawes, *et al.* (2005). 'Rethinking the "Diseases of Affluence" Paradigm: Global Patterns of Nutritional Risks in Relation to Economic Development'. *PLoS Medicine,* vol. 2, no. 5. <medicine.plosjournals.org/perlserv?request=get-document&doi=10.1371/journal.pmed.0020133> (September 2006).

Jha, Prabhat, David Brown, Nico Nagelkerke, *et al.* (2005). 'Five Members of the Global IDEA Scientific Advisory Committee Respond to Dr. Moore and Colleagues' [Letter]. *Canadian Medical Association Journal,* vol. 172, no. 12, pp. 1538–1539.

Lewis, Stephen (2005). *Race against Time: Searching for Hope in AIDS-Ravaged Africa* (Toronto: House of Anansi).

Monteiro, Carlos A., Erly C. Moura, Wolney L. Conde, *et al.* (2004). 'Socioeconomic Status and Obesity in Adult Populations of Developing Countries: A Review'. *Bulletin of the World Health Organization,* vol. 82, no. 12, pp. 940–946.

O'Manique, Colleen (2005). 'The "Securitisation" of HIV/AIDS in Sub-Saharan Africa: A Critical Feminist Lens'. *Policy and Society,* vol. 24, no. 1, pp. 24–47.

United Nations General Assembly (2005). '2005 World Summit Outcome'. 15 September. <www.un.org/summit2005/documents.html> (September 2006).

Whitehead, Margaret, Gïran Dahlgren, and Timothy Evans (2001). 'Equity and Health Sector Reforms: Can Low-Income Countries Escape the Medical Poverty Trap?' *Lancet,* vol. 358, pp. 833–836.

World Health Organization (2006). 'Commission on Social Determinants of Health'. <www.who.int/social_determinants/en> (September 2006).

Appendix

Appendix: The Millennium Development Goals and Targets

Goal No. 1 Eradicate extreme poverty and hunger

Target 1: Halve, between 1990 and 2015, the proportion of people whose income is less than US$1 a day

Target 2: Halve, between 1990 and 2015, the proportion of people who suffer from hunger

Goal No. 2 Achieve universal primary education

Target 3: Ensure that, by 2015, children everywhere, boys and girls alike, will be able to complete a full course of primary schooling

Goal No. 3 Promote gender equality and empower women

Target 4: Eliminate gender disparity in primary and secondary education preferably by 2005 and in all levels of education no later than 2015

Goal No. 4 Reduce child mortality

Target 5: Reduce by two thirds, between 1990 and 2015, the under-five mortality rate

Goal No. 5 Improve maternal health

Target 6: Reduce by three quarters, between 1990 and 2015, the maternal mortality ratio

Goal No. 6 Combat HIV/AIDS, malaria, and other diseases

Target 7: Have halted by 2015 and begun to reverse the spread of HIV/AIDS

Target 8: Have halted by 2015 and begun to reverse the incidence of malaria and other major diseases

Goal No. 7 Ensure environmental sustainability

Target 9: Integrate the principles of sustainable development into country policies and programmes and reverse the loss of environmental resources

Target 10: Halve, by 2015, the proportion of people without sustainable access to safe drinking water and basic sanitation

Target 11: Have achieved, by 2020, a significant improvement in the lives of at least 100 million slum dwellers

Goal No. 8 Develop a global partnership for development

Target 12: Develop further an open, rule-based, predictable, nondiscriminatory trading and financial system (includes a commitment to good governance, development, and poverty reduction — both nationally and internationally)

Some of the indicators listed below will be monitored separately for the least developed countries, Africa, landlocked countries, and small island developing states.

Target 13: Address the special needs of the least developed countries (includes tariff- and quota-free access for exports-enhanced programme of debt relief for heavily indebted poor countries [HIPCs] and cancellation of official bilateral debt, and more generous official development assistance [ODA] for countries committed to poverty reduction)

Target 14: Address the special needs of landlocked countries and small island developing states (through the Programme of Action for the Sustainable Development of Small Island Developing States and 22nd General Assembly provisions)

Target 15: Deal comprehensively with the debt problems of developing countries through national and international measures in order to make debt sustainable in the long term

Target 16: In cooperation with developing countries, develop and implement strategies for decent and productive work for youth

Target 17: In cooperation with pharmaceutical companies, provide access to affordable, essential drugs in developing countries

Target 18: In cooperation with the private sector, make available the benefits of new technologies, especially information and communications

Source: World Bank Group (2006). 'A Complete Listing of the Goals, Targets, and Indicators for MDGs'. <devdata.worldbank.org/gmis/mdg/list_of_goals.htm> (September 2006).

Bibliography

Abbott, Frederick M. (2002). 'The Doha Declaration on the TRIPS Agreement and Public Health: Lighting a Dark Corner at the WTO'. *Journal of International Economic Law,* vol. 5, no. 2, pp. 469–505.

Aginam, Obijifor (2004). 'Salvaging Our Global Neighbourhood: Critical Reflections on the G8 Summit and Global Health Governance in an Interdependent World'. *Law, Social Justice, and Global Development,* vol. 1. <www2.warwick.ac.uk/fac/soc/law/elj/lgd/2004_1/aginam> (September 2006).

Aginam, Obijifor (2005). *Global Health Governance: International Law and Public Health in a Divided World* (Toronto: University of Toronto Press).

'AIDS Creating a Generation of African Orphans: Experts'. (2003). *Agence France Press,* 26 February. <www.aegis.com/news/afp/2003/AF030281.html> (September 2006).

Albrecht, Gary L., Alfred Fitzpatrick, and Susan Scrimshaw, eds. (2000). *Handbook of Social Studies in Health and Medicine* (London: Sage Publications).

Annan, Kofi (2001). 'We the Children: Meeting the Promises of the World Summit for Children'. United Nations, New York. <www.unicef.org/specialsession/about/sg-report.htm> (September 2006).

Araghi, Farshad (1995). 'Global Depeasantization: 1945–1990'. *Sociological Quarterly,* vol. 36, no. 2, pp. 337–368.

Atarah, Linus (2005). 'Playing Chicken: Ghana vs. the IMF'. 14 June, CorpWatch. <www.corpwatch.org/article.php?id=12394> (September 2006).

Audibert, Martine and Jacky Mathonnat (2000). 'Cost Recovery in Mauritania: Initial Lessons'. *Health Policy and Planning,* vol. 15, no. 1, pp. 66–75. <heapol.oxfordjournals.org/cgi/reprint/15/1/66?ck=nck> (September 2006).

AVERT (2006). 'Canada Statistics by Year and Age'. <www.avert.org/canstatr.htm> (September 2006).

AVERT (2006). 'HIV and AIDS: History, Pictures, and Posters'. <www.avert.org/historyi.htm> (September 2006).

AVERT (2006). 'United Kingdom Statistics by Year'. <www.avert.org/statsyr.htm> (September 2006).

AVERT (2006). 'United States AIDS Cases and Deaths by Year'. <www.avert.org/usastaty.htm> (September 2006).

Baeza, Christian and Marcela Cabezas (1999). 'Es necesario el ajuste de riesgo el los mercados de seguros de salud en América Latina?' [Is Risk Adjustment Necessary in Health Insurance Markets in Latin America?]. Centro Latinoamericano de Investigación para Sistemas de Salud, Santiago, Chile.

Bakker, Isabella and Stephen Gill (2003). 'Ontology, Methods, and Hypothesis'. In I. Bakker and S. Gill, eds., *Power, Production, and Social Reproduction: Human*

In/Security in the Global Political Economy, pp. 17–42 (Basingstoke: Palgrave Macmillan).

Barratt Brown, Michael (1995). *Africa's Choices: After Thirty Years of the World Bank* (Boulder: Westview).

Barrientos, Armando and Peter Lloyd-Sherlock (2000). 'Reforming Health Insurance in Argentina and Chile'. *Health Policy and Planning,* vol. 15, no. 4, pp. 417–423.

Bass, Naomi A. (2002). 'Implications of the TRIPS Agreement for Developing Countries: Pharmaceutical Patent Laws in Brazil and South Africa in the 21st Century'. *George Washington International Law Review,* vol. 34, no. 1, pp. 191–223.

Bayne, Nicholas (1999). 'Continuity and Leadership in an Age of Globalisation'. In M.R. Hodges, J.J. Kirton, and J.P. Daniels, eds., *The G8's Role in the New Millennium,* pp. 21–44 (Aldershot: Ashgate).

Bayne, Nicholas (2000). *Hanging In There: The G7 and G8 Summit in Maturity and Renewal* (Aldershot: Ashgate).

Bayne, Nicholas (2001). 'Managing Globalisation and the New Economy: The Contribution of the G8 Summit'. In J.J. Kirton and G.M. von Furstenberg, eds., *New Directions in Global Economic Governance: Managing Globalisation in the Twenty-First Century,* pp. 171–188 (Aldershot: Ashgate).

Bayne, Nicholas (2002). 'Impressions of the Genoa Summit, 20–22 July, 2001'. In M. Fratianni, P. Savona, and J.J. Kirton, eds., *Governing Global Finance: New Challenges, G7 and IMF Contributions,* pp. 199–210 (Aldershot: Ashgate).

Bayne, Nicholas (2003). 'Impressions of the Evian Summit'. G8 Research Group. <www.g8.utoronto.ca/evaluations/2003evian/assess_bayne030603.html> (September 2006).

Bayne, Nicholas (2003). 'Impressions of the Kananaskis Summit'. In M. Fratianni, P. Savona, and J.J. Kirton, eds., *Sustaining Global Growth and Development: G7 and IMF Governance,* pp. 229–240 (Aldershot: Ashgate).

Bayne, Nicholas (2005). *Staying Together: The G8 Summit Confronts the 21st Century* (Aldershot: Ashgate).

Beaglehole, Robert and Derek Yach (2003). 'Globalisation and the Prevention and Control of Non-Communicable Disease: The Neglected Chronic Diseases of Adults'. *Lancet,* vol. 362, pp. 903–908.

Bennett, Sara and Lucy Gilson (2001). 'Health Financing: Designing and Implementing Pro-Poor Policies'. DfID Health Systems Resource Centre, London. <www.dfidhealthrc.org/shared/publications/Issues_papers/Health_financing_pro-poor.pdf> (September 2006).

Biermann, Frank and Steffen Bauer, eds. (2005). *A World Environmental Organization: Solution or Threat for Effective International Environmental Governance* (Aldershot: Ashgate).

Bijlmakers, Leon A., Mary T. Bassett, and David Sanders (1999). *Socioeconomic Stress, Health, and Child Nutritional Status in Zimbabwe at a Time of Economic Structural Adjustment: A Three-Year Longitudinal Study* (Uppsala: Nordiska Afrikainstitutet).

Birnie, Patricia W. and Alan E. Boyle (2002). *International Law and the Environment*, 2nd ed. (Oxford: Oxford University Press).

Blouin, Chantal, Nick Drager, and Richard Smith, eds. (2005). *International Trade in Health Services and the GATS: Current Issues and Debates* (Washington DC: World Bank and World Health Organization).

Blouin, Chantal, Jens Gobrecht, J. Lethridge, et al. (2005). 'Trade in Health Services under the Four Modes of Supply: Review of the Current Trends and Policy Issues'. In C. Blouin, N. Drager, and R. Smith, eds., *International Trade in Health Services and the GATS: Current Issues and Debates* (Washington DC: World Bank and World Health Organization).

Boyce, James K. and Léonce Ndikumana (2001). 'Is Africa a Net Creditor? New Estimates of Capital Flight from Severely Indebted Sub-Saharan African Countries, 1970–96'. *Journal of Development Studies,* vol. 38, no. 2, pp. 27–56.

Bratt, John, Mark Weaver, James Foreit, *et al.* (2002). 'The Impact of Price Changes on Demand for Family Planning and Reproductive Health Services in Ecuador'. *Health Policy and Planning*, vol. 17, no. 3, pp. 281–287.

Broadhead, Robert L. and Adamson S. Muula (2002). 'Creating a Medical School for Malawi: Problems and Achievements'. *British Medical Journal,* vol. 325, no. 7360, pp. 384–387.

Brock, Karen and Rosemary McGee (2004). 'Mapping Trade Policy: Understanding the Challenges of Civil Society Participation'. Institute for Development Studies, Brighton. <www.ids.ac.uk/ids/bookshop/wp/wp225.pdf> (September 2006).

Brodie, Janine (2003). 'Globalization, In/Security, and the Paradoxes of the Social'. In I. Bakker and S. Gill, eds., *Power, Production, and Social Reproduction: Human In/Security in the Global Political Economy,* pp. 47–65 (Basingstoke: Palgrave Macmillan).

Brower, Jennifer and Peter Chalk (2003). *The Global Threat of New and Reemerging Infectious Diseases: Reconciling U.S. National Security and Public Health Policy* (Santa Monica CA: Rand).

Brown, Phil and Stephen Zavestoski (2004). 'Social Movements in Health: An Introduction'. *Sociology of Health and Illness,* vol. 26, no. 6, pp. 679–694.

Brundtland, Gro Harlem (2000). 'Address at the Opening Dinner of the Massive Effort Advocacy Meeting'. 3 October, Winterthur. <www.who.int/director-general/speeches/2000/english/20001003_massive_effort.html> (September 2006).

Bryce, Jennifer, Robert E. Black, Neff Walker, *et al.* (2005). 'Can the World Afford to Save the Lives of 6 Million Children Each Year?' *Lancet,* vol. 365, no. 9478, pp. 2154–2156.

Bryceson, Deborah (1999). 'African Rural Labour, Income Diversification, and Livelihood Approaches: A Long-Term Development Perspective'. *Review of African Political Economy,* vol. 26, no. 80, pp. 171–189.

Brysk, Alison (2005). *Human Rights and Private Wrongs: Constructing Civil Society* (New York: Routledge).

Buddhasri, W., S. Saithanu, and V. Tangcharoensathien (2003). 'Private Hospital Industry in Thailand after the Economic Crisis, 1996–2001'. International Health Policy Programme, Nanthaburi, Thailand.

Centers for Disease Control and Prevention (2006). 'Smallpox Disease Overview'. Atlanta. <www.bt.cdc.gov/agent/smallpox/overview/disease-facts.asp> (September 2006).

Chanda, Rupa (2001). 'Trade in Health Services'. Commission on Macroeconomics and Health Working Paper WG4:5, World Health Organization, Geneva.

Chang, Ha-Joon (2002). *Kicking Away the Ladder: Development Strategy in Historical Perspective* (London: Anthem Press).

Chang, Ha-Joon (2005). 'Policy Space in Historical Perspective, with Special Reference to Trade and Industrial Policies'. Paper presented at Queen Elizabeth House 50th Anniversary Conference on the Development Threats and Promises, 4–5 July, Oxford. <www.qeh.ox.ac.uk/pdf/qehconf/chang.pdf> (September 2006).

Chapman, Audrey R. (2002). 'Core Obligations Related to the Right to Health'. In A.R. Chapman and S. Russell, eds., *Core Obligations: Building a Framework for Economic, Social, and Cultural Rights,* pp. 185–215 (Antwerp: Intersentia).

Chawla, Mukesh and Randall P. Ellis (2000). 'The Impact of Financing and Quality Changes on Health Care Demand in Niger'. *Health Policy and Planning,* vol. 15, no. 1, pp. 76–84.

Chen, Lincoln, Timothy Evans, Sudhir Anand, *et al.* (2004). 'Human Resources for Health: Overcoming the Crisis'. *Lancet,* vol. 364, no. 9449, pp. 1984–1990.

Chen, Shaohua and Martin Ravallion (2004). 'How Have the World's Poorest Fared since the Early 1980s?' *World Bank Research Observer,* vol. 19, no. 2, pp. 141–169.

Cheru, Fantu (1999). 'Effects of Structural Adjustment Policies on the Full Enjoyment of Human Rights'. E/CN.4/1999/50, 24 February, United Nations Economic and Social Council, New York. <www.unhchr.ch/Huridocda/Huridoca.nsf/TestFrame/f991c6c62457a2858025675100348aef?Opendocument> (September 2006).

Cheru, Fantu (2001). 'The Highly Indebted Poor Countries (HIPC) Initiative: A Human Rights Assessment of the Poverty Reduction Strategy Papers (PRSP)'. E/CN.4/2001/56, 19 January, United Nations Economic and Social Council, New York. <www.unhchr.ch/Huridocda/Huridoca.nsf/(Symbol)/E.CN.4.2001.56.En?Opendocument> (September 2006).

Cheru, Fantu (2002). 'Debt, Adjustment, and the Politics of Effective Response to HIV/AIDS in Africa'. *Third World Quarterly,* vol. 23, no. 2, pp. 299–312.

Cheru, Fantu and Colin I. Bradford Jr. (2005). 'The Planet at Risk: Mobilizing Resources for Global Human Security'. Working Paper for the Track on the Global Economic Agenda, Helsinki Process on Globalisation and Democracy, Helsinki.

Christian Aid (2005). 'The Economics of Failure: The Real Cost of "Free" Trade for Poor Countries'. Briefing paper, London <www.christianaid.org.uk/indepth/506liberalisation/Economics%20of%20failure.pdf> (September 2006).

Commission for Africa (2005). 'Our Common Interest'. Report of the Commission for Africa, London. <www.commissionforafrica.org/english/report/thereport/english/11-03-05_cr_report.pdf> (September 2006).

Commission on Human Security (2003). 'Human Security Now: The Final Report of the Commission on Human Security'. New York. <www.humansecurity-chs.org/finalreport/English/FinalReport.pdf> (September 2006).

Commission on Macroeconomics and Health (2001). 'Macroeconomics and Health: Investing in Health for Economic Development'. World Health Organization, Geneva. <www.cid.harvard.edu/cidcmh/CMHReport.pdf> (September 2006).

Conyers, Diana and Rob Mellors (2005). 'Aid Ineffectiveness in Sub-Saharan Africa: The Problem of Donor Capacity'. *IDS Bulletin,* vol. 36, no. 3, pp. 83–89.

Cooper, Richard N. (1989). 'International Cooperation in Public Health as a Prologue to Macroeconomic Cooperation'. In R.N. Cooper, ed., *Can Nations Agree? Issues in International Economic Cooperation,* pp. 183–190 (Washington DC: Brookings Institution).

Cornia, Giovanni Andrea, Frances Stewart, and Richard Jolly, eds. (1987). *Adjustment with a Human Face.* Vol. 1, *Protecting the Vulnerable and Promoting Growth* (Oxford: Clarendon Press).

Correa, Carlos (2004). 'Implementation of the WTO General Council Decision on Paragraph 6 of the Doha Declaration on the TRIPS Agreement and Public Health'. World Health Organization, Geneva. <www.eldis.org/static/DOC17336.htm> (September 2006).

Cousins, Ben (2006). 'Agrarian Reform and the "Two Economies": Transforming South Africa's Countryside'. In L. Ntsebeza and R. Hall, eds., *The Land Question in South Africa: The Challenge of Transformation and Redistribution* (Cape Town: HSRC Press).

CPTech (2006). 'Court Case between 39 Pharmaceutical Firms and the South African Government'. Washington DC. <www.cptech.org/ip/health/sa/pharma-v-sa.html> (September 2006).

Creese, Andrew (1991). 'User Charges for Health Care: A Review of Recent Experience'. *Health Policy and Planning,* vol. 6, no. 4, pp. 309–319.

DATA (2006). 'The DATA Report 2006: Keep the G8 Promise to Africa'. London. <www.thedatareport.org/pdf/dataReportFull.pdf> (September 2006).

Davis, Mike (2004). 'Planet of Slums'. *New Left Review,* vol. 26 (March-April), pp. 5–34. <newleftreview.org/A2496> (September 2006).

Davis, Mike (2005). *Monster at Our Door: The Global Threat of Avian Flu* (New York: New Press).

de Renzio, Paolo (2005). 'Increased Aid vs. Absorptive Capacity: Challenges and Opportunities Towards 2015'. *IDS Bulletin,* vol. 36, no. 3, pp. 20–27.

De Vogli, Roberto and Gretchen L. Birbeck (2005). 'Potential Impact of Adjustment Policies on Vulnerability of Women and Children to HIV/AIDS in Sub-Saharan Africa'. *Journal of Health Population and Nutrition,* vol. 23 no. 2, pp. 105–120.

Dentico, Nicoletta and Nathan Ford (2005). 'The Courage to Change the Rules: A Proposal for an Essential Health R&D Treaty'. *PLoS Medicine,* vol. 2, no. 2. <medicine.plosjournals.org/perlserv/?request=get-document&doi=10.1371/journal.pmed.0020014> (September 2006).

Department for International Development (United Kingdom) (2006). 'Turning Talk into Action: G8 Gleneagles One Year On'. London. <www.dfid.gov.uk/pubs/files/g8-2006.pdf> (September 2006).

Diderichsen, Finn, Timothy Evans, and Margaret Whitehead (2001). 'The Social Basis of Disparities in Health'. In T. Evans, M. Whitehead, F. Diderichsen, *et al.*, eds., *Challenging Inequities in Health: From Ethics to Action,* pp. 12–23 (New York: Oxford University Press).

Dignitas International (2006). 'Harnessing the Power of Community to Fight AIDS'. <www.dignitasinternational.org> (September 2006).

Dimbleby, Jonathan (2005). 'Our Last Chance'. *Observer,* 11 September.

Diop, François, Abdo Yazbeck, and Ricardo Bitran (1995). 'The Impact of Alternative Cost Recovery Schemes on Access and Equity in Niger'. *Health Policy and Planning,* vol. 10, no. 3, pp. 223–240.

Dodgson, Richard, Kelley Lee, and Nick Drager (2002). 'Global Health Governance: A Conceptual Review'. World Health Organization and London School of Hygiene and Tropical Medicine, Geneva.

Drager, Nick and Robert Beaglehole (2001). 'Globalization: Changing the Public Health Landscape'. *Bulletin of the World Health Organization,* vol. 79, no. 9, p. 803. <www.who.int/bulletin/pdf/2001/issue9/bu1488.pdf> (September 2006).

Drohan, Madelaine (2005). 'Broken Promises'. *Literary Review of Canada,* vol. 13, no. 10, pp. 11–12.

Drugs for Neglected Diseases Initiative (2006). <www.dndi.org> (September 2006).

Eberstadt, Nicholas (2002). 'The Future of AIDS'. *Foreign Affairs,* vol. 81, no. 6, pp. 22–45. <www.foreignaffairs.org/20021101faessay9990/nicholas-eberstadt/the-future-of-aids.html> (September 2006).

Eckstein, Susan and Timothy Wickham-Crowley, eds. (2003). *Struggles for Social Rights in Latin America* (New York: Routledge).

Elliott, Larry and Patrick Wintour (2005). 'Biggest African Debt Rescue Saves Nigeria £17.3bn'. *Guardian,* 1 July. <www.guardian.co.uk/hearafrica05/story/0,,1518961,00.html> (September 2006).

Elliott, Richard (2006). 'Global Access to Medicines: Canada's Law on Compulsory Licensing for Export'. Canadian HIV/AIDS Legal Network. <www.aidslaw.ca/publications/publicationsdocEN.php?ref=552> (September 2006).

English, John, Ramesh Thakur, and Andrew F. Cooper (2005). *Reforming from the Top: A Leaders' 20 Summit* (Tokyo: United Nations University).

European Centre for the Epidemiological Monitoring of AIDS (1998). 'HIV/AIDS Surveillance in Europe'. Quarterly Report No. 60, Saint-Maurice, France. <www-aids.med.unibo.it/eustat> (September 2006).

Evans, Robert G. and Gregory L. Stoddart (1990). 'Producing Health, Consuming Health Care'. *Social Science & Medicine,* vol. 31 no. 12, pp. 1347–1363.

Evans, Robert G. and Gregory L. Stoddart (2003). 'Consuming Research, Producing Policy?' *American Journal of Public Health,* vol. 93, no. 3, pp. 371–379.

Evans, Robert G., Morris L. Barer, and Theodore R. Marmor, eds. (1994). *Why Are Some People Healthy and Others Not? The Determinants of Health of Populations* (New York: Aldine DeGruyter).

Evans, Timothy, Margaret Whitehead, Finn Diderichsen, *et al.*, eds. (2001). *Challenging Inequities in Health: From Ethics to Action* (New York: Oxford University Press).

Ezzati, Majid, Stephen Vander Hoorn, Carlene M.M. Lawes, *et al.* (2005). 'Rethinking the "Diseases of Affluence" Paradigm: Global Patterns of Nutritional Risks in Relation to Economic Development'. *PLoS Medicine,* vol. 2, no. 5. <medicine.plosjournals.org/perlserv?request=get-document&doi=10.1371/journal.pmed.0020133> (September 2006).

Falk, Richard A. (1998). 'The Coming Global Civilization: Neo-Liberal or Humanist'. In A. Anghie and G. Sturgess, eds., *Legal Visions of the 21st Century: Essays in Honour of Judge Christopher Weeramantry* (The Hague: Kluwer Law International).

Falk, Richard A. (1998). *Law in an Emerging Global Village: A Post-Westphalian Perspective* (Ardsley NY: Transnational Publishers).

Farmer, Paul (2003). *Pathologies of Power: Health, Human Rights and the New War on the Poor* (Berkeley: University of California Press).

Farmer, Paul and Nicole Gastineau Campos (2004). 'Rethinking Medical Ethics: A View from Below'. *Developing World Bioethics,* vol. 4, no. 1, pp. 17–41.

Feacham, Richard (2004). 'Financing Global Public Health: Innovation and Investment'. Speech given to the World Federation of Public Health Associations Congress and the UK Health Association's Annual Public Health Forum on Sustaining Health in a Changing World: Vision to Action, 20 April, Brighton UK. <www.theglobalfund.org/en/media_center/speeches/speech_feachem_040411.asp> (September 2006).

Feldbaum, Henry and Kelley Lee (2004). 'Public Health and Security'. In A. Ingram, ed., *Health, Foreign Policy, and Security: Towards a Conceptual Framework for Research and Policy,* pp. 19–28 (London: Nuffield Trust).

Fenner, Frank, ed. (1988). *Smallpox and Its Eradication* (Geneva: World Health Organization).

Fidler, David P. (1999). *International Law and Infectious Diseases* (Oxford: Oxford University Press).

Fidler, David P. (2001). 'The Globalization of Public Health: The First 100 Years of International Health Diplomacy'. *Bulletin of the World Health Organization,* vol. 79, no. 9, pp. 842–849.

Fidler, David P. (2002). 'Global Health Governance: Overview of the Role of International Law in Protecting and Promoting Global Public Health'. Discussion Paper No. 3, World Health Organization and London School of Hygiene and Tropical Medicine, Geneva.

Fidler, David P. (2003). 'Public Health and National Security in the Global Age: Infectious Diseases, Bioterrorism, and Realpolitik'. *George Washington International Law Review,* vol. 35, pp. 788–856.

Fidler, David P. (2004). *SARS: Governance and the Globalization of Disease* (New York: Palgrave Macmillan).

Fidler, David P. (2004). 'Caught between Paradise and Power: Public Health, Pathogenic Threats, and the Axis of Illness'. *McGeorge Law Review,* vol. 35, pp. 45–104.

Fidler, David P. (2005). 'From International Sanitary Conventions to Global Health Security: The New International Health Regulations'. *Chinese Journal of International Law,* vol. 4, no. 2, pp. 325–392.

Filmer, Deon (2003). 'The Incidence of Public Expenditures on Health and Education'. Background note for the World Development Report 2004: Making Services Work for Poor People, World Bank, Washington DC.

Findley, Sally, Ahmed Zayan, Maria Kere, *et al.* (1997). 'Stretching the Limits of Health Interventions in Burkina Faso'. *Health Transition Review,* vol. 7, no. 1, pp. 95–107.

Flood, Colleen M., Mark Stabile, and Caroline Tuohy (2002). 'The Borders of Solidarity: How Countries Determine the Public/Private Mix in Spending and the Impact on Health Care'. *Health Matrix,* vol. 12, no. 2, pp. 297–356.

Food and Agriculture Organization (1997). 'The Rural Population of Africa Confronted with AIDS: A Challenge to Development'. Summary of FAO Studies on AIDS, Rome.

Food and Agriculture Organization (2001). 'The Impact of HIV/AIDS on Food Security'. Paper prepared for the 27th Session of the Committee on World Food Security, 28 May–1 June, Rome.

Food and Agriculture Organization (2005). 'The State of Food Insecurity in the World 2005: Eradicating World Hunger — Key to Achieving the Millennium Development Goals'. Rome. <www.fao.org/docrep/008/a0200e/a0200e00.htm> (September 2006).

Foster, John W. (2002). 'Canada and International Health: A Time of Testing on AIDS'. In N. Hillmer and M.A. Molot, eds., *Canada among Nations 2002: A Fading Power,* pp. 191–208 (Toronto: Oxford University Press).

Foster, John W. (2003). 'Canada's Foreign Policy in Health: Signs and Signals from HIV/AIDS'. Paper presented at the workshop on Canadian Foreign Policy and Global Health, Institut québécois des hautes études internationales and the North-South Institute, 5 December, Quebec City. <www.nsi-ins.ca/english/pdf/Cdn_policy_global_health.pdf> (September 2006).

Foster, Mick (2004). 'MDG-Orientated Sector and Poverty Reduction Strategies: Lessons from Experience in Health'. Paper prepared for the High-Level Forum on the Health MDGs, December, Abuja. <www.hlfhealthmdgs.org/Documents/MDGorientedPRSPs-Final.pdf> (September 2006).

Fourcade-Gourinchas, Marion and Sarah L. Babb (2002). 'The Rebirth of the Liberal Creed: Paths to Neoliberalism in Four Countries'. *American Journal of Sociology,* vol. 108, no. 3, pp. 533–379.

France, Tim, Gorik Ooms, and Bernard Rivers (2002). 'The Global Fund: Which Countries Owe How Much?' Aidspan. <www.aidspan.org/Papers/GlobalFundContributions21April2002.htm> (September 2006).

'France's Parliament Approves Airline Tax to Fund HIV/AIDS Programs'. (2006). *Medical News,* 4 January. <www.medicalnewstoday.com/medicalnews.php?newsid=35687> (September 2006).

Friedman, Eric A. (2004). 'An Action Plan to Prevent Brain Drain: Building Equitable Health Systems in Africa'. Physicians for Human Rights, Boston. <www.phrusa.org/campaigns/aids/pdf/braindrain.pdf> (September 2006).

G7 (1979). 'Declaration'. 29 June, Tokyo. <www.g8.utoronto.ca/summit/1979tokyo/communique.html> (September 2006).

G7 (1982). 'Report by François Mitterrand, President of the French Republic at the Summit of the Industrialized Nations' [Rapport de M. le Président de la République au Sommet des pays industrielles: technologie, emploi et croissance]. 10 June, Versailles. <www.g8.utoronto.ca/summit/1982versailles/report_english> (September 2006).

G7 (1987). 'Chairman's Statement on AIDS'. 10 June, Venice. <www.g8.utoronto.ca/summit/1987venice/aids.html> (September 2006).

G7 (1996). 'Economic Communiqué: Making a Success of Globalization for the Benefit of All'. 28 June, Lyon. <www.g8.utoronto.ca/summit/1996lyon/communique.html> (September 2006).

G8 (2000). 'G8 Communiqué Okinawa 2000'. 23 July, Okinawa. <www.g8.utoronto.ca/summit/2000okinawa/finalcom.htm> (September 2006).

G8 (2001). 'Communiqué'. 22 July, Genoa. <www.g8.utoronto.ca/summit/2001genoa/finalcommunique.html> (September 2006).

G8 (2002). 'G8 Africa Action Plan'. 27 June, Kananaskis. <www.g8.utoronto.ca/summit/2002kananaskis/africaplan.html> (September 2006).

G8 (2003). 'Health: A G8 Action Plan'. 2 June, Evian. <www.g8.utoronto.ca/summit/2003evian/health_en.html> (September 2006).

G8 (2004). 'Chair's Summary'. 10 June, Sea Island. <www.g8.utoronto.ca/summit/2004seaisland/summary.html> (September 2006).

G8 (2005). 'Africa'. 8 July, Gleneagles. <www.g8.utoronto.ca/summit/2005gleneagles/africa.html> (September 2006).

G8 (2005). 'Chair's Summary'. 8 July, Gleneagles. <www.g8.utoronto.ca/summit/2005gleneagles/summary.html> (September 2006).

G8 (2005). 'Climate Change, Clean Energy, and Sustainable Development'. 8 July, Gleneagles. <www.g8.utoronto.ca/summit/2005gleneagles/climatechange.html> (September 2006).

G8 (2005). 'Statement on the Final Day of the Summit'. 8 July, Gleneagles. <www.g8.utoronto.ca/summit/2005gleneagles/statement.html> (September 2006).

G8 (2006). 'Fight Against Infectious Disease'. 16 July, St. Petersburg. <www.g8.utoronto.ca/summit/2006stpetersburg/infdis.html> (September 2006).

'G8 Failed to Tackle the Toxic Politics of Drug Making and Selling'. (2003). *East African,* 10 June.

G8 Research Group (2000). '2000 Okinawa Summit Performance Assessments'. <www.g8.utoronto.ca/evaluations/2000okinawa/country.htm#issues> (September 2006).

G8 Research Group (2004). '2003 Evian Final Compliance Report'. <www.g8.utoronto.ca/evaluations/2003evian_comp_final> (September 2006).

G8 Research Group (2004). '2003 Evian Interim Compliance Report'. <www.g8.utoronto.ca/evaluations/2003evian_comp_interim> (September 2006).

G8 Research Group (2005). '2004 Sea Island Final Compliance Report'. Toronto. <www.g8.utoronto.ca/evaluations/2004seaisland_final> (September 2006).

G8 Research Group (2005). 'The G8 and Africa Final Report: An Overview of the G8's Ongoing Relationship with African Development from the 2001 Genoa Summit to the 2005 Gleneagles Summit'. <www.g8.utoronto.ca/evaluations/csed/g8africa_050624.html> (September 2006).

G8 Research Group (2006). '2005 Gleneagles Final Compliance Report'. <www.g8.utoronto.ca/evaluations/2005compliance_final> (September 2006).

G8 Research Group (2006). 'All G7/8 Commitments, 1975–2006'. <www.g8.utoronto.ca/evaluations/G8_commitments.pdf> (September 2006).

G8 Research Group (2006). 'The Prospective Agenda for the 2007 G8 Heiligendamm Summit'. <www.g8.utoronto.ca/evaluations/2007heiligendamm/2007agenda061215.html> (September 2006).

G8 Research Group (2006). 'What Is the G8'. <www.g8.utoronto.ca/what_is_g8.html> (September 2006).

Gagel, Sabine and Elodie Niederlaender (2004). 'VIH et SIDA dans l'Union europeénne' [HIV and AIDS in the European Union]. Eurostat. <epp.eurostat.cec.eu.int/cache/ITY_OFFPUB/KS-NK-04-018/FR/KS-NK-04-018-FR.PDF> (September 2006).

Garcia, Frank J. (2004). 'Beyond Special and Differential Treatment'. *Boston College International and Comparative Law Review,* vol. 27 no. 2, pp. 291–317.

Garrett, Laurie (1994). *The Coming Plague: Newly Emerging Diseases in a World Out of Balance* (New York: Farrar, Strauss and Giroux).

Garrett, Laurie (2000). *Betrayal of Trust The Collapse of Global Public Health* (New York: Hyperion).

Garrett, Laurie (2005). 'HIV and National Security: Where Are the Links?' Council on Foreign Relations, New York. <www.cfr.org/content/publications/attachments/HIV_National_Security.pdf> (September 2006).

Gathii, James Thuo (2002). 'The Legal Status of the Doha Declaration on TRIPS and Public Health under the Vienna Convention on the Law of Treaties'. *Harvard Journal of Law and Technology,* vol. 15, no. 2, pp. 291–317.

GAVI Alliance (2006). 'Questions and Answers about GAVI and the GAVI Fund'. Geneva. <www.gavialliance.org/General_Information/About_alliance/FAQ/qanda.php> (September 2006).

General Agreement on Tariffs and Trade (1947). <www.wto.org/english/docs_e/legal_e/gatt47_01_e.htm> (September 2006).

Gertler, Paul J. and Jeffrey S. Hammer (1997). 'Strategies for Pricing Publicly Provided Health Services'. World Bank Policy Research Working Paper No. 1762. <ssrn.com/abstract=615024> (September 2006).

Giacomini, Mita, Jeremiah Hurley, Irving Gold, *et al.* (2004). 'The Policy Analysis of "Values Talk": Lessons from Canadian Health Reform'. *Health Policy,* vol. 67, no. 1, pp. 15–24.

Gilson, Lucy (1997). 'The Lessons of User Fee Experience in Africa'. *Health Policy and Planning,* vol. 12, no. 4, pp. 273–285.

Gilson, Lucy and Anne Mills (1995). 'Health Sector Reforms in Sub-Saharan Africa'. *Health Policy,* vol. 32, no. 1, pp. 215–243.

Gilson, Lucy, Denny Kalyalya, Felix Kuchler, *et al.* (2001). 'Strategies for Promoting Equity: Experience with Community Financing in Three African Countries'. *Health Policy,* vol. 58, no. 1, pp. 37–67.

Global Fund to Fight AIDS, Tuberculosis, and Malaria (2004). 'Confirmation of U.S. Pledge for 2004 Boosts Global Fund Resources for Fourth Proposal Round to $900 Million'. Press release, 26 February. <www.theglobalfund.org/en/media_center/press/pr_040226.asp> (September 2006).

Global Fund to Fight AIDS, Tuberculosis, and Malaria (2005). 'Addressing HIV/AIDS, Malaria, and Tuberculosis: The Resource Needs of the Global Fund 2005–2007'. Geneva. <www.theglobalfund.org/en/files/about/replenishment/Resource%20Needs%20-%20February%202005.pdf> (September 2006).

Global Fund to Fight AIDS, Tuberculosis, and Malaria (2005). 'Global Fund Receives Pledges of US$3.7 Billion for 2006–2007'. Press release, 6 September, Geneva. <www.theglobalfund.org/en/media_center/press/pr_050906.asp> (September 2006).

Global Fund to Fight AIDS, Tuberculosis, and Malaria (2006). 'Distribution of Funding after Five Rounds'. Geneva. <www.theglobalfund.org/en/funds%5Fraised/distribution> (September 2006).

Global Fund to Fight AIDS, Tuberculosis, and Malaria (2006). 'Guide to the Global Fund's Policies on Procurement and Supply Management'. Geneva. <www.theglobalfund.org/en/about/procurement/policies> (September 2006).

Global Fund to Fight AIDS, Tuberculosis, and Malaria (2006). 'Pledges and Contributions to the Global Fund'. Geneva. <www.theglobalfund.org/en/files/pledges&contributions.xls> (July 2005).

Global Fund to Fight AIDS, Tuberculosis, and Malaria (2006). Geneva. <www.theglobalfund.org/en> (September 2006).

Global Markets Institute (2006). 'G8 Summit in St. Petersburg'. Poll conducted for the 2006 St. Petersburg Summit, Goldman Sachs, New York.

Godlee, Fiona (1994). 'WHO in Retreat: Is It Losing Its Influence?' *British Medical Journal,* vol. 309, no. 6967, pp. 1491–1495.

Goodman, Neville M. (1971). *International Health Organizations and Their Work*, 2nd ed. (Edinburgh: Churchill Livingstone).

Gostin, Laurence O. and Zita Lazzarini (1997). *Human Rights in Public Health in the AIDS Pandemic* (London: Oxford University Press).

Gottschalk, Ricardo (2004). 'The Macroeconomic Policy Content of PRSPs: How Much Pro-Growth, How Much Pro-Poor?' Paper prepared for the North-South Institute. <www.ids.ac.uk/ids/global/pdfs/RGPRSPpaper.pdf> (September 2006).

Gow, David (2006). 'British Government Accused of Inflating Aid Figures'. *Guardian,* 4 April.<politics.guardian.co.uk/development/story/0,,1746398,00.html> (September 2006).

Grabowski, Henry (2002). 'Patents, Innovation, and Access to New Pharmaceuticals'. *Journal of International Economic Law,* vol. 5, no. 4, pp. 849–860.

Grein, Thomas W., Kande-Bure O. Kamara, Guénaël Rodier, *et al.* (2000). 'Rumors of Disease in the Global Village: Outbreak Verification'. *Emerging Infectious Diseases,* vol. 6, no. 2, pp. 97–102. <www.cdc.gov/ncidod/eid/vol6no2/grein.htm> (September 2006).

Gruskin, Sofia and Daniel Tarantola (2000). 'Health and Human Rights'. Working Paper No. 10, François-Xavier Bagnoud Center, Boston. <www.hsph.harvard.edu/fxbcenter/FXBC_WP10—Gruskin_and_Tarantola.pdf> (September 2006).

Gupta, Sanjeev, Benedict Clements, Maria Teresa Guin-Siu, *et al.* (2002). 'Debt Relief and Public Health Spending in Heavily Indebted Poor Countries'. *Bulletin of the World Health Organization,* vol. 80 no. 2, pp. 151–157.

Gwatkin, Davidson, Shea Rutstein, Kiersten Johnson, *et al.* (2005). *Socioeconomic Differences in Health, Nutrition, and Population*, 2nd ed. (Washington DC: World Bank).

Haddad, Slim and Pierre Fournier (1995). 'Quality, Cost, and Utilization of Health Services in Developing Countries: A Longitudinal Study in Zaire'. *Social Science and Medicine,* vol. 40, no. 6, pp. 743–753.

Hajnal, Peter I. (1999). *The G7/G8 System: Evolution, Role, and Documentation* (Aldershot: Ashgate).

Hardeman, Wim, Wim Van Damme, Maurits Van Pelt, *et al.* (2004). 'Access to Health Care for All? User Fees plus a Health Equity Fund in Sotnikum, Cambodia'. *Health Policy and Planning,* vol. 19, no. 1, pp. 22–32.

Hardon, Anita (2001). 'Immunisation for All? A Critical Look at the First GAVI Partners Meeting'. *HAI-Lights,* vol. 6, no. 1. <www.haiweb.org/pubs/hailights/mar2001/mar01_lead.html> (September 2006).

Harries, Anthony D., Erik Schouten, and Edwin Libamba (2006). 'Scaling Up Antiretroviral Treatment in Resource-Poor Settings'. *Lancet,* vol. 376, pp. 1870–1872.

Health Canada (2000). 'HIV and AIDS in Canada: Surveillance Report to December 31, 1999'. Ottawa. <www.phac-aspc.gc.ca/publicat/aids-sida/aic04-00/pdf/aic0400e.pdf> (September 2006).

Health Services Working Group (2003). 'Developing Singapore as the Compelling Hub for Healthcare Services in Asia: Potential Implications on Domestic Policy Objectives'. Ministry of Trade and Industry, Singapore. <app.mti.gov.sg/data/pages/507/doc/ERC_SVS_HEA_Annex2.pdf> (September 2006).

Held, David (2003). 'The Changing Structure of International Law: Sovereignty Transformed?' In D. Held and A. McGrew, eds., *The Global Transformations Reader,* pp. 162–166 (Cambridge: Polity Press).

Held, David and Anthony McGrew (2002). 'Introduction'. In D. Held and A. McGrew, eds., *Governing Globalization: Power, Authority, and Global Governance* (Cambridge: Polity Press).

Heymann, David L. (2003). 'Evolving Infectious Disease Threats to National and Global Security'. In L. Chen, J. Learning, and V. Narasimhan, eds., *Global Health Challenges for Human Security,* pp. 105–124 (Cambridge MA: Harvard University Press).

Heymann, David L. and Guénaël Rodier (1998). 'Global Surveillance of Communicable Diseases'. *Emerging Infectious Diseases,* vol. 4, no. 3, pp. 362–365. <www.cdc.gov/ncidod/eid/vol4no3/heymann.htm> (September 2006).

Heymann, David L. and Guénaël Rodier (2001). 'Hot Spots in a Wired World: WHO Surveillance of Emerging and Re-emerging Infectious Diseases'. *Lancet,* vol. 1, no. 5, pp. 345–353.

Heymann, Jody, Clyde Hertzman, Morris L. Barer, *et al.* (2005). *Healthier Societies: From Analysis to Action* (New York: Oxford University Press).

Hodges, Michael (1999). 'The G8 and the New Political Economy'. In M.R. Hodges, J.J. Kirton, and J.P. Daniels, eds., *The G8's Role in the New Millennium,* pp. 69–74 (Aldershot: Ashgate).

Hoekman, Bernard (2004). 'Policy Space, Coherence, and Economic Development: Options for the WTO'. Mimeo, Yale University, New Haven. <www.ycsg.yale.edu/core/forms/Project_terms_Reference.doc> (September 2006).

Hoogvelt, Ankie (2001). *Globalization and the Postcolonial World: The New Political Economy of Development* (Baltimore: Johns Hopkins University Press).

Howard, Lee (1989). 'The Evolution of Bilateral and Multilateral Cooperation for Health in Developing Countries'. In M.R. Reich and E. Marui, eds., *International Cooperation for Health: Problems, Prospects, and Priorities* (Dover MA: Auburn House).

Howard-Jones, Norman (1950). 'Origins of International Health Work'. *British Medical Journal,* vol. 1, no. 4661, pp. 1032–1037.

Howard-Jones, Norman (1975). *The International Scientific Background of the International Sanitary Conferences* (Geneva: World Health Organization).

Howard-Jones, Norman (1975). *The Scientific Background of the International Sanitary Conferences, 1851–1938* (Geneva: World Health Organization).

Howard-Jones, Norman (1978). *International Public Health between the Two Wars: The Organizational Problems* (Geneva: World Health Organization).

Howell, John (2005). 'Farm Subsidies: A Problem for Africa Too'. Opinions, September, Overseas Development Institute, London. <www.odi.org.uk/publications/opinions/47_farm_subsidies_sept05.pdf> (September 2006).

Howse, Robert and Makau Mutua (2000). 'Protecting Human Rights in a Global Economy: Challenges for the World Trade Organization'. International Centre for Human Rights and Democratic Development, Montreal.

Hsu, Lee-Nah (2004). 'Building Dynamic Democratic Governance and HIV-Resilient Societies'. Paper presented at the Oslo Governance Centre, 3 November 2003, United Nations Development Programme.

Hunt, Paul (2003). 'Economic, Social, and Cultural Rights: The Right of Everyone to the Enjoyment of the Highest Attainable Standard of Physical and Mental Health'. 13 February, E/CN.4/2003/58, United Nations Economic and Social Council, New York. <www.unhchr.ch/Huridocda/Huridoca.nsf/0/9854302995c2c86fc1256cec005a18d7> (September 2006).

Hunt, Paul (2004). 'Economic, Social, and Cultural Rights: The Right of Everyone to the Enjoyment of the Highest Attainable Standard of Physical and Mental Health — Addendum'. 8 March, E/CN.4/2004/49/Add.1, United Nations Economic and Social Council, New York. <www.unhchr.ch/Huridocda/Huridoca.nsf/(Symbol)/E.CN.4.2004.49.Add.1.En?Opendocument> (September 2006).

Hunt, Paul (2005). 'The Right of Everyone to the Enjoyment of the Highest Attainable Standard of Physical and Mental Health'. Report to the United Nations General Assembly. 12 September, A/60/348, United Nations Economic and Social Council, New York. <daccess-ods.un.org/access.nsf/Get?Open&DS=A/60/348&Lang=E> (September 2006).

'In the Twilight of Doha' (2006). *Economist*, 29 July, pp. 63–64.

Infectious Disease Surveillance Center (Japan) (2006). 'Index of IASR Topics'. <idsc.nih.go.jp/iasr/iasr-ge1.html> (September 2006).

Initiative on Public-Private Partnerships for Health (2006). Geneva. <www.ippph.org> (September 2006).

International Centre for Trade and Sustainable Development (2003). 'Making Special and Differential Treatment More Effective and Responsive to Development Needs'. Chavannes-de-Bogis, Switzerland, 6–7 May. Draft meeting report, Geneva. <www.ictsd.org/dlogue/2003-05-06/Dialogue-draft-meeting-report.pdf> (September 2006).

International Centre for Trade and Sustainable Development (2004). 'Special and Different Treatment'. Doha Round Briefing Series: Developments since the Cancun Ministerial Conference, Vol. 3, No. 13. <www.ictsd.org/pubs/dohabriefings/Vol3/V3_13.pdf> (September 2006).

International Centre for Trade and Sustainable Development (2005). 'Special and Differential Treatment in the Multilateral Trading System'. ICTSD-FES Independent Analytical Track Meeting, 1–2 July, Lausanne. <www.ictsd.org/dlogue/2005-07-01/2005-07-01-docu.htm> (September 2006).

International Centre for Trade and Sustainable Development (2006). 'Doha Round Suspended Indefinitely After G6 Talks Collapse'. *Bridges Weekly,* vol. 10, no. 27. <www.ictsd.org/weekly/06-07-26/story1.htm> (September 2006).

International Conference on Primary Health Care (1978). 'Declaration of Alma-Ata'. 12 September, Alma-Ata, Kazakhstan. <www.euro.who.int/AboutWHO/Policy/20010827_1> (September 2006).

International Court of Justice (1996). 'Legality of the Use by a State of Nuclear Weapons in Armed Conflict'. Advisory Opinion of 8 July 1996: Dissenting Opinion of Judge Weeramantry. <www.icj-cij.org/icjwww/icases/ianw/ianwframe.htm> (September 2006).

International Labour Organization (2003). 'The HIV/AIDS Epidemic in the Russian Federation'. <www.ilo.ru/aids/docs/dec02/cis/Russia-eng.pdf> (September 2006).

International Monetary Fund (2005). 'Development Committee Communiqué'. 25 September, Washington DC. <www.imf.org/external/np/cm/2005/092505.htm> (September 2006).

International Monetary Fund and World Bank (2005). 'Zambia: Enhanced Initiative for Heavily Indebted Poor Countries — Completion Point Document'. IMF Country Report No. 05/137, Washington DC. <www.imf.org/external/pubs/ft/scr/2005/cr05137.pdf> (September 2006).

International Society for Infectious Diseases (2006). 'ProMED-mail'. Brookline MA. <www.promedmail.org> (September 2006).

Italy [G8 Host] (2001). 'Beyond Debt Relief'. Genoa. <www.g8.utoronto.ca/summit/2001genoa/pres_docs/pres_doc2.html> (September 2006).

Jackson, John (1998). *The World Trade Organization: Constitution and Jurisprudence* (London: Royal Institute of International Affairs).

Jaggar, Alison (2002). 'Vulnerable Women and Neo-Liberal Globalization: Debt Burdens Undermine Women's Health in the Global South'. *Theoretical Medicine,* vol. 23, no. 6, pp. 425–440.

Jawara, Fatoumata and Eileen Kwa (2003). *Behind the Scenes at the WTO: The Real World of International Trade Negotiations* (London: Zed Books).

Jeter, Jon (2002). 'The Dumping Ground: As Zambia Courts Western Markets, Used Goods Arrive at a Heavy Price'. *Washington Post,* 22 April.

Jha, Prabhat, David Brown, Nico Nagelkerke, *et al.* (2005). 'Five Members of the Global IDEA Scientific Advisory Committee Respond to Dr. Moore and Colleagues' [Letter]. *Canadian Medical Association Journal,* vol. 172, no. 12, pp. 1538–1539.

Jha, Prabhat, Anne Mills, Kara Hanson, *et al.* (2002). 'Improving the Health of the Global Poor'. *Science, Technology, and Human Values,* vol. 295, no. 5562, pp. 2036–2039.

Joint Learning Initiative (2004). 'Human Resources for Health: Overcoming the Crisis'. Global Equity Initiative, Harvard University, Cambridge MA. <www.globalhealthtrust.org/report/Human_Resources_for_Health.pdf> (September 2006).

Jubilee Research (2005). 'The G8 2005: What Are the Lessons?' 11 July. <www.jubileeresearch.org/latest/g8110705.htm> (September 2006).

Karsenty, Guy (2002). 'Trends in International Trade in Services'. Assessment of GATS and Trade in Health Services: An International Consultation on Monitoring and Research Priorities. World Health Organization, Geneva.

Kawachi, Ichiro and Sarah Wamala, eds. (2006). *Globalization and Health* (Oxford: Oxford University Press).

Keck, Margaret E. and Kathryn Sikkink (1998). *Activists Beyond Borders: Advocacy Networks in International Politics* (Ithaca: Cornell University Press).

Kickbusch, Ilona (2000). 'The Development of International Health Policies — Accountability Intact?' *Social Science and Medicine,* vol. 51, no. 6, pp. 979–989.

Kickbusch, Ilona (2003). 'The Contribution of the World Health Organization to a New Public Health and Health Promotion'. *American Journal of Public Health,* vol. 93, no. 3, pp. 383–388. <www.ajph.org/cgi/content/full/93/3/383> (September 2006).

Killick, Tony (2004). 'Politics, Evidence, and the New Aid Agenda'. *Development Policy Review,* vol. 22, no. 1, pp. 5–29.

Killick, Tony (2005). 'Don't Throw Money at Africa'. *IDS Bulletin,* vol. 36, no. 3, pp. 14–19.

Kim, Jim Yong, Joyce V. Millen, John Gershman, *et al.*, eds. (2000). *Dying for Growth: Global Inequality and the Health of the Poor* (Monroe ME: Common Courage Press).

Kim, Jim Yong, Aaron Shakow, Jaime Bayona, *et al.* (2000). 'Sickness Amidst Recovery: Public Debt and Private Suffering in Peru'. In J.Y. Kim, J.V. Millen, J. Gershman, *et al.*, eds., *Dying for Growth: Global Inequality and the Health of the Poor,* pp. 127–154 (Monroe ME: Common Courage Press).

King, Jeff, Ashfaq Khalfan, and Bryan Thomas (2003). 'Advancing the Odious Debt Doctrine'. CISDL Working Paper, Centre for International Sustainable Development Law, Montreal <www.odiousdebts.org/odiousdebts/publications/Advancing_the_Odious_Debt_Doctrine.pdf> (September 2006).

Kipp, Walter, Jimmy Kamugisha, Phil Jacobs, *et al.* (2001). 'User Fees, Health Staff Incentives, and Service Utilization in Kabarole District, Uganda'. *Bulletin of the World Health Organization,* vol. 79, no. 11, pp. 1032–1037.

Kirton, John J. (2004). 'Explaining G8 Effectiveness: A Concert of Vulnerable Equals in a Globalizing World'. Paper prepared for the International Studies Association conference, 17–20 March, Montreal. <www.g8.utoronto.ca/scholar/kirton2004/kirton_isa_040304.pdf> (September 2006).

Kirton, John J. (2005). 'A Promising Push: Complying with the Gleneagles G8 Africa Commitments and Parliamentarians' Role'. Paper prepared for a conference on Partnership Beyond 2005: The Role of Parliamentarians in Implementing NEPAD Commitments, Parliamentary Seminar on Africa, 19–22 October, London. <www.g8.utoronto.ca/scholar/kirton2005/kirton_london2005.pdf> (September 2006).

Kirton, John J. (2005). 'America at the G8: From Vulnerability to Victory at the Sea Island Summit'. In M. Fratianni, J.J. Kirton, A.M. Rugman, *et al.*, eds., *New perspectives on Global Governance: Why America Needs the G8,* pp. 31–50 (Aldershot: Ashgate).

Kirton, John J. (2005). 'Gleneagles G8 Boosts Blair at Home'. 1 August, G8 Research Group, Toronto. <www.g8.utoronto.ca/evaluations/2005gleneagles/coverage.html> (September 2006).

Kirton, John J. (2006). 'Explaining Compliance with G8 Finance Commitments: Agency, Institutionalizaton, and Structure'. *Open Economies Review,* vol. 17, no. 4.

Kirton, John J. (2006). 'The G8 and Global Health Governance: The Case for a 2006 Eurasian HIV/AIDS Initiative'. Paper prepared for the International Parliamentary Conference in Conjunction with Russia's G8 Presidency on HIV/AIDS in Eurasia and the Role of the G8, sponsored by the Transatlantic Partners Against AIDS, 8 June, Moscow. <www.g8.utoronto.ca/scholar/kirton2006/kirton_health_060609.pdf> (September 2006).

Kirton, John J. and Ella Kokotsis (2005). 'Keeping Faith with Africa: Assessing Compliance with the G8's Commitments at Kananaskis and Evian'. In J.B. Atwood, R.S. Brown, and P. Lyman, eds., *Freedom, Prosperity, and Security: G8 Partnership with Africa, Sea Island 2004 and Beyond,* pp. 11–33 (Washington DC: Council on Foreign Relations).

Klare, Michael (2004). 'Blood for Oil: The Bush-Cheney Energy Strategy'. In L. Panitch and C. Leys, eds., *Socialist Register 2004: The New Imperial Challenge,* pp. 166–185 (Monmouth: Merlin Press).

Kleen, Peter and Sheila Page (2005). 'Special and Differential Treatment of Developing Countries in the World Trade Organization'. Ministry for Foreign Affairs, Sweden, Stockholm. <www.egdi.gov.se/pdf/study/40725_Gl%20Dev%20Stud%202.pdf> (September 2006).

Knobler, Stacey, Adel Mahmoud, Stanley Lemon, *et al.*, eds. (2004). *Learning from SARS: Preparing for the Next Disease Outbreak* (Washington DC: National Academies Press).

Kober, Katerina and Wim Van Damme (2004). 'Scaling Up Access to Antiretroviral Treatment in Southern Africa: Who Will Do the Job?' *Lancet,* vol. 364, pp. 103–107.

Koivusalo, Meri (2003). 'Assessing the Health Policy Implications of WTO Trade and Investment Agreements'. In K. Lee, ed., *Health Impacts of Globalization,* pp. 161–176 (London: Palgrave Macmillan).

Kokotsis, Eleanore (1999). *Keeping International Commitments: Compliance, Credibility, and the G7, 1988–1995* (New York: Garland).

Kokotsis, Ella and Joseph P. Daniels (1999). 'G8 Summits and Compliance'. In M.R. Hodges, J.J. Kirton, and J.P. Daniels, eds., *The G8's Role in the New Millennium,* pp. 75–91 (Aldershot: Ashgate).

Kraev, Egor (2005). 'Estimating GDP Effects of Trade Liberalisation on Developing Countries'. Centre for Development, Policy and Research, School of Oriental and African Studies, London <www.christianaid.org.uk/indepth/506liberalisation/FinalPaper4.pdf> (September 2006).

Kremer, Michael and Seema Jayachandran (2002). 'Odious Debt'. April. International Monetary Fund, Washington DC. <www.imf.org/external/np/res/seminars/2002/poverty/mksj.pdf> (September 2006).

Krieger, Nancy and Anne-Emanuelle Birne (1988). 'A Vision of Social Justice as the Foundation of Public Health: Commemorating 150 Years of the Spirit of 1848'. *American Journal of Public Health,* vol. 88, no. 11, pp. 1603–1606.

Kwaramba, P. (1997). 'The Socio-Economic Impact of HIV/AIDS on Communal Agricultural Production Systems in Zimbabwe'. Working Paper 19, Economic Advisory Project, Friedrich Ebert Stiftung Foundation.

Labonté, Ronald and Ted Schrecker (2004). 'Committed to Health for All? How the G7/8 Rate'. *Social Science and Medicine,* vol. 59, no. 8, pp. 1661–1676.

Labonté, Ronald and Ted Schrecker (2005). *The G8, Africa, and Global Health: A Platform for Global Health Equity for the 2005 Summit* (London: Nuffield Trust).

Labonté, Ronald and Ted Schrecker (2006). 'The G8 and Global Health: What Now? What Next?' *Canadian Journal of Public Health,* vol. 97, no. 1, pp. 35–38.

Labonté, Ronald, Corinne Packer, and Nathan Klassen (2006). 'The "Brain Drain" of Health Professionals from Sub-Saharan Africa to Canada: Findings and Options'. South African Migration Project, Queen's University, Kingston.

Labonté, Ronald, Ted Schrecker, David Sanders, *et al.* (2004). *Fatal Indifference: The G8, Africa, and Global Health* (Cape Town: University of Cape Town Press).

Lebel, Jean (2003). *Health: An Ecosystem Approach* (Ottawa: International Development Research Centre).

Lederberg, Joshua, Robert E. Shope, and Stanley C. Oaks, eds. (1992). *Emerging Infections: Microbial Threats to Health in the United States* (Washington DC: National Academies Press).

Lee, Kelley, Kent Buse, and Suzanne Fustukian, eds. (2001). *Health Policy in a Globalising World* (New York: Cambridge University Press).

Lee, Kelley and Richard Dodgson (2000). 'Globalization and Cholera: Implications for Global Governance'. *Global Goverance,* vol. 6, no. 2, pp. 213–236.

Lee, Kelley, Gill Walt, and Andy Haines (2004). 'The Challenge to Improve Global Health: Financing the Millennium Development Goals'. *Journal of the American Medical Association,* vol. 291, no. 2, pp. 2636–2638.

León, Francisco (2003). 'The Case of the Chilean Health System, 1983–2003'. Paper presented at the World Health Organization Workshop on Trade in Health Services, Ottawa.

Lethridge, J. (2004). 'Trade in Health Services under the Four Modes of Supply: Review of Current Trends and Policy Issues'. World Health Organization, Geneva.

Lewis, Stephen (2005). *Race against Time: Searching for Hope in AIDS-Ravaged Africa* (Toronto: House of Anansi).

Lewis, Stephen (2006). 'Press Conference by Stephen Lewis on HIV/AIDS in Africa'. 17 March, United Nations, New York. <www.un.org/News/briefings/docs/2006/060317_Lewis.doc.htm> (September 2006).

Li, Quan (2001). 'Commitment Compliance in G7 Summit Macroeconomic Policy Coordination'. *Political Research Quarterly,* vol. 54, no. 2, pp. 355–378.

Lister, John (2005). *Driving the Wrong Way? A Critical Guide to the Global 'Health Reform' Industry* (London: Middlesex University Press).

Lomborg, Bjørn, ed. (2004). *Global Crises, Global Solutions* (Cambridge: Cambridge University Press).

Lucas, Adetokunbo O. (2002). 'Public-Private Partnerships: Illustrative Examples'. In M.R. Reich, ed., *Public-Private Partnerships for Public Health,* pp. 19–39 (Cambridge MA: Harvard Center for Population and Development Studies).

MacInnis, Ron (2006). 'The International AIDS Conference: A Retrospective'. Global AIDSLink. <www.internews.org/articles/2006/20060800_aidslink_macinnis.htm> (September 2006).

'Malawi: AIDS Deaths Fuelling Orphan Numbers'. (2005). *IRIN News,* 5 October. <www.irinnews.org/AIDSreport.asp?ReportID=5286&SelectRegion=Southern_Africa&SelectCountry=MALAWI> (September 2006).

Martin, Matthew (2004). 'Assessing the HIPC Initiative: The Key HIPC Debates'. In J.J. Teunissen and A. Akkerman, eds., *HIPC Debt Relief: Myths and Realities* (The Hague: FONDAD).

Matthews, Duncan (2002). *Globalizing Intellectual Property Rights: The TRIPS Agreement* (London: Routledge).

Matthews, Duncan (2004). 'WTO Decision on Implementation of Paragraph 6 of the Doha Declaration on the TRIPS Agreement and Public Health: A Solution to the Access to Essential Medicines Problems?' *Journal of International Economic Law,* vol. 7, no. 1, pp. 73–107.

McChesney, Robert W. and Dan Schiller (2003). 'The Political Economy of International Communications: Foundations for the Emerging Global Debate about Media Ownership and Regulation'. Technology, Business, and Society Programme Paper No. 11, United Nations Research Institute for Social Development.

McInnes, Colin (2004). 'Health and Foreign Policy'. In A. Ingram, ed., *Health, Foreign Policy, and Security: Towards a Conceptual Framework for Research and Policy,* pp. 29–42 (London: Nuffield Trust).

McKie, John and Jeff Richardson (1982). 'The Rule of Rescue'. *Social Science and Medicine,* vol. 56, no. 1212, pp. 2407–2419.

McMichael, Philip (2003). 'Food Security and Social Reproduction: Issues and Contradictions'. In I. Bakker and S. Gill, eds., *Power, Production, and Social Reproduction: Human In/Security in the Global Political Economy,* pp. 169–188 (Basingstoke: Palgrave Macmillan).

McMichael, Philip (2005). 'Global Development and the Corporate Food Regime'. In F.H. Buttel and P. McMichael, eds., *New Directions in the Sociology of Global Development* (Amsterdam: Elsevier).

McPake, Barbara, Kara Hanson, and Anne Mills (1993). 'Community Financing of Health Care in Africa: An Evaluation of the Bamako Initiative'. *Social Science and Medicine,* vol. 36, no. 11, pp. 1383–1395.

Médecins Sans Frontières (1999). 'Amsterdam Statement to WTO Member States on Access to Medicine'. 26 November, Amsterdam. <www.accessmed-msf.org/prod/publications.asp?scntid=17122001173935&contenttype=PARA&> (September 2006).

Médecins Sans Frontières (2006). 'Campaign for Access to Essential Medicines'. <www.accessmed-msf.org> (September 2006).

'Medical Tourism in India: Get Well Away' (2004). *Economist*, 7 October.

Mehrotra, Santosh and Stephen Jarett (2002). 'Improving Basic Health Service Delivery in Low-Income Countries: "Voice" to the Poor'. *Social Science and Medicine,* vol. 54, no. 11, pp. 1685–1690.

Merianos, Angela and Malik Peiris (2005). 'International Health Regulations'. *Lancet,* vol. 366, pp. 1249–1251.

Meuwissen, Liesbeth Emm (2002). 'Problems of Cost Recovery Implementation in District Health Care: A Case Study from Niger'. *Health Policy and Planning,* vol. 17, no. 3, pp. 304–313.

Meyer, David S. and Sidney Tarrow (1998). 'A Movement Society: Contentious Politics for a New Century'. In D.S. Meyer and S. Tarrow, eds., *The Social Movement Society: Contentious Politics for a New Century* (New York: Rowman and Littlefield).

Millen, Joyce V. and Timothy H. Holtz (2000). 'Dying for Growth, Part 1: Transnational Corporations and the Health of the Poor'. In J.Y. Kim, J.V. Millen, J. Gershman, *et al.*, eds., *Dying for Growth: Global Inequality and the Health of the Poor,* pp. 177–223 (Monroe ME: Common Courage Press).

Mills, Anne (1998). 'To Contract or Not to Contract? Issues for Low and Middle Income Countries'. *Health Policy and Planning,* vol. 13, no. 1, pp. 32–40.

Monteiro, Carlos A., Erly C. Moura, Wolney L. Conde, *et al.* (2004). 'Socioeconomic Status and Obesity in Adult Populations of Developing Countries: A Review'. *Bulletin of the World Health Organization,* vol. 82, no. 12, pp. 940–946.

Moses, Stephen, F. Manji, J.E. Bradley, *et al.* (1992). 'Impact of User Fees on Attendance at a Referral Centre for Sexually Transmitted Diseases in Kenya'. *Lancet,* vol. 340, no. 8817, pp. 463–466.

Moss, Todd (2005). 'Ten Myths of the International Finance Facility'. Working Paper No. 60, Center for Global Development. <ssrn.com/abstract=800706> (September 2006).

Mullan, Fitzhugh (2005). 'The Metrics of the Physician Brain Drain'. *New England Journal of Medicine,* vol. 353, no. 17, pp. 1810–1818.

Mwabu, Germano, James Mwanzia, and Wilson Liambila (1995). 'User Charges in Government Health Facilities in Kenya: Effect on Attendance and Revenue'. *Health Policy and Planning,* vol. 10, no. 2, pp. 164–170.

'NAFTA Report Cites Dana Corp. in Small Step for Justice in Mexico'. (1999). *PR Newswire,* 22 March.

Nakajima, Hiroshi (1997). 'Global Disease Threats and Foreign Policy'. *Brown Journal of World Affairs,* vol. 4, no. 1, pp. 319–332.

Nanda, Priya (2002). 'Gender Dimensions of User Fees: Implications for Women's Utilization of Health Care'. *Reproductive Health Matters,* vol. 10, no. 20, pp. 127–134.

National Advisory Committee on SARS and Public Health (2003). 'Learning from SARS: Renewal of Public Health in Canada'. Health Canada, Ottawa. <www.phac-aspc.gc.ca/publicat/sars-sras/naylor> (September 2006).

National Intelligence Estimate (2000). 'The Global Infectious Disease Threat and Its Implications for the United States'. NIE 99-17D. National Intelligence Council, Washington DC. <www.ciaonet.org/wps/dod109/dod109.pdf> (September 2006).

Nussbaum, Martha (2000). *Women and Human Development: A Capabilities Approach* (New York: Cambridge University Press).

Nye, Joseph S. and John Donahue, eds. (2000). *Governance in a Globalizing World* (Washington DC: Brookings Institution Press).

Obi, Cyril I. (2001). 'Global, State, and Local Intersections: Power, Authority, and Conflict in the Niger Delta Oil Communities'. In T. Callaghy, R. Kassimir, and R. Latham, eds., *Interventions and Transnationalism in Africa: Global–Local Networks of Power,* pp. 173–196 (Cambridge: Cambridge University Press).

Office of the High Commissioner for Human Rights (1966). 'International Covenant on Economic, Social, and Cultural Rights'. <www.unhchr.ch/html/menu3/b/a_cescr.htm> (September 2006).

Office of the High Commissioner for Human Rights (1989). 'Convention on the Rights of the Child'. <www.unhchr.ch/html/menu3/b/k2crc.htm> (September 2006).

Office of the High Commissioner for Human Rights (2006). 'Special Rapporteur of the Commission on Human Rights on the Right of Everyone to the Enjoyment of the Highest Attainable Standard of Physical and Mental Health'. <www.ohchr.org/english/issues/health/right> (September 2006).

O'Manique, Colleen (2005). 'The "Securitisation" of HIV/AIDS in Sub-Saharan Africa: A Critical Feminist Lens'. *Policy and Society,* vol. 24, no. 1, pp. 24–47.

O'Manique, John (1990). 'Universal and Inalienable Rights: A Search for Foundations'. *Human Rights Quarterly,* vol. 12, no. 4, pp. 465–485.

O'Manique, John (2003). *The Origins of Justice* (Philadelphia: University of Pennsylvania Press).

One World (2005). 'Malawi Guide'. <uk.oneworld.net/guides/malawi/development> (September 2006).

Orbinski, James (2002). 'AIDS, Médecins Sans Frontières, and Access to Essential Medicines'. In P.I. Hajnal, ed., *Civil Society in the Information Age,* pp. 127–135 (Aldershot: Ashgate).

Orbinski, James (2004). 'Access to Medicines and Global Health: Will Canada Lead or Flounder'. *Canadian Medical Association Journal,* vol. 170, no. 2, pp. 224–226. <www.cmaj.ca/cgi/content/full/170/2/224> (September 2006).

Organisation for Economic Co-operation and Development (2004). *Agricultural Policies in OECD Countries at a Glance* (Paris: Organisation for Economic Co-operation and Development).

Overseas Development Institute (2005). 'Scaling Up versus Absorptive Capacity: Challenges and Opportunities for Reaching the MDGs in Africa'. Briefing paper, London. <www.odi.org.uk/publications/briefing/bp_may05_absorptive_capacity.pdf> (September 2006).

Pachanee, Cha-aim and Suwit Wibulpolprasert (2003). 'Trade in Health Services and GATS: The Case of Thailand'. Paper presented at the World Health Organization Workshop on Trade in Health Services, Ottawa.

Paluzzi, Joan E. and Paul Farmer (2005). 'The Wrong Question'. *Development,* vol. 48, no. 1, pp. 12–18.

Pannenborg, Charles O. (1979). *A New International Health Order: An Inquiry into the International Relations of World Health and Medical Care* (Alphen aan den Rijn, Netherlands: Sijthoff and Noordhoff).

Panova, Victoria (2005). 'Impressions of the 2005 Gleneagles Summit'. 18 July, G8 Research Group. <www.g8.utoronto.ca/evaluations/2005gleneagles/panova2005-0718.html> (September 2006).

Paphassarang, Chanthakath, Khampienne Philavong, Boungnong Boupha, *et al.* (2002). 'Equity, Privatization, and Cost Recovery in Urban Health Care: The Care of Lao PDR'. *Health Policy and Planning,* vol. 17 (Suppl. 1), pp. 72–84.

Petchesky, Rosalind (2003). *Global Prescriptions: Gendering Health and Human Rights* (London: Zed Books).

Picard, André (2001). 'Malaria Cases Soar in Canada'. *Globe and Mail,* 6 March.

Pirages, Dennis (1997). 'Ecological Theory and International Relations'. *Indiana Journal of Global Legal Studies,* vol. 5, no. 1, pp. 53–63.

Plahe, Jagjit Kaur (2005). 'Globalizing Trade in Agriculture: The Implications of the WTO Agricultural Agreement on the Right to Food in Developing Countries'. Paper prepared for a conference on Human Rights in a Globalizing Era?, 4–6 August, Windsor ON.

Pogge, Thomas (2001). 'Priorities of Global Justice'. *Metaphilosophy,* vol. 32, no. 1/2, pp. 6–24.

Pogge, Thomas (2002). *World Poverty and Human Rights* (Cambridge: Polity Press).

Pogge, Thomas (2005). 'Human Rights and Global Health'. *Metaphilosophy,* vol. 36, no. 1-2, pp. 182–209.

Pogge, Thomas (2005). 'World Poverty and Human Rights'. *Ethics and International Affairs,* vol. 19, no. 1.

Pogge, Thomas (2006). 'Human Rights and Global Health: A Research Program'. In C. Barry and T.W. Pogge, eds., *Global Institutions and Responsibilities: Achieving Global Justice,* pp. 190–217 (Oxford: Blackwell Publishing).

Price-Smith, Andrew (2001). *Plagues and Politics: Infectious Disease and International Policy* (New York: Palgrave).

Price-Smith, Andrew (2002). *The Health of Nations: Infectious Disease, Environmental Change, and Their Effects on National Security and Development* (Cambridge MA: MIT Press).

Princeton Project on National Security (2005). 'Report of the Working Group on State Security and Transnational Threats'. Woodrow Wilson School of Public and International Affairs, Princeton. <www.wws.princeton.edu/ppns/conferences/reports/fall/SSTT.pdf> (September 2006).

Public Health Agency of Canada (2004). 'Global Public Health Intelligence Network'. Ottawa. <www.phac-aspc.gc.ca/media/nr-rp/2004/2004_gphin-rmispbk_e.html> (September 2006).

Reddy, Sanjay G. and Thomas W. Pogge (2005). 'How Not to Count the Poor'. Columbia University, New York. <papers.ssrn.com/sol3/papers.cfm?abstract_id=893159> (September 2006).

Reich, Michael R. (2002). 'Introduction'. In M.R. Reich, ed., *Public-Private Partnerships for Public Health,* pp. 1–16 (Cambridge MA: Harvard Center for Population and Development Studies).

Ridde, Valéry (2003). 'Fees for Services, Cost Recovery, and Equity in a District of Burkina Faso Operating the Bamako Initiative'. *Bulletin of the World Health Organization,* vol. 81, no. 7, pp. 532–538.

Russell, Sabin (2005). 'Bird Flu Capable of Causing "Incalculable" Misery: 100-Nation Meeting Focuses on Plans to Contain Outbreak'. *San Francisco Chronicle,* 8 November. <sfgate.com/cgi-bin/article.cgi?f=/c/a/2005/11/08/MNGGAFKKU51.DTL&type=science> (September 2006).

Sachs, Jeffrey (2005). 'The End of Poverty'. *Time*, 14 March, pp. 44–54.

Sachs, Jeffrey and J.W. McArthur (2005). 'The Millennium Project: A Plan for Meeting the Millennium Development Goals'. *Lancet,* vol. 365, pp. 347–353.

Salleh, Ariel (2000). 'The Meta-Industrial Class and Why We Need It'. *Democracy and Nature,* vol. 6, no. 1, pp. 27–36.

Salvador, Soledad and Cintia Quiliconi (2003). 'Argentina Trade in Health Services and GATS: The Argintinean Case Study'. Paper presented at the World Health Organization Workshop on Trade in Health Services, Ottawa.

Sanders, David and Abdulrahman Sambo (1991). 'AIDS in Africa: The Implications of Economic Recession and Structural Adjustment'. *Health Policy and Planning,* vol. 6, no. 2, pp. 157–165.

Sanders, David, Mickey Chopra, and Charles Todd (2005). 'Confronting Africa's Health Crisis: More of the Same Will Not Be Enough'. *British Medical Journal,* vol. 331, no. 7519, pp. 755–758.

Sanhueza, Ricardo and Jaime Ruiz-Tagle (2002). 'Choosing Health Insurance in a Dual Health Care System: The Chilean Case'. *Journal of Applied Economics*, vol. 5 (May), pp. 157–184.

Satterthwaite, David (2003). 'The Millennium Development Goals and Urban Poverty Reduction: Great Expectations and Nonsense Statistics'. *Environment and Urbanization,* vol. 15 no. 2, pp. 181–190.

Savona, Paolo and Chiara Oldani (2003). 'Globalisation: The Private Sector Perspective'. In M. Fratianni, P. Savona, and J.J. Kirton, eds., *Sustaining Global Growth and Development: G7 and IMF Governance,* pp. 99–112 (Aldershot: Ashgate).

Savostiyanov, Mikhail (2005). 'Presentation at the Pre-G8 Summit Academic Conference'. Paper presented at the conference on Development, Sustainability and Finance: The Role of the G8 and the Gleneagles Summit, University of Glasgow, 29–30 June, Glasgow. <www.g8.utoronto.ca/conferences/2005/conf/savostiyanov.html> (September 2006).

Schmidt, Rodney and Roy Culpeper (2003). 'Private Foreign Investment in the Poorest Countries'. North-South Institute, Ottawa. <www.nsi-ins.ca/english/pdf/FDI_policy_brief.pdf> (September 2006).

Schoepf, Brooke G., Claude Schoepf, Joyce V. Millen, *et al.* (2000). 'Theoretical Therapies, Remote Remedies: SAPs and the Political Ecology of Poverty and Health in Africa'. In J.Y. Kim, J.V. Millen, J. Gershman, *et al.*, eds., *Dying for Growth: Global Inequality and the Health of the Poor,* pp. 91–126 (Monroe ME: Common Courage Press).

Scholte, Jan Aart (2000). *Globalization: A Critical Introduction* (Houndsmills: Palgrave).

Sell, Susan K. (2003). *Private Power, Public Law: The Globalization of Intellectual Property Rights* (Cambridge: Cambridge University Press).

Sell, Susan K. (2004). 'The Quest for Global Governance in Intellectual Property and Public Health: Structural, Discursive, and Institutional Dimensions'. *Temple Law Review,* vol. 77, no. 2, pp. 363–400.

Sen, Amartya (2005). 'Foreword'. In P. Farmer, ed., *Pathologies of Power: Health, Human Rights, and the New War on the Poor* (Berkeley: University of California Press).

Shadlen, Kenneth C. (2005). 'Exchanging Development for Market Access? Deep Integration and Industrial Policy under Multilateral and Regional-Bilateral Trade Agreements'. *Review of International Political Economy,* vol. 12, no. 5, pp. 750–775.

Shafir, Gershon (2004). 'Citizenship and Human Rights in an Era of Globalization'. In A. Brysk and G. Shafir, eds., *People out of Place: Globalization, Human Rights, and the Citizenship Gap,* pp. 11–25 (New Haven: Routledge).

Shi Guang (2003). 'Trade in Health Services and GATS in China: Preliminary Observation and Analysis'. Paper presented at the World Health Organization Workshop on Trade in Health Services, Ottawa.

Shue, Henry (1996). 'Environmental Change and the Varieties of Justice'. In F.O. Hampson and J. Reppy, eds., *Earthly Goods: Environmental Change and Social Justice,* pp. 9–29 (Ithaca: Cornell University Press).

Simon, David, Wim van Spengen, Chris Dixon, *et al.*, eds. (1995). *Structurally Adjusted Africa: Poverty, Debt, and Basic Needs* (London: Pluto Press).

Slaughter, Anne-Marie (2005). 'Government Networks, World Order, and the L20'. In J. English, R. Thakur, and A.F. Cooper, eds., *Reforming from the Top: A Leaders' 20 Summit,* pp. 281–295 (Tokyo: United Nations University Press).

'Sleep Less in Seattle' (1999). *Lancet,* vol. 354, no. 9194, p. 1917.

Smolinski, Mark S., Margaret A. Hamburg, and Joshua Lederberg, eds. (2003). *Microbial Threats to Health: Emergence, Detection, and Response* (Washington DC: National Academies Press).

Solar, Orielle and Alec Irwin (2005). 'Towards a Conceptual Framework for Analysis and Action on the Social Determinants of Health'. Discussion paper for the Commission on Social Determinants of Health, World Health Organization, Geneva. <www.who.int/entity/social_determinants/resources/framework.pdf> (September 2006).

Somerville, Keith (2002). 'U.S. Looks to Africa for "Secure Oil"'. BBC News Online. <news.bbc.co.uk/2/hi/africa/2255297.stm> (September 2006).

South Centre (2005). 'Policy Space for the Development of the South'. Trade Policy Brief No. 1, November, Geneva. <www.southcentre.org/info/policybrief/01PolicySpace.pdf> (September 2006).

Stevens, Christopher and Jane Kennan (2005). 'EU-ACP Economic Partnership Agreements: The Effects of Reciprocity'. Institute of Development Studies, Sussex. <www.dfid.gov.uk/aboutdfid/organisation/epas-effects-reciprocity.pdf> (September 2006).

Stiglitz, Joseph and Andrew H. Charlton (2004). 'Common Values for the Development Round'. *World Trade Review,* vol. 3, no. 3, pp. 495–506.

Stiglitz, Joseph and Andrew H. Charlton (2005). 'A Development Round of Trade Negotiations?' In F. Bourguignon, B. Pleskovic, and A. Sapir, eds., *Are We on Track to Achieve the Millennium Development Goals? Annual World Bank Conference on Development Economics: Europe 2005,* pp. 31–60 (New York: Oxford University Press).

Sykes, Alan (2002). 'TRIPS, Pharmaceuticals, Developing Countries and the "Doha Solution"'. *Chicago Journal of International Law,* vol. 3, no. 1, pp. 47–68.

t'Hoen, Ellen (2002). 'TRIPS, Pharmaceutical Patents, and Access to Essential Medicines: A Long Way from Seattle to Doha'. *Chicago Journal of International Law,* vol. 3, no. 1, pp. 27–46.

Tanzi, Vito (2002). 'Globalization and the Future of Social Protection'. *Scottish Journal of Political Economy,* vol. 49, no. 1, pp. 116–127.

Teeple, Gary (2005). 'Honoured in the Breach: Human Rights as Principles of a Past Age'. Paper prepared for the conference on Human Rights in a Globalizing Era?, 4–6 August, Windsor ON.

Thakur, Ramesh and Thomas George Weiss (forthcoming). *The United Nations and Global Governance: An Idea and Its Prospects* (Bloomington IN: University of Indiana Press).

'The AIDS Fund Gets Going'. (2002). *Washington Post,* 29 April.

Thomas, Caroline (2002). 'Trade Policy and the Politics of Access to Drugs'. *Third World Quarterly,* vol. 23, no. 2, pp. 251–264.

Travis, Phylida, Sara Bennett, Andy Haines, *et al.* (2004). 'Overcoming Health-Systems Constraints to Achieve the Millennium Development Goals'. *Lancet,* vol. 364, no. 9437, pp. 900–906.

Trebilcock, Michael J. and Robert Howse (1999). *The Regulation of International Trade*, 2nd ed. (New York: Routledge).

UNAIDS (2005). 'AIDS Epidemic Update: December 2005'. <www.unaids.org/epi/2005/doc/EPIupdate2005_html_en/epi05_00_en.htm> (September 2006).

UNAIDS (2005). 'Equatorial Guinea'. <www.unaids.org/en/geographical+area/by+country?equatorial+guinea.asp> (June 2005).

UNAIDS (2006). '2006 Report on the Global AIDS Epidemic'. Geneva. <www.unaids.org/en/HIV_data/2006GlobalReport/default.asp> (September 2006).

UNICEF (2005). 'Children under Threat: The State of the World's Children 2005'. <www.unicef.org/sowc05> (September 2006).

United Kingdom (2000). 'Eliminating World Poverty: Making Globalisation Work for the World's Poor'. White Paper on International Development. <www.dfid.gov.uk/pubs/files/whitepaper2000.pdf> (September 2006).

United Nations (1948). 'Universal Declaration of Human Rights'. <www.un.org/Overview/rights.html> (September 2006).

United Nations (1999). 'Declaration on the Right and Responsibility of Individuals, Groups, and Organs of Society to Promote and Protect Universally Recognized Human Rights and Freedoms'. A/RES/53/144, 8 March. <www.unhchr.ch/

huridocda/huridoca.nsf/(Symbol)/A.RES.53.144.En?OpenDocument> (September 2006).

United Nations (2002). 'Final Outcome of the International Conference on Financing for Development'. A/CONF/198. 1 March. Monterrey. <www.un.org/esa/ffd/0302finalMonterreyConsensus.pdf> (September 2006).

United Nations (2004). 'A More Secure World: Our Shared Responsibility'. Report of the Secretary General's High-Level Panel on Threats, Challenges, and Change. New York. <www.un.org/secureworld> (September 2006).

United Nations (2005). 'In Larger Freedom: Towards Security, Development, and Human Rights for All'. Report of the Secretary General of the United Nations for Decision by Heads of State and Government in September 2005. New York. <www.un.org/largerfreedom> (September 2006).

United Nations (2005). 'Population, Development, and HIV/AIDS with Particular Emphasis on Poverty: The Concise Report'. ST/ESA/SER.A/247. <www.un.org/esa/population/publications/concise2005/PopdevHIVAIDS.pdf> (September 2006).

United Nations (2005). 'The Millennium Development Goals Report 2005'. New York. <millenniumindicators.un.org/unsd/mi/pdf/MDG%20Book.pdf> (September 2006).

United Nations Conference on Trade and Development (1998). 'World Investment Report 1998: Trends and Determinants'. United Nations Conference on Trade and Development, Geneva.

United Nations Conference on Trade and Development (2004). 'Economic Development in Africa: Debt Sustainability, Oasis, or Mirage?' <www.unctad.org/Templates/Download.asp?docid=5457&lang=1&intItemID=3246> (September 2006).

United Nations Conference on Trade and Development (2004). 'World Investment Report 2004: The Shift Toward Services'. United Nations Conference on Trade and Development, Geneva. <www.unctad.org/en/docs/wir2004_en.pdf> (September 2006).

United Nations Department of Economic and Social Affairs (2005). 'World Economic and Social Survey 2005: Financing for Development'. United Nations, New York.

United Nations Development Programme (1994). *Human Development Report* (New York: United Nations Development Programme).

United Nations Development Programme (1999). 'Governance for Sustainable Development'. Policy document, New York.

United Nations Development Programme (2002). 'Introducing Governance into HIV/AIDS Programmes: People's Republic of China, Lao PDR, and Viet Nam'. <www.undp.org/hiv/docs/alldocs/Asia%20-%20Introducing%20Governance%20into%20HIV-AIDS%20Programmes%20(2002).pdf> (September 2006).

United Nations Development Programme (2003). *Human Development Report 2003 Millennium Development Goals: A Compact among Nations to End Human Poverty* (New York: Oxford University Press) <hdr.undp.org/reports/global/2003/?CFID=2670336&CFTOKEN=65436232> (September 2006).

United Nations Economic and Social Council (2000). 'The Right to the Highest Attainable Standard of Health'. E/C.12/2000/4, 11 August. <www.unhchr.ch/tbs/doc.nsf/(symbol)/E.C.12.2000.4.En?OpenDocument> (September 2006).

United Nations General Assembly (2005). '2005 World Summit Outcome'. 15 September. <www.un.org/summit2005/documents.html> (September 2006).

United Nations Millennium Project (2005). 'Investing in Development: A Practical Plan to Achieve the Millennium Development Goals'. United Nations Development Programme, New York. <www.unmillenniumproject.org/reports/fullreport.htm> (September 2006).

United Nations Millennium Project (2005). *Preparing National Strategies to Achieve the Millennium Development Goals: A Handbook* (New York: United Nations Development Programme).

United Nations Security Council (2000). 'Resolution 1308 (2000) on the Responsibility of the Security Council in the Maintenance of International Peace and Security: HIV/AIDS and International Peacekeeping Operations'. <daccess-ods.un.org/access.nsf/Get?Open&DS=S/RES/1308%20(2000)&Lang=E&Area=UNDOC> (September 2006).

United Nations Security Council (2005). 'Security Council Presidential Statement Recognizes "Significant Progress" Addressing HIV/AIDS among Peacekeepers, But Says Many Challenges Remain'. Press release SC/8450, 18 July, New York. <www.un.org/News/Press/docs/2005/sc8450.doc.htm> (September 2006).

United Nations Standing Committee on Nutrition (2000). 'Fourth Report on the World Nutrition Situation: Nutrition Throughout the Life Cycle'. <www.unsystem.org/scn/Publications/rwns/4RWNS.html> (September 2006).

United States (2002). 'The National Security Strategy of the United States of America'. Washington DC. <www.whitehouse.gov/nsc/nss.html> (September 2006).

United States General Accounting Office (2004). 'Emerging Infectious Diseases: Asian SARS Outbreak Challenged International and National Responses'. GAO-04-564. Report to the Chairman, Subcommittee on Asia and the Pacific, Committee on International Relations, House of Representatives. United States General Accounting Office, Washington DC. <www.gao.gov/cgi-bin/getrpt?GAO-04-564> (September 2006).

van de Walle, Nicolas (2001). *African Economies and the Politics of Permanent Crisis, 1979–1999* (Cambridge: Cambridge University Press).

Vandemoortele, Jan (2003). 'The MDGs and Pro-Poor Policies: Can External Partners Make a Difference?' Paper prepared for the annual Global Development Conference of the Global Development Network on Understanding Reform, 28–30 January, New Delhi. <www.gdnet.org/pdf2/gdn_library/annual_conferences/fifth_annual_conference/vandemoortele_paper.pdf> (September 2006).

Versi, Anver (2005). 'The G8 Pledges: What Happens Next?' *African Business*, August/September, pp. 14–20.

Vidal, John and Tim Radford (2005). 'One in Six Countries Facing Food Shortage'. *Guardian,* 30 June.

Virchow, Rudolph (1848). 'Die offentliche gesundheitspflege' [The Public Health Service]. *Medizinische Reform,* vol. 5, pp. 21–22.

von Furstenberg, George M. and Joseph P. Daniels (1991). 'Policy Undertakings by the Seven "Summit" Countries: Ascertaining the Degree of Compliance'. *Carnegie-Rochester Conference Series on Public Policy,* vol. 35, pp. 267–308.

Wagstaff, Adam and Mariam Claeson (2004). 'The Millennium Development Goals for Health: Rising to the Challenges'. World Bank, Washington, DC

Wagstaff, Adam, Naoko Watanabe, and Eddy van Doorslaer (2001). 'Impoverishment, Insurance, and Health Care Payments'. Health, Nutrition, and Population Network, World Bank, Washington DC.

Weatherspoon, Dave D. and Thomas Reardon (2003). 'The Rise of Supermarkets in Africa: Implications for Agrifood Systems and the Rural Poor'. *Development Policy Review,* vol. 21, no. 3, pp. 333–355. <papers.ssrn.com/sol3/papers.cfm?abstract_id=410968> (September 2006).

Webb, Michael (2000). 'The Group of Seven and Political Management of the Global Economy'. In R. Stubbs and G. Underhill, eds., *Political Economy and the Changing Global Order,* pp. 141–151 (Don Mills: Oxford University Press Canada).

White, Howard (2005). 'The Case for Doubling Aid'. *IDS Bulletin,* vol. 36, no. 3, pp. 8–12.

Whitehead, Margaret, Gïran Dahlgren, and Timothy Evans (2001). 'Equity and Health Sector Reforms: Can Low-Income Countries Escape the Medical Poverty Trap?' *Lancet,* vol. 358, pp. 833–836.

Widdus, Roy (2001). 'Public-Private Partnerships for Health: Their Main Targets, Their Diversity, and Their Future Directions'. *Bulletin of the World Health Organization,* vol. 79, no. 8, pp. 713–720.

Williamson, John (1990). 'What Washington Means by Policy Reform'. In J. Williamson, ed., *Latin American Adjustment: How Much Has Happened?,* pp. 5–38 (Washington DC: Institute for International Economics).

Wise, Timothy A. (2004). 'The Paradox of Agricultural Subsidies: Measurement Issues, Agricultural Dumping, and Policy Reform'. Tufts University, Medford MA. <ase.tufts.edu/gdae/Pubs/wp/04-02AgSubsidies.pdf> (September 2006).

Wolf, Martin (2004). *Why Globalization Works* (New Haven: Yale University Press).

Woodward, David, Nick Drager, Robert Beaglehole, *et al.* (2001). 'Globalization and Health: A Framework for Analysis and Action'. *Bulletin of the World Health Organization,* vol. 79, no. 9, pp. 847–881. <www.who.int/bulletin/pdf/2001/issue9/bu1329.pdf> (September 2006).

World Bank (1993). *World Development Report 1993: Investing in Health* (Washington DC: World Bank).

World Bank (2002). 'Health, Nutrition, and Population Sector Strategy Paper'. World Bank, Washington DC. <www.worldbank.org/html/extdr/hnp/sector_strategy/download.htm> (September 2006).

World Bank (2004). *World Development Report 2004: Making Services Work for Poor People* (Washington DC: World Bank and Oxford University Press).

World Bank (2004). *Global Economic Prospects 2005: Trade, Regionalism, and Development* (Washington DC: World Bank).

World Bank (2005). 'With World Bank Assistance, Stolen Funds Deposited in Swiss Banks Are Returned to Nigeria'. News, 27 September, Washington DC.

World Bank (2006). 'HNP Comparative Data' [Database]. <devdata.worldbank.org/hnpstats/cd3.asp> (September 2006).

World Bank (2006). 'The Multilateral Debt Relief Initiative'. 29 June, Washington DC. <www.worldbank.org/html/extdr/thematic.htm » Debt Issues> (September 2006).

World Bank Group (2006). 'A Complete Listing of the Goals, Targets, and Indicators for MDGs'. <devdata.worldbank.org/gmis/mdg/list_of_goals.htm> (September 2006).

World Health Organization (1994). 'Constitution of the World Health Organization'. Geneva. <www.who.int/about/en » WHO Constitution> (September 2006).

World Health Organization (1997). 'The Denver G8 Summit Highlights Infectious Disease'. Press release WHO/50, 24 June, Geneva.

World Health Organization (1997). 'Health and Environment in Sustainable Development 1997: Five Years after the Earth Summit'. WHO/EHG/97.8. Geneva.

World Health Organization (2000). 'World Health Report 2000 — Health Systems: Improving Performance'. World Health Organization, Geneva.

World Health Organization (2001). 'Global Health Security: Epidemic Alert and Response'. World Health Assembly Resolution WHA54.14, 21 May, Geneva. <ftp.who.int/gb/pdf_files/WHA54/ea54r14.pdf> (September 2006).

World Health Organization (2002). '25 Questions and Answers on Health and Human Rights'. World Health Organization, Geneva.

World Health Organization (2002). *Global Crisis, Global Solutions: Managing Public Health Emergencies of International Concern through the Revised International Health Regulations* (Geneva: World Health Organization).

World Health Organization (2003). 'World Health Report 2003: Shaping the Future'. World Health Organization, Geneva. <www.who.int/whr/2003/en> (September 2006).

World Health Organization (2005). 'Global and Regional Immunization Profile: African Region'. <www.who.int/immunization_monitoring/data/data_AFR/en> (September 2006).

World Health Organization (2005). 'Avian Influenza and the Pandemic Threat in Africa: Risk Assessment for Africa'. 28 October, Geneva. <www.who.int/csr/disease/avian_influenza/riskassessmentAfrica/en> (September 2006).

World Health Organization (2005). 'Ecosystems and Human Well-Being: Health Synthesis'. Geneva. <www.who.int/entity/globalchange/ecosystems/ecosys.pdf> (September 2006).

World Health Organization (2005). 'Health in the Millennium Development Goals'. Geneva. <www.who.int/entity/mdg/publications/MDG_Report_revised.pdf> (September 2006).

World Health Organization (2005). 'Revision of the International Health Regulations'. WHA58.3. Geneva. <www.who.int/entity/csr/ihr/IHRWHA58_3-en.pdf> (September 2006).

World Health Organization (2005). 'World Health Assembly Official Records'. <policy.who.int/cgi-bin/om_isapi.dll?infobase=wharec-e&softpage=Browse_Frame_Pg42> (September 2006).

World Health Organization (2006). 'Commission on Social Determinants of Health'. <www.who.int/social_determinants/en> (September 2006).

World Health Organization (2006). 'Cumulative Number of Reported Probably Cases of Severe Acute Respiratory Syndrome (SARS)'. Geneva. <www.who.int/csr/sars/country/en> (September 2006).

World Health Organization (2006). 'Global Outbreak Alert and Response Network'. Geneva. <www.who.int/csr/outbreaknetwork/en/> (September 2006).

World Health Organization (2006). 'Globalization, Trade, and Health'. Geneva. <www.who.int/trade> (September 2006).

World Health Organization (2006). 'International Health Regulations'. Geneva. <www.who.int/csr/ihr/en> (September 2006).

World Health Organization (2006). 'International Trade and Health'. WHA59.26, 27 May, Geneva. <www.who.int/gb/ebwha/pdf_files/WHA59/A59_R26-en.pdf> (September 2006).

World Health Organization (2006). 'Reports on Global HIV/AIDS Situation'. Geneva. <www.who.int/hiv/epiupdates/en> (September 2006).

World Health Organization (2006). 'Situation Updates — Avian Influenza'. Geneva. <www.who.int/csr/disease/avian_influenza/updates/en> (September 2006).

World Health Organization (2006). 'WHO and the Millennium Development Goals'. Geneva. <www.who.int/mdg/en> (September 2006).

World Health Organization (2006). 'Why Is Tobacco a Public Health Priority?' Geneva. <www.who.int/tobacco/health_priority/en> (September 2006).

World Health Organization (2006). 'World Health Report 2006: Working Together for Health'. World Health Organization, Geneva. <www.who.int/whr/2006/en> (September 2006).

World Health Organization and World Trade Organization (2002). 'WTO Agreements and Public Health: A Joint Study by WHO and the WTO Secretariat'. Geneva. <www.wto.org/English/res_e/booksp_e/who_wto_e.pdf> (September 2006).

World Trade Organization (1994). 'Trade-Related Aspects of Intellectual Property Rights'. Annex IC of the Marrakesh Agreement Establishing the World Trade Organization. 15 April, Marrakesh. <www.wto.org/english/docs_e/legal_e/27-trips_01_e.htm> (September 2006).

World Trade Organization (2001). 'Ministerial Declaration'. 14 November, Doha. <www.wto.org/english/thewto_e/minist_e/min01_e/mindecl_e.htm> (September 2006).

World Trade Organization (2001). 'Declaration on the TRIPS Agreement and Public Health'. WT/MIN(01)/DEC/2. 14 November. <www.wto.org/English/thewto_e/minist_e/min01_e/mindecl_trips_e.htm> (September 2006).

World Trade Organization (2003). 'Implementation of Paragraph 6 of the Doha Declaration of the TRIPS Agreement and Public Health'. Decision of the General

Council of 30 August. <www.wto.org/english/tratop_e/trips_e/implem_para6_e.htm> (September 2006).

Wouters, Annemarie (1995). 'Improving Quality Through Cost Recovery in Niger'. *Health Policy and Planning,* vol. 10, no. 3, pp. 257–270.

Wroughton, Lesley (2005). 'World Bank Report Calls for Changes to G8 Debt Plan'. *Reuters,* 3 August.

'WTO Chief Says Drugs Row May Scuttle Trade Round'. (2001). *Agence France-Presse,* 8 November.

Xingzhu Lui and Anne Mills (2002). 'Financing Reforms of Public Health Services in China: Lessons for Other Nations'. *Social Science and Medicine,* vol. 54, no. 11, pp. 1691–1698.

Yach, Derek and Douglas Bettcher (1998). 'The Globalization of Public Health I: Threats and Opportunities'. *American Journal of Public Health,* vol. 88, no. 5, pp. 735–738.

Yach, Derek and Douglas Bettcher (1998). 'The Globalization of Public Health II: The Convergence of Self-Interest and Altruism'. *American Journal of Public Health,* vol. 88, no. 5, pp. 738–741.

Yale Center for the Study of Globalization (2003). 'A Discussion on Ethical Globalization'. 15 January. <www.yaleglobal.yale.edu/article.print?id=751> (September 2006).

Yoder, Richard (1989). 'Are People Willing and Able to Pay for Health Services?' *Social Science and Medicine,* vol. 29, no. 1, pp. 35–42.

Zacher, Mark W. (1999). 'Global Epidemiological Surveillance: International Cooperation to Monitor Infectious Diseases'. In I. Kaul, I. Grunberg, and M.A. Stern, eds., *Global Public Goods: International Cooperation in the 21st Century,* pp. 266–283 (New York: Oxford University Press for the United Nations Development Programme).

Zupi, Marco (2001). 'The Genoa G8 Summit: Great Expectations, Disappointing Results'. *International Spectator,* vol. 36, no. 3, p. 59.

Index

Global Environmental Governance

Also published in the series

Agricultural Policy Reform
Wayne Moyer and Tim Josling
ISBN 978-0-7546-3050-0

Hard Choices, Soft Law
Edited by John J. Kirton and Michael J. Trebilcock
ISBN 978-0-7546-0966-7

Linking Trade, Environment, and Social Cohesion
Edited by John J. Kirton and Virginia W. Maclaren
ISBN 978-0-7546-1934-5

International Equity and Global Environmental Politics
Paul G. Harris
ISBN 978-0-7546-1735-8

Governing Global Biodiversity
Edited by Philippe G. Le Prestre
ISBN 978-0-7546-1744-0

The Politics of Irrigation Reform
Edited by Peter P. Mollinga and Alex Bolding
ISBN 978-0-7546-3515-4